THE
WELL-MANAGED
Healthcare
Organization

THE WELL-MANAGED

Healthcare Organization

EIGHTH EDITION

Kenneth R. White
John R. Griffith

AUPHA

Health Administration Press, Chicago, Illinois
Association of University Programs in Health Administration, Arlington, Virginia

Your board, staff, or clients may also benefit from this book's insight. For more information on quantity discounts, contact the Health Administration Press Marketing Manager at (312) 424-9470.

20   19   18   17   16   5   4   3   2   1

Library of Congress Cataloging-in-Publication Data

White, Kenneth R. (Kenneth Ray), 1956-
The well-managed healthcare organization / Kenneth R. White, John R. Griffith. --
Eighth edition.
     pages cm
Includes bibliographical references and index.
ISBN 978-1-56793-721-3 (alk. paper)
1. Health services administration. I. Griffith, John R. II. Title.
RA971.G77 2016
362.1068--dc23
                          2015010231

The paper used in this publication meets the minimum requirements of American National Standard for Information Sciences—Permanence of Paper for Printed Library Materials, ANSI Z39.48-1984. ♾ ™

Acquisitions editor: Janet Davis; Project manager: Joyce Dunne; Cover designer: Marisa Jackson; Layout: Cepheus Edmondson

Found an error or a typo? We want to know! Please e-mail it to hapbooks@ache.org, and put "Book Error" in the subject line.

For photocopying and copyright information, please contact Copyright Clearance Center at www.copyright.com or at (978) 750-8400.

Health Administration Press
A division of the Foundation of the American
   College of Healthcare Executives
One North Franklin Street, Suite 1700
Chicago, IL 60606-3529
(312) 424-2800

Association of University Programs
   in Health Administration
2000 North 14th Street
Suite 780
Arlington, VA 22201
(703) 894-0940

BRIEF CONTENTS

DETAILED CONTENTS

EXHIBITS

PREFACE

The *Well-Managed Healthcare Organization*, now in its eighth edition, is a text for students pursuing professional careers in managing healthcare organizations (HCOs). It describes actual practices that lead to high performance, based on our careful analysis of a small but reasonably representative set of HCOs that have been studied by competent peers and have produced auditable evidence of excellence. We believe the evidence of the superiority of these practices passes both academic and professional challenge. The footnotes in each chapter support our belief. There may be other ways to achieve excellence, but they have not been documented and quite possibly have not been discovered. Healthcare organizations that follow the methods we describe are positioned to thrive under the Affordable Care Act and other health reforms. Indirectly, health reform initiatives reinforce our message and are consistent with managing and leading excellent HCOs on the basis of evidence, best practices, benchmarks, and a culture of continuous improvement.

The common theme in these organizations is that a specific culture (one that is transformational and embraces evidence-based management) and certain management activities (listening, measurement, benchmarking, negotiated goal setting, and continuous improvement) are essential to high performance. Specialized teams must complete specified tasks correctly to measured standards. These teams include those involved in not only patient care but also clinical support (e.g., laboratory, pharmacy, imaging), logistics (e.g., information, personnel, training, supplies), or strategic planning (e.g., finance, internal consulting, enterprise-level goals). Chapters 2 through 15 have the following structure: Purpose, Functions, People, Measures, and Managerial Issues. The Functions section describes the unit's essential contribution to the whole, and the Measures section identifies opportunities to improve that contribution.

The challenge in managing HCOs is to sustain excellence over all the teams, and the solution to this challenge lies in two core thrusts:

1. Maintaining a culture that empowers each associate (transformational management)
2. Supporting continuous improvement with measurement, process analysis, negotiated goals, and rewards (evidence-based management)

In excellent HCOs, measurement is central, improvement is constant, leaders respond to associates and patients, professionals communicate as equals, everyone is treated with respect, and authority is derived from knowledge rather than rank. These are the foundations of high performance. The record of excellent HCOs shows quite clearly that the transformational management approach produces excellence in all the sites that now constitute the healthcare industry. High-performing HCOs successfully operate the full gamut of healthcare, including doctors' offices, general and specialty hospitals, continuing care, home care, and hospices.

Using *The Well-Managed Healthcare Organization*

Any organization is a collaboration to do what an individual alone cannot do. This collaboration succeeds by division of labor—assigning tasks for individuals and small teams to complete to achieve the goals of collaboration. The text begins (Chapter 1) with a description of the collaborators, called *stakeholders*.

Performance excellence is built on a comprehensive and well-supported theory of management (Chapter 1). The elements of that theory are as follows:

1. An HCO is supported by many stakeholders who, in turn, benefit from its success. In general, stakeholders are either *customers* or *providers*, and a key organizational issue is balancing and optimizing the rewards to each group.
2. The goals of the HCO are stated in its mission. Missions of HCOs are similar because all stakeholders share the common purposes of extending the length and quality of life and providing safe, effective, patient-centered, timely, efficient, and equitable care.
3. Goal achievement is evidence based, using objective measures of performance, comparison to competitors and best practices, goal setting, and continuous improvement.
4. The rewards of improvement are shared among the stakeholders so that both customer and provider stakeholders view the organization as their preferred affiliation.

These elements constitute cross-cutting themes that recur throughout the text.

From chapter 1 through 15, the text describes the activities of an HCO in three divisions—corporate, clinical, and logistic/strategic. Each chapter identifies an activity and the functions it must perform for the whole to succeed, its organization structures and personnel, its measures of performance, and some of the critical areas in which it needs managerial support. Each chapter addresses (1) *what this activity must do well for the whole to succeed* and (2) *how this activity measures and improves its performance*. Each chapter begins with Critical Issues, an outline that emphasizes the distinctions associated with excellence, and Questions for Discussion, five important and easily misunderstood application topics.

Chapter 2 describes leadership and the activities required of senior management to build and sustain the HCO's cultural foundations. Chapter 3 expands the discussion on the operational foundation, exploring the activities that identify opportunities for improvement (OFIs) and lead to improved work processes. Chapter 4 addresses governance, the strategic decision making that provides effective long-term responsiveness to stakeholder needs. Chapters 5 through 9 describe the operation of the various clinical and clinical support teams. Chapters 10 through 15 discuss the logistic and strategic support activities.

Each chapter addresses purpose, functions, people, measures, and managerial issues associated with the activity. The content of these chapters gives the student the ability to engage in meaningful dialogue with members of any activity or team, to understand how well a team or an activity is currently performing and what its current OFIs are, and to assist in translating those OFIs to actual improvement. That pattern of listening, learning, and supporting improvement is what twenty-first-century healthcare managers do for a living.

HCO managers build excellent organizations by ensuring that the functions are carried out as a whole. The theory demands comprehensiveness, as failure in one activity contributes to failure in another. The three divisions must all perform; an HCO cannot have clinical excellence without corporate excellence and logistic excellence. The learning manager, therefore, must grasp the totality and interdependence of the HCO as well as the contributions expected of each activity. He or she must also understand the application of the cross-cutting themes—the role of the mission, evidence-based decisions, measured performance, continuous improvement, and reward. The test of learning is the ability to explain these issues to others, such as customer stakeholders, beginning supervisors, and new employees.

We believe one effective path to mastery is to use the book partly as a text and partly as a reference. Some of the detail should be memorized, for immediate recall in conversations with others. The functions of the governing board (Chapter 4), the way budgets are developed (primarily chapters 3, 4, 7, and 12), and the use of the epidemiologic planning model (every chapter from 4 through 15) are prime examples. Other matters are not unimportant, but when they arise, they can be accessed through the index and table of contents and reviewed.

A beginning student might best master the text not by reading from page 1 to page 548 but rather by interacting with each chapter:

1. Study the Critical Issues, making an effort to relate them to her prior experience.
2. Review the details of the functions to understand how each element contributes to the whole and how each is best implemented.
3. Study the exhibit that shows the performance measures, and review the Measures section to understand how the measures are defined and used.
4. Check the Managerial Issues section for important elements that relate the activity to management in the organization as a whole and to sustaining high performance.

5. Review the Questions for Discussion in relation to her or his prior experience, striving to understand both the importance of the question and the best way it can be answered in real HCOs.
6. Consider how the material in the chapter can be effectively conveyed to the right people in an HCO—that is, how it can be best summarized in formal policies and procedures, in training programs, and in day-to-day interactions.

The text can certainly be mastered in self-study. We believe a class or discussion group and a mentor or teacher can help substantially, particularly in the latter steps.

Suite of Online Learning Resources

Support for instructors and multiple learning resources for students are available online. All the components will integrate easily into most universities' learning management systems.

The learning resources suite includes the following materials to increase students' application skills and support instructors in a lecture-free, interactive classroom:

- Real-world application questions with instant feedback and answer rationales

- Instructor's tips for the book's discussion questions, highlighting how real managers apply best practices in real healthcare organizations

- Gradable essay questions with grading checklists

- PowerPoint slides of this book's exhibits and chapter-opening material

- Instructor and student guides on how to use the book in combination with its online resources

- Glossary of technical terms

For access, instructors will please apply by e-mailing hapbooks@ache.org. In your e-mail, include course and university information and a contact name and phone number/e-mail address for verification of all requests.

Acknowledgments

As the editions of *The Well-Managed Healthcare Organization* mount, keeping track of all who have contributed to this text by their examples becomes difficult. The applications of the HCO recipients of the Malcolm Baldrige National Quality Award are the most comprehensive documentation of the transformational and evidence-based approach. Our visits to Catholic Health Initiatives, Henry Ford Health System, Intermountain Healthcare, Legacy Health, MediCorp Health System, MedStar Health, Moses Cone Health System (now Cone Health), and Sentara Healthcare have helped us understand how leading practices are designed and implemented.

Over a period of time, both of us have worked with specific organizations, including Summa Health System in Akron, Ohio; Allegiance Corporation (a physician hospital organization) in Ann Arbor, Michigan; Mercy Health Center in Oklahoma City, Oklahoma; Mercy International Health Services in Farmington Hills, Michigan; and Bon Secours Health System in Marriottsville, Maryland. We are grateful to these HCOs. We are also grateful for the assistance of our colleagues at the University of Michigan, Virginia Commonwealth University, and the University of Virginia.

We are especially grateful to Christy Harris Lemak, PhD, FACHE, for her contribution to Chapter 1 and for her many helpful comments and suggestions for revising the eighth edition.

Kenneth R. White, PhD, APRN-BC, FACHE, FAAN
The University of Virginia
Charlottesville, Virginia

John R. Griffith, MBA, FACHE
The University of Michigan
Ann Arbor, Michigan

I

INTRODUCTION AND OVERVIEW

1 FOUNDATIONS OF HIGH-PERFORMING HEALTHCARE ORGANIZATIONS

Critical Issues for Excellence

1. *Emphasizing mission and vision.* Make the contribution and importance of care itself a shared value among all the organization's associates.

2. *Understanding and meeting the needs of all stakeholders.* Extend the listening activities so that every major customer, associate, competitor, or other affiliate has a point of contact and is assured of fairness and responsiveness.

3. *Building a culture that listens, empowers, trains, and rewards.* Begin a program that identifies what associates see as barriers to their work and remove them.

4. *Measuring performance, seeking benchmarks, and continuously improving.* Negotiate realistic goals for every work unit that adds quality, customer satisfaction, and associated satisfaction measures.

5. *Protecting the corporate capability.* Ensure that the organization's physical assets and information are protected and that the rights of its stakeholders are fulfilled.

Questions for Discussion

These questions are about applying the chapter content. It is often helpful to discuss them with classmates or mentors, gaining different perspectives on the issues.

1. This chapter outlines a transformational style of management, emphasizing values, empowerment, communication, trust/accountability, and rewards. Some people say that transformation is completely unrealistic; you must enforce order, they say, to have accountability. How is accountability achieved in high-performing, transformational HCOs?

2. HCOs are strongly oriented to healing the sick, one person at a time. The first word of this chapter—*patient*—is consistent with that tradition. Some say that the real role of HCOs is population health, including but going well beyond healing the sick. (Contrast the missions of SSM Health Care, Bronson Healthcare, and Saint Luke's Hospital with those of

Baptist Healthcare, RWJ University Hospital, and North Mississippi Health System in Exhibit 1.7.) Should this chapter have started with, "Building healthy communities is the focus of HCOs, including patient care but going well beyond"?

3. What happens to an HCO (or any organization) that fails in its strategic positioning (see Exhibit 1.14)? Can you name an example or two, and then identify with hindsight where they failed?

4. Mercy Health System has two staff awards: "Above and Beyond the Call of Duty" (ABCD) and "Someone to Admire and Respect" (STAR). Both are intended to recognize individuals for exceptional effort. Nominations come from patients, colleagues, or guests. A committee reviews and ranks them. Personal letters are sent to the awardees' home address, and recipients are identified in departmental meetings. Similar programs (they have various names) often involve small prizes, like a dinner-for-two gift certificate. Bronson has a gift drawing for recipients. Should every well-managed healthcare organization have a similar program? Can you describe to a customer stakeholder why the program is (or is not) a good idea?

5. Evidence-based management relies heavily on numbers. The benchmarks, strategic and unit scorecards, and goals are all quantitative. A number of questions arise about such a quantitative approach. A competent professional manager has to be able to answer them at several levels of sophistication. (The chief of surgery and the chair of the board will expect more specifics than the kitchen workers, but servant leadership obligates leaders to answer both to the questioners' satisfaction.) For Chapter 1, let's answer them at the simplest level, say for a smart high school graduate.
   a. Are these the right measures?
   b. How do I know my team can influence the measures? (Don't they include a lot of things outside our control?)
   c. Can we really get better? (If we set a goal, how do we know we can reach it?)
   d. Will the leadership punish us for not reaching our goals?

Purpose

Patient care—meeting the diagnostic and therapeutic needs of individuals—is the primary focus of healthcare organizations (HCOs). The purpose of any HCO is

to provide care to individual patients.

It is usually stated as the HCO's "mission." The purpose can be expanded to "population health," but the larger purpose depends upon excellence in care to individual patients.

Patient care is also an important contributor to a broader purpose—the health of individuals and populations. An extensive social structure influences health, including schools, environmental sanitation, public safety, public health, and other activities. HCOs are an important part of this structure. The healthy population that the structure achieves is central to "life, liberty, and the pursuit of happiness," the shared goals of American society.

Any HCO delivers care through one or more caregiving teams, as shown in the top triangle of Exhibit 1.1. Caregiving teams are backed by three levels of support—clinical, logistic, and strategic—that are themselves composed of teams. A small HCO has one or a few caregiving teams and often contracts with other organizations for support; a large HCO has a broad array of patient care and support teams. A healthcare system is an organization of HCOs, often meeting a wide range of needs and operating in several geographic locations.

HCO teams are usually housed in purpose-built spaces (e.g., clinics, operating rooms, business offices) so that facilities reflect the activities depicted in Exhibit 1.1. With the growth of electronic communication, many facilities and their teams can be geographically dispersed. A primary care team needs timely laboratory results, but they might come from a centralized laboratory serving dozens of teams. All teams require strategic capability, but it might be provided from the system headquarters in another state.

Many HCOs work to improve the health of patients and communities.[1,2] A population health mission requires excellence in patient care, so the population health mission is an addition to the overall mission. There are four steps in improving **population health**: defining the population (by geography, sociodemographic factors, disease state, risk, insurance coverage, or in some other way), measuring the current state of health in the population, setting goals for improvement, and directing resources toward making improvements.[3] The U.S. Department of Health and Human Services specifies national goals and objectives for population health in the Healthy People 2020 program.[4]

Population health
The health outcomes of a defined group of individuals.

EXHIBIT 1.1 Components of Healthcare Organizations

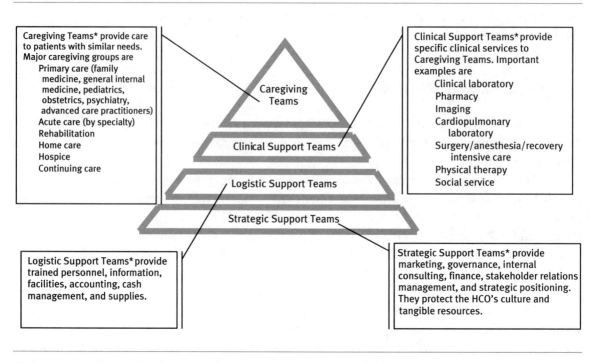

Caregiving Teams* provide care to patients with similar needs. Major caregiving groups are
Primary care (family medicine, general internal medicine, pediatrics, obstetrics, psychiatry, advanced care practitioners)
Acute care (by specialty)
Rehabilitation
Home care
Hospice
Continuing care

Caregiving Teams

Clinical Support Teams* provide specific clinical services to Caregiving Teams. Important examples are
Clinical laboratory
Pharmacy
Imaging
Cardiopulmonary laboratory
Surgery/anesthesia/recovery intensive care
Physical therapy
Social service

Clinical Support Teams

Logistic Support Teams

Strategic Support Teams

Logistic Support Teams* provide trained personnel, information, facilities, accounting, cash management, and supplies.

Strategic Support Teams* provide marketing, governance, internal consulting, finance, stakeholder relations management, and strategic positioning. They protect the HCO's culture and tangible resources.

*HCOs can contract for clinical and logistic support activities, retaining control of their strategic activities. Large HCOs, integrating many different care teams, dominate the healthcare marketplace and have been growing.

Improving population health requires identifying and overcoming determinants of health, typically through collaborative relationships among HCOs and across a variety of other organizations in a given community, including public health, community development, education, and social service sectors. Evidence suggests that medical care represents a relatively small influence on population health, but personal care provided by HCOs is a critical part of improving population health.[5]

As shown in Exhibit 1.2, an HCO directly influences population health by investing in a full range of personal health services. Many HCOs that formerly focused on acute inpatient care ("hospitals") have moved to broaden their scope, adding primary and rehabilitation services. Population health expands beyond Exhibit 1.2, to community-wide activities to promote healthy behavior and deliberate efforts to promote safety and reduce environmental hazards. More indirect influence can result from an HCO creating partnerships with local community health centers in order to improve access to immunizations and healthy behaviors for pregnant women.

The Collaborative, Dynamic Nature of HCOs

The HCO creates, supports, and coordinates the caregiving and support teams. HCOs involve extensive collaboration within and across teams. Within a single hospital, for example, one team of caregivers works together

EXHIBIT 1.2
Personal
Services for
Community
Health

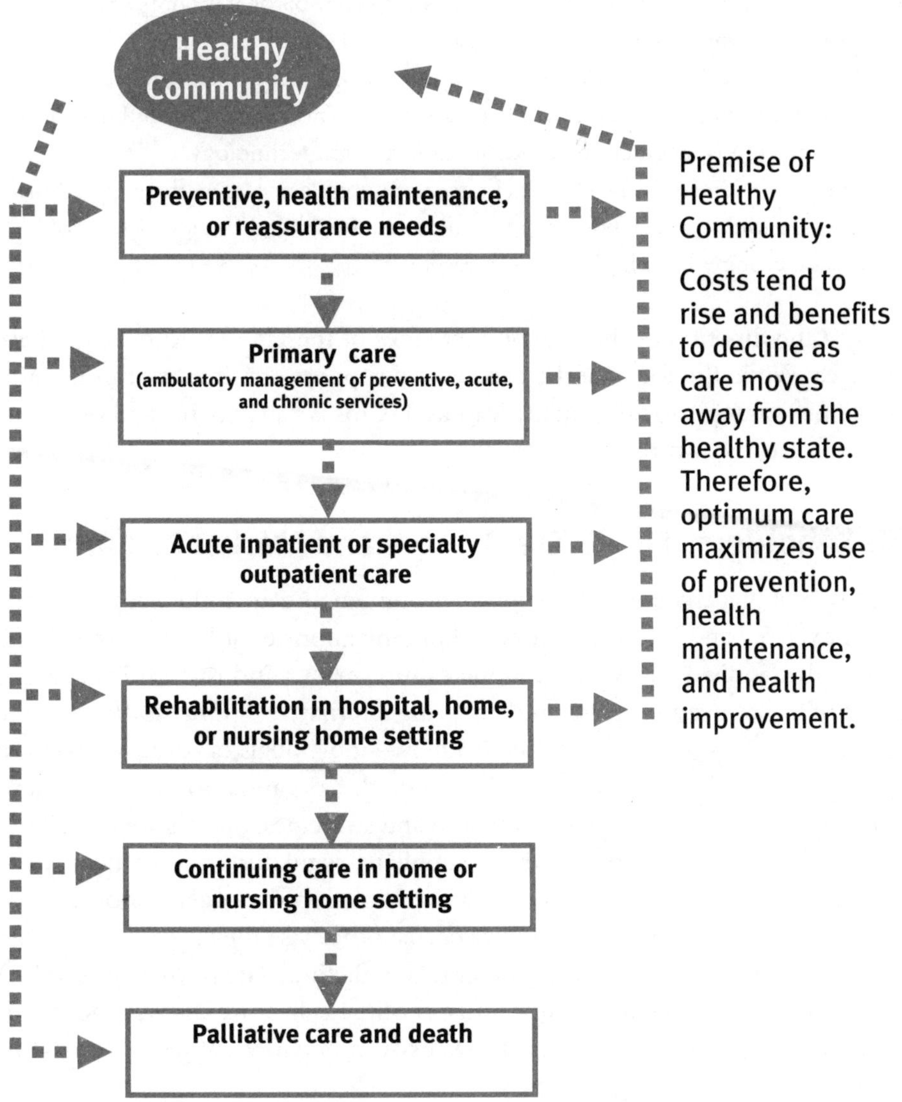

Healthy Community

Premise of Healthy Community:

Preventive, health maintenance, or reassurance needs

Costs tend to rise and benefits to decline as care moves away from the healthy state. Therefore, optimum care maximizes use of prevention, health maintenance, and health improvement.

Primary care (ambulatory management of preventive, acute, and chronic services)

Acute inpatient or specialty outpatient care

Rehabilitation in hospital, home, or nursing home setting

Continuing care in home or nursing home setting

Palliative care and death

to perform a surgical procedure and several teams manage the patient's care before and after surgery. Exhibit 1.2 extends that model to comprehensive individual patient care, beginning with the prevention of illness and extending to end-of-life care. The various teams are grouped in **service lines**, patient care teams coordinated around a set of similar diseases or patient needs.

Service lines
Patient care teams organized and coordinated around a set of similar diseases or patient needs.

Large not-for-profit HCOs now provide a comprehensive array of service lines, coordinating primary care, inpatient and outpatient acute care, rehabilitation, and follow-up care to support the treatment and recovery.

Exhibit 1.2 is static. Any real HCO is highly dynamic in three ways:

1. The HCO constantly responds to the changing array of patients and their changing needs. This makes most HCOs a 24/7/365 operation, prepared for more than will happen in any given day.
2. The HCO evolves as medicine, health, and management change, reflecting the latest scientifically proven treatments, activities to prevent illness, and new developments in management practices and information technology.
3. The HCO adjusts to the changes in its community's needs. As the population grows, shrinks, and changes in age and ethnic diversity, the epidemiology of disease changes and the HCO must respond.

One function of the strategic activities of the HCO is to manage these changes. While the focus of the clinical and support activities is "this patient, now," the strategic focus of many leading HCOs is "all patients and our community, into the future."

Stakeholders: The HCO's Owners and Market Partners

HCOs exist in a changing, complex environment and are influenced by a variety of external and internal factors. All organizations exist because they fulfill a need that individuals working alone cannot meet,[6] and they thrive because they fulfill that need better than competing alternatives.[7] Organizations serve many **stakeholders**—individuals or groups who have a direct interest in the organization's success and shape its mission and strategies. Stakeholders are buyers, workers, suppliers, regulators, and owners. They can choose to participate in the organization or not.

Stakeholders
Individuals or groups who have a direct interest in the organization's success.

Organizations must meet stakeholder needs; otherwise they fail and disappear.

Stakeholders' desires are inherently conflicting. The buyer wants to buy inexpensively, the supplier to maximize profit. Each of us is a stakeholder in many organizations. Our organizations exist in networks of negotiated solutions to those conflicting desires.

A summary of the stakeholder environment for HCOs is shown in Exhibit 1.3. Because of the intimate and life-changing nature of healthcare services, their cost, and the complex structure to finance the costs, HCOs represent one of the most complex applications of the stakeholder model. HCOs become "excellent" or "high performing" because they are able to negotiate effective solutions among their stakeholders.

Customer Partners

Patients and Families

Patients are the most important HCO stakeholders. They expect and deserve care that meets the goals summarized in the Institute of Medicine's report *Crossing the Quality Chasm*: safe, effective, patient centered, timely, efficient,

EXHIBIT 1.3 Model of Stakeholder–HCO Interaction

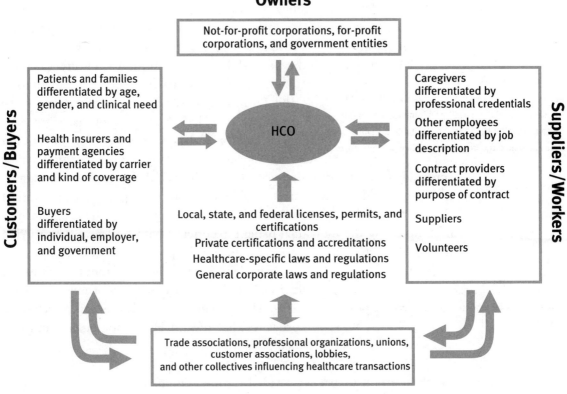

and equitable.[8] They also expect reasonably comfortable amenities and confidentiality. Friends and family accompany most patients, and many family members serve as important caregivers, so HCOs must establish close and direct relations with them. HCOs are increasingly focusing on **patient-centered care** and involving patients and families in care planning and decision making so that they can provide "care that is respectful [of] and responsive to individual patient preferences, needs, and values."[9]

Patient-centered care
Care that is respectful of and responsive to individual patient preferences, needs, and values.

Health Insurers and Payment Agencies

Patients rely on a variety of mechanisms to pay for care, which can easily cost a large fraction of a family's annual income. Health insurers and **fiscal intermediaries** provide most of the revenue to HCOs, making them essential stakeholders. Private health insurers are agents for buyers, which include governments, employers, and citizens at large. Two large governmental insurance programs—Medicare

Fiscal intermediary
An outside contractor that processes claims for U.S. government programs such as Medicare and Medicaid.

and Medicaid—are exchange partners with most HCOs. The federal Medicare program deals with HCOs through fiscal intermediaries.[10] Medicaid, a combination state and federal program that finances care for the poor, is run by the state Medicaid agency or an intermediary. Representing the buyers, payment organizations use contractual requirements, regulatory support, and incentive payments to improve the quality, safety, and cost of care.

The insurance industry and HCOs' relations to it were dramatically changed by the passage and implementation of the **Patient Protection and Affordable Care Act (ACA)**. This historic legislation has significant implications for healthcare organizations, including increased insurance coverage for many patients, new approaches to support those with chronic disease, and greater accountability for the cost and quality of care.[11,12] The ACA was developed in part to support the the "Triple Aim"—three goals for transforming the health system, including improving the individual patient experience with healthcare, improving the health of the population, and reducing the per capita cost of care.[13]

Patient Protection and Affordable Care Act (ACA)
A federal law (P.L. 111-148) providing for a fundamental reform of the U.S. healthcare and health insurance system, signed by President Barack Obama in 2010.

The ACA has increased the number of insured individuals and created new payer arrangements for HCOs. These changes use **value-based purchasing** approaches that reward HCOs for quality and sustained patient health.[14]

Value-based purchasing
Linking financial incentives to the quality of care provided.

Buyers   Much health insurance is provided through employment, making employers important stakeholders. Historically, unions played a major role in establishing health insurance as an employee benefit. Federal, state, and local governments purchase care for special groups of citizens and also buy insurance as employers. Insurance buyers, who must meet the demands of their own exchange networks, have taken action to restrict the growth of costs, acting principally through value-based purchasing, which is expected to become a major force in shaping most HCOs.

Regulatory Agencies

Government regulatory agencies are stakeholders that at least nominally act on behalf of the patient and buyer. State licensing agencies are common, not only for hospitals and healthcare professionals but sometimes also for other facilities such as ambulatory care centers. Many states have **certificate-of-need** laws, requiring HCOs to seek permission for construction or expansion. Quality improvement organizations (QIOs) are external agencies that review the quality of care and use of insurance benefits by individual physicians and patients for Medicare and other insurers. The QIOs have been instrumental in the national Surgical Care Improvement Project, a national quality partnership of organizations

Certificate of need
Certificate or approval for new services and construction or renovation of hospitals or related facilities; issued in many states.

interested in improving surgical care by significantly reducing surgical complications.[15] The project has almost universal endorsement among regulatory and healthcare trade associations, and an important record in reducing the hazards of surgical care.[16] HCOs are subject to many consumer-protection laws, including the Health Insurance Portability and Accountability Act (HIPAA), which addresses major issues of privacy and security of protected health information. The **Emergency Medical Treatment and Active Labor Act (EMTALA)** requires all HCOs providing emergency care to accept all patients, regardless of ability to pay, until they are stabilized and can be safely moved. Provisions of the ACA require not-for-profit hospitals to review community needs and report the **community benefit** value of the HCO contribution.[17]

Emergency Medical Treatment and Active Labor Act (EMTALA)
The act requires all HCOs providing emergency care to accept all patients, regardless of ability to pay, until they are stabilized and can be safely moved.

Most payment organizations mandate external reviews of HCO performance through accreditation and financial audits. Accreditation is voluntary, but HCOs must have accreditation by a Centers for Medicare & Medicaid Services (CMS) deemed-status organization, such as **The Joint Commission**, in order to receive funds from Medicare. Most payment organizations also require annual audits by the accounting firm of the HCO's choice. Some insurance plans are accredited by the National Committee for Quality Assurance (NCQA), which also accredits ambulatory care and disease management programs.

Community benefit
Current law requires hospitals to satisfy the community benefit standard in order to qualify as tax-exempt charities under section 501(c)(3) of the Internal Revenue Code.[18] The standard addresses charitable care, educational services, and other benefits HCOs provide to their communities.[19]

The Joint Commission
A voluntary consortium of professional provider organizations that evaluates and accredits a wide range of different HCOs.

HCOs require land-use and zoning permits; they use water, sewer, traffic, electronic communications, fire protection, and police services and thus are subject to environmental regulations. HCOs often present unique needs in these areas that must be negotiated with their local government.

The courts can also be viewed as regulatory agencies. HCOs may be sued for malpractice or negligence—harmful conduct that is unintentional but avoidable with reasonable care. Suits are brought by individuals in specific cases, but the court findings establish the rules of conduct for future actions. Thus the courts can also be viewed as regulatory organizations.

Community Groups

HCOs make numerous, varied, and far-reaching exchanges with community agencies and groups. They facilitate infant adoption; receive the victims of accidents and violence; and attract the homeless, the mentally ill, and those with chronic substance abuse concerns. These activities draw HCOs into exchanges with law enforcement and social service agencies.

In addition, HCOs work with United Way and other charities. HCOs facilitate baptisms, ritual circumcisions, group religious observances, individual spiritual activity, and rites for the dying. They provide educational facilities for caregivers and services to improve community health and well-being, such as health education and disease prevention programs, assistance to support groups, and mobile clinics. Such activities often make HCOs partners of cultural, religious, educational, and charitable organizations. Prevention and outreach activities draw HCOs into alliances with governmental organizations, such as public health departments and school boards, and with local employers, churches, and civic organizations.

Not-for-profit HCOs often occupy facilities that, if taxed, would add noticeably to local tax revenues. The community may hold the organization to certain conditions, such as a certain level of charity care, in return for nonprofit status.[20] Communication with stakeholders often involves the media—print, radio, television, and Internet coverage—and purchased advertising. Web-based public sources such as HealthGrades and WhyNotTheBest are increasingly influential in forming customer opinion, although they may not give consistent results.[21]

Provider Partners

Associates

The second most fundamental exchange, next to patients, is between the HCO and its **associates**—people who give their time and energy to the organization. HCO associates are employees, trustees and other volunteers, and medical staff members. The term *associates* is intentional and reflects the concept of servant leadership, which will be discussed in Chapter 2.

Employees are compensated by salaries and wages. Trustees and a great many others volunteer their time to not-for-profit HCOs; their only compensation is the satisfaction they achieve from the work. Medical staff members receive monetary compensation from either patients and insurance intermediaries or the HCO. **Licensed independent practitioners (LIPs)** are caregivers granted legal status to provide specific kinds of healthcare, categorized as primary care or specialist providers who are usually physicians or advanced practice nurses (nurse practitioners, nurse midwives). **Primary care practitioners** include physicians and advanced practice nurses specializing in family medicine, general internal medicine, pediatrics, obstetrics, and psychiatry and are the most common initial contacts for patients. **Specialist practitioners** tend to see patients referred by primary care

---

Associates
People (employees, trustees and other volunteers, and medical staff members) who give their time and energy to the HCO and its activities.

Licensed independent practitioners (LIPs)
Caregivers granted legal status to provide specific kinds of healthcare.

Primary care practitioners
Initial contact providers, including physicians, nurse practitioners, midwives in family medicine, general internal medicine, pediatrics, obstetrics, and psychiatry; often a longitudinal relationship.

Specialist practitioners
Licensed independent practitioners who care for patients referred by primary care practitioners on a limited or transient basis; likely to manage episodes of inpatient care.

practitioners and to care for these patients on a more limited and transient basis. They are more likely to manage episodes of inpatient hospital care. **Hospitalists** accept relatively broad categories of patients and manage inpatient care only. Other LIPs (e.g., dentists, psychologists, podiatrists) may also be members or associates of the HCO's medical staff.

Hospitalists
Physicians who manage broad categories of hospitalized patients.

Associate Organizations

Associates are often organized into groups that manage their exchanges to varying extents. Unions, or collective bargaining units, sometimes represent employed associates. Physicians and advanced practice nurses often form professional associations and practice groups. Neurologists, for example, can become a group to represent their interests to the organization as a whole.

Government agencies of various kinds monitor the rights of associate groups. Occupational safety, professional licensure, and equal employment opportunity agencies are among those entitled access to the HCO and its records. The National Labor Relations Board and various state agencies define which organizations are unions and establish rules for their relations with employers.

Suppliers and Financing Agencies

HCOs use goods and services—from artificial implants to food to banking to utilities—purchased from outside suppliers. Financing partners help HCOs acquire capital through a variety of equity, loan, and lease arrangements. HCOs often enter into strategic partnerships with suppliers and other provider partners.

Other Provider Organizations

In the course of meeting patient needs, HCOs have considerable contact with other HCOs, such as primary care clinics, mental health and substance abuse services, home care agencies, hospices, and rehabilitation and long-term care facilities. Many large HCOs incorporate and own these services. Others may have formal relationships with organizations, such as referral agreements, affiliations, strategic partnerships, and joint ventures. It is not uncommon for two HCOs to collaborate in some activities, such as medical education or care of the poor, and to compete actively on other activities.

Sources of Stakeholder Influence

The ultimate source of stakeholders' power is the marketplace—their ability to participate or choose not to participate in the exchange. In reality, influence is exercised in four ways that achieve ongoing negotiation rather than discontinued participation.

Participation and Market Pressure

Successful HCOs work steadily and systematically to increase the loyalty of their stakeholders. Their goal is to identify stakeholder needs and design effective responses before unmet needs become points of contention. Stakeholder participation is carefully measured. Customer participation is measured by market share, and provider participation is measured by retention and shortages. Surveys monitor satisfaction of both. Loyal customers and associates are vital assets of any HCO.

Negotiation

Stakeholders often present their concerns for negotiation, usually through organized representation. Desires frequently conflict and can easily become adversarial, as in the traditional relationship between unions and management. High-performing HCOs strive to minimize adversarial relationships by building a record of responsiveness and truth telling, making a diligent effort to find and understand relevant facts, maintaining respect and decorum in the debate, and searching diligently for win-win solutions. The goal is to have the stakeholders leave the discussion feeling that their concerns were heard, that the decision was fair, and that no realistic opportunity to improve the decision exists.

Networking and Coalition Building

Each exchange partner of the HCO has relationships with exchange partners of their own. Individuals and families affiliate with employers, businesses, schools, churches, and community groups. Stakeholder coalitions form among these relationships based on shared values or common needs. Many are more or less permanent, while others are temporary alliances to forward a specific goal.

Buyer- and consumer-oriented networks, such as the National Business Group on Health and the AARP, are coalitions that allow stakeholders to address complicated social problems, such as healthcare's uninsured and health promotion. The Joint Commission is a provider coalition that has been accepted as a central quality monitor for HCOs. The National Quality Forum (NQF) is a coalition of buyer and provider organizations that evaluates and standardizes measures of quality.[22] The measures become a central component for measuring HCO performance and for contracting with insurers.

Social Controls

Stakeholders can imbed their viewpoints into law, regulation, and contract. They can also sue in courts. These actions are social controls on HCOs. They create the various regulatory mechanisms. For example, The Joint Commission has been given extraordinary power by CMS through Medicare and

Medicaid, which withhold payment unless its standards are met. As a result, it can effectively shut down any HCO by denying accreditation. Medicare and private insurance programs now use the NQF measures in pay-for-performance programs to improve quality,[23] and The Joint Commission has added the measures to its criteria.[24]

Social controls almost always reflect good intentions—safety, quality, individual rights, equity, and efficiency. Accomplishment is another matter. It is fair to conclude that both the regulatory agencies dealing with healthcare delivery and the contracts of the health insurers and intermediaries have generally fallen short of expectations. Safety, quality, access, and cost remain problems despite decades of activity in these areas. In part, this reflects the complexity of the goal and the difficulty of measurement. In part, it reflects the limitations of the market and governmental systems.

The American Healthcare Marketplace

HCOs constitute one of the largest sectors in the U.S. economy. They are geographically universal but organizationally diverse. Every community has HCOs—typically one or more hospitals, several physicians' offices, and various continuing care and specialty services—but how those HCOs are organized differs from community to community.

Ownership and Centralization

This section describes HCOs—hospitals, primary care, post-acute care—by the services provided, ownership type, and extent of centralization.

Hospitals

Acute care hospitals are the largest single group of HCOs in terms of dollars. They are licensed corporate entities and also the largest and oldest components of most large health systems. Hospitals consume 30 percent of all healthcare expenditures; an additional 20 percent is spent on their affiliated physicians. Other expenditure is dispersed among a variety of vendors, utility providers, and others.[25] In combination, hospitals and physicians are the focus of most stakeholder efforts to control cost and quality. The organization of hospitals is shown in Exhibit 1.4. The 4,800 "general" or "community" hospitals account for 90 percent of hospital expenditures. These hospitals typically provide acute, inpatient medical, surgical, and obstetrical care. Fifteen hundred specialty hospitals consume only 10 percent of expenditures.

Hospital ownership is dominated by nonreligious and religious not-for-profit corporations. The not-for-profit structure has afforded substantial tax advantages to not-for-profit organizations, recognizing that their services would otherwise be required of government to fulfill.[26] Community hospitals operated by local government are organizationally similar.

EXHIBIT 1.4 Ownership and Specialization of U.S. Hospitals, 2010

Ownership	General Medical/ Surgical Hospitals Expenditures (billion $)	Count	Other Hospitals Expenditures (billion $)	Count	Total Expenditures (billion $)	Count
Federal	$ 49	197	$ 4	18	$ 53	215
For-profit	$ 63	794	$17	793	$ 80	1,587
Nonreligious not-for-profit	$395	2,250	$38	341	$433	2,591
Religious not-for-profit	$ 85	501	$ 2	45	$ 87	546
State/local government	$ 97	1,082	$17	290	$114	1,372
Grand total	$689	4,824	$77	1,487	$766	6,311

Source: Data from American Hospital Association Annual Survey Database, fiscal year 2010.

Exhibit 1.5 shows the relative expenditures of hospitals by owner-ship. Religious, other not-for-profit, and local government hospitals, often called *community hospitals*, provide about 80 percent of the total care. Federal and for-profit hospitals provide about 10 percent each. Virtually all federal hospitals were under the purview of four systems: Department of Defense, Veterans Affairs, Indian Health Service for Native American healthcare, and

EXHIBIT 1.5
Hospital
Expenditures
by Ownership

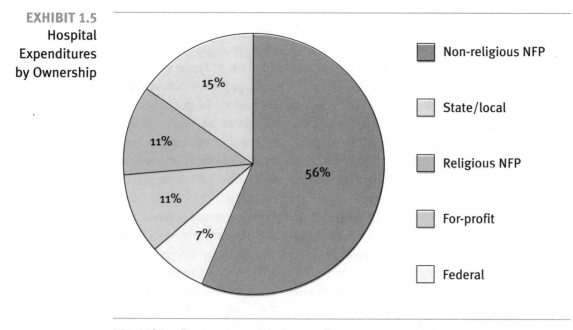

NFP: not-for-profit
Source: Data from American Hospital Association Annual Survey Database, fiscal year 2010.

federal prison hospitals. In the 1970s, a movement to for-profit ownership quickly reached about 10 percent of all community hospitals, and expenditures plateaued at that level. For-profit, or investor-owned, hospitals are heavily concentrated in specialty hospitals rather than community hospitals, and they tend to be small.

The trend has been toward larger HCOs, integrating both hospitals and other HCOs into **healthcare systems**. Most for-profit hospitals are in large systems. More than two thirds of community hospitals are in systems, by either count or expenditures. The median size of healthcare systems was $2 billion per year in 2010; the median size of independent hospitals was $30 million.

Healthcare system
A corporate or governmental structure including one or more hospitals and often other HCO services.

Many healthcare systems operate in multiple states; most provide a range of services beyond acute hospital care. Their size difference provides a number of operating advantages over independent hospitals. The typical HCO system is now almost 10 times the size of the typical independent hospital. Small organizations must purchase many clinical and logistic support services from independent vendors and obtain strategic advice from consultants. Larger systems can own and coordinate these activities more effectively. It is likely that they will grow, becoming the dominant source of personal healthcare. Specialty hospitals (such as cancer hospitals) and specialized services (such as urgent care centers, retail clinics, nursing homes, and hospices) will still exist as "niche" businesses targeting special patient needs and populations.

Primary Care

Primary care HCOs were traditionally organized around one or a few practitioners—doctors' offices, or urgent care centers, for example—generally tax-paying limited liability corporations, only slightly different from an owner-operated business. Larger groups of caregivers have steadily increased in popularity and expanded rapidly after passage of the ACA. Many individual practitioners affiliate with hospitals through a contract called "privileges." Privileges define quality and service obligations but allow a wide variety of financial arrangements. The traditional independent fee-for-service medical practice has largely yielded to larger corporate structures, including jointly owned physician hospital corporations and employment contracts. The joint corporations are generally for-profit. They employ physicians but permit practitioner owners to take an equity (ownership) position and participate directly in strategic decisions. Many physicians and other caregivers are now directly employed by large HCOs. Community health centers, often **federally qualified health centers**, which are not-for-profit clinics addressing the needs of the poor and uninsured, have grown in recent decades.

Federally qualified health center
Services for underserved areas or populations that offer a sliding fee scale, provide comprehensive services, have an ongoing quality program, and seat a board of directors; funded with grants under section 330 of the Public Health Service Act.

They have independent local governing boards but often affiliate with local hospitals. **Accountable care organizations (ACOs)**, created by the ACA, expand the concept of a **patient-centered medical home**. ACOs will largely be run by large HCOs, affiliating with group practices and community health centers, although other models are developing.[27,28]

Post-acute and Specialty Care

Many patients require extended support at less intense levels than acute inpatient care. The HCOs filling these needs can have any of a variety of corporate structures. Post-acute rehabilitation facilities are operated both by hospitals and by national for-profit chains that also operate nursing homes. They expanded rapidly in the late twentieth century, but growth has slowed. DaVita, a national chain of kidney dialysis centers, and several corporations operating bariatric surgery facilities are specialized, publicly owned, for-profit systems. It is not clear that they or similar systems will grow.

Chronic care facilities, or nursing homes, are operated both by not-for-profit hospitals and by a few large national for-profit chains. Independent local corporations are declining in number.

Palliative care and hospice services have been provided by hospitals and small independent not-for-profit corporations. It is likely that large HCOs will own or joint venture with many of these organizations.

Designing Excellence in an HCO

The better an HCO is managed, the greater the total advantages it produces. Excellence is achieved when the needs of both customer and provider stakeholders are optimally met:

- Patient care is safe, effective, patient centered, timely, efficient, and equitable.[31]
- The HCO participates actively with other community organizations to meet population health needs.
- Caregivers and other associates are attracted to the HCO, and they are given support to do their best.
- Expenditures are controlled so that the total cost is within the community's economic reach.

The Well-Managed Healthcare Organization describes how excellence is achieved by large HCOs. It identifies the essential functions, their integration, and the measures that document their performance. It is based not on average or typical HCOs but on the work of HCOs that have achieved excellence and documented it with objective measures.

The teams shown in Exhibit 1.1 can work as independent units in a marketplace where each team is a vendor, selling either to the patient or to another vendor. Much of American healthcare was essentially that. Small HCOs—doctors' offices, pharmacies, hospitals, equipment vendors, nursing homes, etc.—traditionally operated without any permanent relationship to each other. They bought logistic services from other vendors. There was no overarching strategy; the patients and their care teams selected each vendor as they needed them. Leading HCOs and healthcare systems have a very different vision, called **vertical integration**. They will integrate and support a large group of care teams, most commonly in acute care and rehabilitation but increasingly also primary care and long-term care. Many also pursue the same kinds of care teams in multiple sites, known as **horizontal integration**.

Vertical integration
The affiliation of organizations that provide different kinds of service, such as hospital care, ambulatory care, long-term care, and social services.

Horizontal integration
Integration of organizations that provide the same kind of service, such as two hospitals or two clinics.

As shown in Exhibit 1.6, excellence has three major foundations:

1. *Cultural*, a commitment to values that attract the respect and support of stakeholders as individuals
2. *Operational*, a system that seeks out, evaluates, and implements opportunities to improve stakeholder returns
3. *Strategic*, a system that deliberately monitors the long-term relationship between stakeholders and responds to changing needs

Cultural Foundation of Excellence: Transformational Management

The history of organizations in all industries suggests that stakeholders must build a cultural foundation that consists of five major elements: shared values, empowerment, communication, service excellence, and rewards for success. Excellent HCOs make major investments in clarifying, publicizing, and implementing their commitments to these elements. Their investments create a culture sometimes called *transformational management* that is highly satisfactory to both customer and associate stakeholders.

The transformational culture provides team members with important but intangible rewards—a sense of contribution to critical values, empowerment to shape the work, and partnership with like-minded individuals. The power of transformational management has been extensively documented.[32,33,34] It produces substantially better performance for two reasons:

1. Associates' insights about the job frequently improve the processes used, eliminating waste and inefficiency.
2. Associates are psychologically committed to the goal, rather than simply acting as sellers of their services. Also, when they are well trained, they can adjust to changes that arise, enabling them to avoid many causes of failure.[35]

EXHIBIT 1.6
Foundations
of Excellence
in Healthcare
Organizations

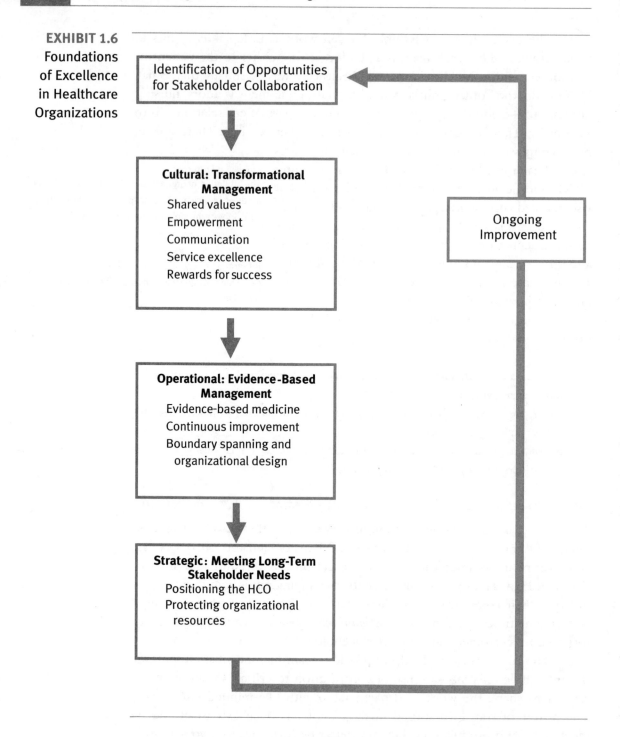

Shared Values

HCOs state that their **mission** is the central purpose of stakeholder collaboration. The fact that that mission is one of humanity's highest callings makes work in an HCO inherently attractive to many people. The mission to serve the sick provides a common bond that crosses many of the usual separations in society, and it is strongly endorsed by most of the world's religions. It is consistent with the ethical foundation of the care-giving professions. It is frequently mentioned as a personal commitment and source of satisfaction by HCO associates at all levels. Excellent HCOs build deliberately on a strong, visible commitment to this mission.

The mission is supplemented with a shared **vision**, an idealistic goal such as universal healthcare. The mission and vision are, in turn, supplemented by a commitment to **values**, shared rules of conduct. Values reflect the humanistic consensus of American thought: respect for all, compassion, honesty, trust, stewardship, and improvement.

The mission, vision, and values of an HCO are usually written by multiple teams with broad stake-holder representation so that many associates and customers can take part in the discussion and commit to the concepts. As a result, the wording of mission, vision, and values statements differs from HCO to HCO, but common threads are obvious among them.[36] The moral concepts behind the mission, vision, and values are often stated as *autonomy* (commitment to the patient's right to decide his or her own course), *benefi-cence* (commitment to serve the patient's needs), *nonmaleficence* (commitment to "do no harm"), and *justice* (commitment to equity and respect for all).[37] They can easily be expanded into the twenty-first-century goals for care delivery: safe, effective, patient centered, timely, efficient, and equitable. Exhibit 1.7 shows the mission and vision statements of HCOs that have documented their excellence for the Malcolm Baldrige National Quality Award.

Excellent HCOs publicize and display their mission, vision, and values widely, often on every associate's badge and always on every major entrance path, including the website. The mission, vision, and values are extensively advertised to the community at large and are an attractive statement to customers, communicating that "This HCO is here to meet your health needs."

Mission
A statement of purpose—the good or benefit the HCO intends to contribute—couched in terms of an identi-fied community, a set of services, and a specific level of cost or finance. Missions were frequently vague, such as "Excellence in care." Now many leading HCOs are moving to population health missions, ex-plicitly accepting responsibility for the broader goal.

Vision
An expansion of the mission that expresses inten-tions, philosophy, and organizational self-image.

Values
An expansion of the mission that expresses basic rules of acceptable conduct, such as respect for human dignity or acceptance of equality.

Empowerment

One purpose of transformational management is to create an environment where every associate can feel comfortable to think: "I will treat patients with compassion and be confident that members of my team and those in other teams will do the same. I will do my job, and I can trust others to do theirs. I can rely on what I'm told. My needs will be met. I won't be ignored, let alone harassed. And we will get better over time." This comfort level reflects **empowerment**.

Empowerment
The ability of an associate to control his or her work situation in ways consistent with the organization's mission.

Empowerment is particularly important in healthcare, where caregiving professionals must respond rapidly and correctly to patient needs. It improves

EXHIBIT 1.7

Mission and Vision Statements of HCO Baldrige National Quality Award Recipients

Year	Organization (State)	Mission	Vision
2002	SSM Health Care (MO) www.ssmhealth.com/ system	Through our exceptional health care services, we reveal the healing presence of God.	Through our participation in the healing ministry of Jesus Christ, communities, especially those that are economically, physically and socially marginalized, will experience improved health in mind, body, spirit, and environment within the financial limits of the system.
2003	Baptist Healthcare (FL) www.ebaptisthealth care.org/	To provide superior service based on Christian values to improve the quality of life for people and communities served.	To be the best health system in America.
2003	Saint Luke's Health System (MO) www.saintlukes healthsystem.org/	[A] faith-based, not-for-profit, aligned health system committed to the highest levels of excellence in providing health care and health-related services in a caring environment. We are dedicated to enhancing the physical, mental, and spiritual health of the diverse communities we serve.	The best place to get care. The best place to give care.
2004	RWJ University Hospital Hamilton (NJ) http://rwjhamilton .org/	[C]ommitted to excellence through service. We exist to promote, preserve and restore the health of our community.	[B]e a Quality Driven Center for Health that is nationally recognized for passionately exceeding the needs of our patients, employees, physicians and community.
2005	Bronson Healthcare (MI) www.bronsonhealth. com	Provide excellent healthcare services.	To be a national leader in healthcare quality.
2007	Mercy Health System (WI) www.mercyhealth system.org	[P]rovide exceptional health care services resulting in healing in the broadest sense.	Mercy's many service lines have individual visions. See, for example, the Trauma Center: "We are committed to provide: Regional trauma leadership Community injury prevention education Education to those who care for the injured The highest quality of care through continuous quality improvement" (www.mercyhealthsystem.org/body. cfm?id=487)

EXHIBIT 1.7

Mission and Vision Statements of HCO Baldrige National Quality Award Recipients *(continued)*

Year	Organization (State)	Mission	Vision
2007	Sharp HealthCare (CA) www.sharp.com	[I]mprove the health of those we serve with a commitment to excellence in all that we do.	[B]e the best health system in the universe. Sharp will attain this position by transforming the health care experience through a culture of caring, quality, service, innovation and excellence. Sharp will be recognized by employees, physicians, patients, volunteers and the community as the best place to work, the best place to practice medicine and the best place to receive care. Sharp is known as an excellent community citizen embodying an organization of people working together to do the right thing every day to improve the health and well-being of those we serve.
2008	Poudre Valley (CO) (now part of UC Health) www.uchealth.org/	Putting patients first. Leading the way in academic medicine, building healthier communities.	We improve lives. In big ways through learning, healing and discovery. In small, personal ways through human connection. But in all ways, we improve lives.
2009	AtlantiCare (NJ) www.atlanticare.org/	We deliver health and healing to all people through trusting relationships.	AtlantiCare builds healthy communities.
2009	Heartland Health (MO) (now Mosaic Lifecare) www.mymosaiclife care.org	To improve the health of individuals and communities located in the Heartland Health region and provide the right care, at the right time, in the right place, at the right cost with outcomes second to none.	To make Heartland Health and our service area the best and safest place in America to receive health care and live a healthy and productive life.
2010	Advocate Good Samaritan (IL) www.advocatehealth. com/gsam/	To serve the health needs of individuals, families and communities through a wholistic philosophy rooted in our fundamental undertanding of human beings as created in the image of God.	
2011	Henry Ford Health System (MI) www.henryford.com/	To improve people's lives through excellence in the science and art of health care and healing.	Transforming lives and communities through health and wellness—one person at at time.

(continued)

EXHIBIT 1.7

Mission and Vision Statements of HCO Baldrige National Quality Award Recipients *(continued)*

Year	Organization (State)	Mission	Vision
2011	Schneck Medical Center (IN) www.schneckmed.org/	To provide quality health care to all we serve.	To be a healthcare organization of excellence: every person, every time.
2011	Southcentral Foundation (AK) www.southcentralfoundation.com	Working together with the Native Community to achieve wellness through health and related services.	A Native Community that enjoys physical, mental, emotional, and spiritual wellness.
2013	Sutter Davis Hospital (CA) www.sutterdavis.org/	To enhance the health and well-being of people in the communities we serve, through a not-for-profit commitment to compassion and excellence in health care services.	Sutter Health leads the transformation of health care to achieve the highest levels of quality, access and affordability.
2012 and 2006	North Mississippi Health System (MS) www.nmhs.net/	To continuously improve the health of the people of our region.	What We Want to Be: The provider of the best patient-centered care and health services in America.

Source: Information from Malcolm Baldrige National Quality Award website. [Online information; retrieved 8/11/14.] www.baldrige.nist.gov/Contacts_Profiles.htm.

overall performance because associates (1) are not distracted or frustrated by their work situation and (2) feel empowered to meet patient needs. Empowered workers are known to be more effective.[38] Empowerment has long been a concern of the caregiving profession. Excellent HCOs ensure that their doctors, nurses, and other caregivers are empowered, but they also extend the same support to all associates.

Communication

Failures of communication are an obvious source of difficulty. "I didn't know you needed that" is a clear and frequent example. Transformational management addresses communication in several ways, some of which are discussed in this section. Excellent HCOs pursue all such methods, making frequent, candid, and useful communication a hallmark of their organizations and a strength in improving performance.

For example, Exhibit 1.8 shows the planned communication and training approaches at Bronson Methodist Hospital in Kalamazoo, Michigan. Bronson, a Malcolm Baldrige National Quality Award recipient in 2005, explains in its Baldrige application that managers are expected to dedicate much effort to ensuring that these processes are completed frequently and

Pre-hire and selection process (C, SK, TT)	Competency assessments (C, SK, TT)	**EXHIBIT 1.8** Bronson Methodist Hospital: Mechanisms for Communication, Skill Sharing, and Knowledge Transfer
New hire orientation (C, SK, TT)	Workshops and educational courses (C, SK, TT)	
Nursing core orientation (C, SK, TT)		
Leadership communication process (C)	Employee forums and focus groups (C, TT)	
Leadership communication forums (C)	Employee neighborhood meetings (C, TT)	
Knowledge-sharing documents (C, SK)	Computer-based learning modules (C, SK)	
Department meetings (C, SK, TT)	Leader rounds (C, SK, TT)	
Bulletin boards (C)	Self-study modules (C, SK)	
Communication books (C)	Skills fairs and learning labs (C, SK, TT)	
E-mail for all employees (C, TT)	Safety champions (C, SK, TT)	
Instant messaging (C, TT)	Preceptors (C, SK, TT)	
InsideBronson intranet (C, SK, TT)	Externships/internships (C, SK, TT)	
Department-specific newsletters (C)	Management mentor program (C, SK, TT)	
Shared directories (C)	Shared governance (C, SK, TT)	
Daily huddles (C, SK, TT)	Teams, work groups, councils, and committees (C, SK, TT)	
Healthlines newsletter (C)		
CEO/CNE open office hours (C, TT)	Staff performance management system (C, SK, TT)	
Leadership (C, SK, TT)		

C: communication; SK: skill sharing and knowledge; TT: two-way transfer
Source: Information from Bronson Methodist Hospital application to the Malcolm Baldrige National Quality Award. 2006. "Bronson Methodist Hospital." [Online information; retrieved 8/11/14.] www.baldrige.nist.gov/Contacts_Profiles.htm.

well. Each senior manager is expected to spend five hours per week listening to caregiving, logistic, and clinical teams.

Listening

Much of modern healthcare (more than most people think) can be quantified, but much remains subjective. Excellent HCOs formally and informally listen to all stakeholders to complement and strengthen their measured performance. Listening means deliberately soliciting stakeholder input through various communication methods, such as surveys, positive and negative event reports, group and individual interviews, direct conversations, e-mails, and blogs. The results of listening are systematically described, tallied, and analyzed to identify trends and opportunities for improvement.

Negotiating

Empowerment requires that organization goals and plans be discussed in advance of implementation to gain widespread understanding and commitment. Understanding and commitment are not automatic. Their achievement requires exploring implications, identifying concerns and barriers, and finding ways to remove those barriers. From the manager's perspective, conflicting stakeholder needs must be negotiated and a mutually acceptable settlement reached.

Negotiation is a major shift in organizational thought. The bureaucratic organization, going back to Machiavelli's time and before that, operated under the command from superior to subordinate. In excellent HCOs, however, commands are used only in extreme emergency situations, where a team leader must coordinate the team quickly through uncharted territory. All other interactions are established by implicit or explicit negotiation.

Teaching   The activities shown in Exhibit 1.1 are learned. They follow prescribed scripts that are replicable for every process but can be adapted to individual patient needs and unanticipated events. Patient care follows **protocols**—from greeting a patient ("Good morning, may I check your armband?") to administering an intravenous drip to performing a surgical "time-out" whereby the circulating nurse verifies the patient, procedure, location, and any unusual risks. Specific **procedures** or **processes** are also followed for nonclinical activities, such as cleaning washrooms, posting payments to patient accounts, and conducting meetings of the governing board.

Protocols
Agreed-on procedures for each task in the care process.

Procedures or *processes*
Actions or steps that transform inputs to outputs.

All processes are learned, and most are taught by the organization. High-performing organizations invest heavily in teaching (using a variety of approaches), measuring learning, and rewarding correct application. Bronson Methodist, for example, documents an average of more than 100 hours of teaching for each full-time employee.[39]

Modeling   Actions inevitably speak louder than words. Everyone in leadership positions must model the behaviors that support the organizational values. High-performing HCOs expect their managers' professional actions to personify and implement the mission, vision, and values. Training programs help managers understand how to respond to common problems in ways that encourage associates. These programs often include coaching and mentoring to improve skills and counseling when specific problems arise. Managers at all levels are expected to point out to each other anything that falls short of model behavior. Managers undergo a multi-rater review, a system that allows subordinates, coworkers, customers, and supervisors to evaluate the managers anonymously.

Service Excellence

Agency or *accountability*
The notion that the organization can rely on an individual or a team to fulfill a specific, prearranged expectation.

Every team and organization functions under a contract or an agreement; that is, team members are agents who agree to carry out individual acts and to share accountability for the results. Caregiving teams are agents for patients who are unable to act for themselves. The concept of **agency** or **accountability** (also called *stewardship*) is essential to building trust within the organization. HCOs reinforce trust and stewardship by building team spirit and by modeling and rewarding correct behaviors.

Trust and accountability, agency, and stewardship are difficult to sustain. They are subject to moral hazard; any member can do less than her share, free-riding on the efforts of others. High-performing HCOs build trust and stewardship with a program of **service excellence**, recognizing that associates will work to meet customer needs if their own needs are met.[40] That is, if management shares the values of its workers, listens to them, responds to the issues they raise (empowering them), trains them, and supports them logistically, the workers perform to the extent that customers' needs are satisfied.

Service excellence
Concept whereby associates anticipate and meet or exceed customer needs and expectations on the basis of the mission and values.

Service excellence has gained wide support, particularly in service industries.[41] It is a universal practice among high-performing HCOs.[42] In addition, team evaluations and team pressure help make free-riding unattractive or difficult. An important motivator among workers is the belief that their colleagues will not let them down, so they will not let their colleagues down in return.

Rewards for Success

The most important reward for most associates is the satisfaction of having done a good job. Excellent HCOs not only provide that reward but also strengthen and complement it. Success at continuous improvement provides measurable gains in achieving stakeholder goals. HCO operations become safer, more pleasant, more responsive, and more efficient. The new processes developed are better than the ones they replaced. The negotiated goals are almost always achieved. Patients and families express their gratitude.

High-performing HCOs distribute a substantial portion of the gains back to the associates who helped produce those gains. HCOs do this in two ways—celebrations and incentive pay. Celebrations include parties, meals, various tokens of recognition, and prizes such as gift certificates or small amounts of cash. They are frequent, usually informal, and can be put together quickly. Often, first-line supervisors are given a budget explicitly for celebrations. Incentive compensation links employee performance to the HCO goals. Substantial financial rewards are provided to associates in return for achieving continuous improvement goals.[43]

The reward system of Mercy Health System in Janesville, Wisconsin, is shown in Exhibit 1.9. The six celebrations offer prizes for various individual achievements that embody the organization's vision and values, such as offering extra help to a patient or family, serving on a demanding committee, contributing a useful solution or a new idea, or reaching out to a coworker. The incentive compensation is open to all but is tailored to specific professions and economic situations. Mercy's retirement program is designed to retain its best associates.

Reward	Award/Incentive Programs	Objectives
Celebrations	"Above and Beyond the Call of Duty" Partner* Recognition Dinner Quest for the Best Baskets for Champions Partner Idea Program "Someone to Admire and Respect"	Promote excellent services by rewarding/recognizing best practices, quality outcomes, innovation, teamwork, or partnering initiatives
Incentive Compensation	Report cards/performance appraisals; bonuses dependent on organizational and individual achievement of targets Physician incentive program Individual merit increases Matched savings retirement plan	Reward best-practice achievers of individual targets, tied to Four Pillars of Excellence** Reward superior customer service performance

Partners are all employees, including managers and senior management.
**The *Four Pillars of Excellence* is Mercy Health System's dimensions of strategic measurement: Quality—excellence in patient care and service; Exceptional Patient and Customer Service; Partnering—best place to work; and Cost—long-term financial success.
Source: Adapted from Mercy Health System's application to the Malcolm Baldrige National Quality Award, 2007, p. 22. [Online information; retrieved 8/11/14.] www.baldrige.nist.gov.

Operational Foundation of Excellence: Evidence-Based Management

Evidence-based management
Relies heavily on performance measurement, identification of best practices, and formal process specification.

The operational foundation reflects a major shift in thinking that began in the 1990s[44] and continues today in more than half of the nation's hospitals.[45] This model, often called **evidence-based management**, relies heavily on performance measurement, identification of best practices, and formal process specification. Evidence-based management deliberately parallels *evidence-based medicine*, a similar shift in medical thinking toward the systematic use of science to identify clinical best practices.

Patient care guidelines
Formally established, scientifically based expectations that specify what must be done, by whom, how, and when, subject to the caregiver's judgment regarding the individual patient.

The core concept of evidence-based medicine is that scientific knowledge should drive as many clinical decisions as possible.[46] Much of medicine is judgmental, but as the diagnosis is clarified, evidence can be drawn from existing similar cases. **Patient care guidelines** define the scientifically proven steps appropriate for treating most patients with a specific disease or condition. They are translated to **patient care protocols** that can be implemented in specific

Patient care protocols
Guidelines that have been tested and accepted for use by a specific HCO.

HCOs. **Functional protocols** detail the specific steps for performing individual clinical procedures, such as admission interviews and subcutaneous injections. These protocols make explicit the agency and stewardship obligations behind service excellence.

Functional protocols
Formally established, scientifically based expectations that specify how and by whom specific care activities are carried out.

Protocols are not rules; the empowered caregiver has the obligation to depart from the protocol when the patient's condition requires it.

Evidence-based medicine has become the standard of practice. Many professional organizations and academic medical centers prepare patient care guidelines, and more than 2,000 are listed on Guideline.gov, the federal website recording them.[47] Evidence-based medicine is deeply embedded in both graduate and continuing clinical education.[48,49]

Evidence-based management applies the scientific method to managing organizations. It is widely recognized in other industrial sectors, and it requires a thoughtful, thorough, and professionally disciplined approach.[50] In HCOs, it is built around the following elements:

1. *Boundary spanning:* establishing and maintaining effective relationships with all stakeholders, and adapting the HCO to the needs of its community
2. *Knowledge management:* maintaining a detailed fact base about the organization, including performance measures, benchmarks, and work processes, and making that fact base accessible to associates through training and communication
3. *Accountability and organizational design:* identifying and integrating the contribution and goals of each HCO component
4. *Continuous improvement:* continually analyzing and improving all work processes following a systematic cycle of measurement, opportunity identification, analysis, trial, goal setting, and training for implementation

Evidence-based management is a major philosophic change. Like the advances in web communication, it is one of the latest steps in the centuries-long growth of empiricism and science in human enterprise. Used with transformational management and evidence-based medicine, evidence-based management creates HCOs that can achieve performance previously thought to be beyond reach.

Boundary Spanning

An excellent HCO must be able to provide reliable and timely answers to several recurring questions:

1. What are the opportunities for improvement as seen by customer stakeholders?
2. What are the demands and restrictions imposed by regulatory agencies?
3. What services should be available to our customers?

4. Which services should our HCO own and operate, and which should it acquire by contract?
5. How big should each service be?
6. What are the formal links between services and with the enterprise as a whole?
7. How do we acquire capital?
8. How do we acquire new technology and replace outdated facilities?
9. How do we ensure an adequate group of associates?

These questions identify the components of the HCO, relate them to each other, and relate the HCO to external suppliers and stakeholder networks. They are strategic questions, but the operational foundation must include substantial information gathering and analytic activity to ensure that the best alternatives are fully prepared and understood. Listening to customer stakeholders is an important part of this activity. Understanding and influencing the thinking of insurers, buyers, and regulators allow proactive instead of reactive relations. Quantitative analyses and forecasts of external data, such as population trends, economic trends, and epidemiology, support proposals that are economically realistic and that identify and reduce risks.

Knowledge Management

Data Warehouse

Facts, usually numbers, drive evidence-based decisions. Excellent HCOs build and maintain a **data warehouse**, a large library of work processes, protocols, and performance measures; a reporting system that keeps all associates current on measured performance and goal achievement; and a communication system to relay information relevant to immediate applications. The warehouse is web-accessed. It typically contains several hundred protocols and procedures and several thousand individual data sets. (An acute care HCO needs several hundred measures to implement its operational scorecards, described below.)

Data warehouse
Web-accessible library of work processes, protocols, and performance measures available to all associates.

There is a "way we do things" for most activities in HCOs—from how the governing board is selected to how a new patient is greeted to how a spontaneous obstetric delivery is managed. Many different associates will be involved in most of these processes, and consistency is important. The processes will change, and the changes must be recorded. In evidence-based management, change is deliberately sought using performance measures.

Strategic and Operational Scorecards

As shown in Exhibit 1.10, six dimensions of measurement are necessary to guide the individual teams listed in Exhibit 1.1. This set is called an **operational scorecard**. It is usually generated monthly and reports three dimensions of inputs or resources—demand for service; physical resources or costs; and status of resources, such as the satisfaction and commitment of the unit's

Input Oriented	Output Oriented	
Demand	*Output and productivity*	**EXHIBIT 1.10**
Requests for service	Counts of services rendered	Operational
Market share	Productivity (resources/treatment or	Scorecard:
Appropriateness of demand	service)	Performance
Unmet need		Measures for
Demand logistics	*Quality*	Individual
Demand errors	Clinical outcomes	Teams and
	Procedural quality	Work Units
Cost and resources	Structural quality	
Physical counts		
Costs	*Customer satisfaction*	
Resource conditions	Patients	
	Referring physicians	
Human resources	Other customers	
Supply		
Development		
Satisfaction		
Loyalty		

associates—and three dimensions of results—output and productivity (ratio of resource to output), quality of service or product, and customer satisfaction. The actual measures can differ by unit, but enough common measures must be used to allow similar units to be aggregated into service lines.

Success for the whole is more than the sum of success of individual teams. The measures must be carefully aggregated to progressively higher levels of accountability. Certain measures—chiefly income and financial position—cannot be calculated at the individual team level but are critical for the HCO as a whole. The **strategic scorecard**, sometimes called *balanced scorecard*, measures the enterprise as a whole or in large components, particularly those with independent financial structure, such as joint venture corporations. As shown in Exhibit 1.11, they are carefully aggregated from operational measures to reflect the needs of major stakeholder groups. About 30 measures are used, grouped in major dimensions—customers, associates and suppliers, operations (quality and cost), and finance.

In the next chapters, the templates in exhibits 1.10 and 1.11 are expanded to show the kinds of measures used by excellent HCOs in each activity and in the aggregate. The system of measures described in these

Operational scorecard
Performance report for a single work unit or an aggregate of several related units, reporting three dimensions of inputs or resources—demand for service; physical resources or costs; and status of resources, such as the satisfaction and commitment of the unit's associates—and three dimensions of results—output and productivity (ratio of resource to output), quality of service or product, and customer satisfaction. The actual measures can differ by unit, but enough common measures must be used to allow similar units to be aggregated into service lines.

Strategic scorecard
Measures of overall enterprise performance grouped in major dimensions—customers, associates and suppliers, operations (quality and cost), and finance. The strategic scorecard is reported to the governing board and is appropriate for service lines, the HCO as a whole, or its major components.

EXHIBIT 1.11
Template of
Strategic
Measures
of HCO
Performance

Dimension	Major Concepts	Healthcare Examples
Financial performance	Ability to acquire, support, and effectively reinvest essential resources	Profit and cash flow Days' cash on hand Credit rating and financial structure
Internal operations, including quality and safety	Ability to provide competitive service Quality, efficiency, safety, and availability of service	Unit cost of care Measures of safety and quality of care Processes and outcomes of care Timeliness of service
Market performance and customer satisfaction	Reflects all aspects of relationship to customers	Market share Patient and family satisfaction Measures of access for disadvantaged groups
Associate satisfaction and ability to adapt and improve	Ability to attract and retain an effective associate group Learning and motivation of workforce Response to change in technology, customer attitudes, and economic environment	Physician and employee satisfaction Associate safety and retention Training program participation and skill development Availability of emerging methods of care Trends in service and market performance Ability to implement changes in timely fashion

exhibits tracks the stakeholder relations and mission achievement for each unit of the HCO, making clear what the unit's critical contributions are and allowing for negotiated goals with measured achievement. Quantified goals and measures substantially reduce ambiguity and clarify each team's and associate's obligation. Frequently posted results discourage procrastination. When customers frequently post ratings of your work and attitude, the ratings are difficult to ignore.

Training   Work processes and protocols must be learned by all users. Web-based outlines are helpful, but many healthcare protocols require users to master specific manual, verbal, and observational skills by practicing these processes regularly. Exhibit 1.8 includes a number of training activities, or "knowledge transfer" in Bronson's terminology. Bronson and other high-performing systems and hospitals invest about twice as much time—two to two-and-a-half weeks per associate per year—in training. Much of this training is made available through organized sessions, but much is provided "just in time," supplied on site by coaches, consultants, or leaders.

The culture of high-performing HCOs emphasizes listening, which requires facts and information such as patient orders, patient conditions, supplies used, and hours worked. Part of knowledge management is supplying this information promptly and accurately. Electronic medical records, e-mail, web access, telephone systems, newsletters, posters, and memos create a network through which time-dependent information can be exchanged.

Communications Networks

Accountability and Organizational Design

Integrating an HCO requires careful planning to combine the caregiving and support teams into an effective whole. This means creating effective networks of accountability. Each team must know its contribution, and within the team, each member. In a transformational culture, these contributions are negotiated, but they must still be integrated into the whole.

A framework must exist for the negotiation and integration. The framework, called an **accountability hierarchy**, is a communications network that promotes factual exchange among related work teams and links each work team to the governing board. In addition to negotiating performance goals, the accountability hierarchy facilitates review of investment opportunities.

Accountability hierarchy
A reporting and communication system that links each operating unit to the governing board, usually by grouping similar centers together under middle management.

Not all patient needs are filled by associates; many are met by contractual partners, and some services are provided by remote organizations. Various legal structures are available to manage these relationships. Most large HCOs now have subsidiary corporations, joint ventures, and long-term contracts, which are sometimes called *strategic partnerships*. The accountability hierarchy of associates is supplemented with a designed array of other relationships.

Continuous Improvement

Continuous improvement depends on performance measurement and commits the HCO to systematic change; what was done last year is no longer the automatic standard for the future. Continuous improvement was recognized in the 1980s, largely as a result of the work of W. Edwards Deming.[51] It had widespread acceptance and is now a foundation for high-performing organizations in all industries. It is universal among excellent HCOs.[52,53,54]

Systematic change is built on establishing goals, reporting actual results, and comparing actual outcome against goal and goal against **benchmark**. This comparison identifies **opportunities for improvement** (**OFIs**, pronounced "oafies") and involves all teams, ideally all associates. OFIs also arise

Benchmark
The best-known value for a specific measure, from any source.

Opportunities for improvement (OFIs)
Result of comparing actual outcome against goal and goal against benchmark; also arise from qualitative assessments, including listening.

from qualitative assessments, including listening. Systematic change entails determining OFIs to design and implement changes in the work processes to achieve better performance. Exhibit 1.12 shows how processes are analyzed to translate OFIs to actual performance improvement.

The analysis is carried out by a **process improvement team (PIT)**. Successfully translating OFIs to improvement requires finding the **root causes**, the underlying factors that must be changed to yield consistently better outcomes. Root causes almost always lie in the methods, tools, equipment, supplies, information, training, and rewards provided the team, and almost never in issues of individual effort or attitude. The proposition that opportunities to improve performance lie with process rather than with people has been proven countless times in all kinds of organizations.[55]

Process improvement team (PIT)
A group that analyzes processes and translates OFIs to actual performance improvement.

Root causes
The underlying factors that must be changed to yield consistently better outcomes.

Systematic change is a four-step process that applies to any OFI:

1. *Identify:* find improvable processes or OFIs.
2. *Analyze:* uncover root causes or possible corrections.
3. *Test:* develop alternative solutions and select the best for implementation.
4. *Evaluate:* implement the best solution, establish new goals, and monitor progress.

An older version of this concept is the Shewhart cycle, which labels these four steps as Plan, Do, Check, and Act.

The process, shown as the circle in Exhibit 1.12, can be quite elaborate, involving hundreds of associates and steps. A number of formal approaches to analysis are popular, including Lean management, Six Sigma, and GE Work-Out; these are rigorous, objective, and thorough work processes for continuous improvement.

Performance improvement council (PIC)
A formal coordinating structure composed of representatives from all major activities or activity groups; the PIC's first job is to prioritize the OFIs.

OFIs that apply to only one team can often be addressed by that team, but most OFIs are complicated and need a formal coordinating structure called the **performance improvement council (PIC)**. The PIC is composed of representatives from all major activities or activity groups and is usually closely linked to senior management. The PIC's first job is to prioritize the OFIs, and top priority are the OFIs that have the highest potential impact on mission achievement and the strategic scorecard (Exhibit 1.11). The PIC pursues as many OFIs as possible, limited only by the ability of the organization to staff the PITs. An important part of PIC activity is coordinating multiple PITs and keeping them aligned with the annual goal-setting activity.

EXHIBIT 1.12 Process Analysis: Translating OFIs to Improved Performance

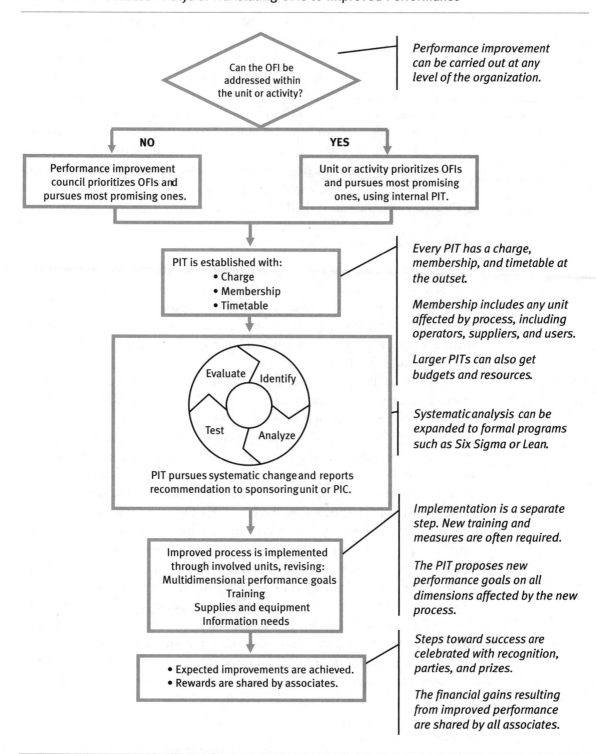

OFI: opportunity for improvement; PIC: performance improvement council; PIT: process improvement team

Strategic Foundation of Excellence: Positioning and Protection

Strategy
A systematic response to a specific stakeholder need.

Strategic positioning
The set of decisions about mission, ownership, scope of activity, location, and partners that defines the organization and relates it to stakeholder needs.

Strategic protection
Activities to safeguard the assets of the organization.

An HCO must support its cultural and operational foundations with a **strategy** or process for matching the activities and resources to stakeholder needs. **Strategic positioning** is an integrative activity that seeks maximum return from the resources available. Its success is measured by improvement in the strategic measures (Exhibit 1.11). Decision making provides definitive answers to boundary-spanning questions. **Strategic protection** safeguards the assets of the organization, including ensuring the reliability and validity of the data and information used for patient care and continuous improvement.

Strategic Positioning

Strategic positioning has two major components. The first component is data intensive and analytical. Boundary spanning (externally oriented) and organization OFIs (internally oriented) generate proposals for responding to the most important questions. The second component is the decision to implement specific proposals. Decision making requires experience, imagination, diligence, and risk taking.

Excellent HCOs use their governing boards, managers, and internal and external consultants for strategic positioning. Planning committees are established to pursue specific opportunities. They operate much like PITs in that they usually follow an iterative review process, such as the competitive tests for investment opportunities (see Exhibit 1.13). But planning committees have a broader agenda and greater license to consider innovation. They evaluate the impact of alternative actions on the strategic performance measures.

Exhibit 1.14 shows how excellent HCOs coordinate their strategic activity using an annual cycle of review that integrates analysis, proposals, and ongoing operations data to establish specific plans. These plans forecast expectations for the strategic performance measures several years into the future on the basis of the planning committee's analyses. The forecast is refined as time passes, and for the immediate next year it becomes the initial proposal for strategic goals. The governing board and its committees review the forecast and establish the annual goals, which guide internal goal negotiations. Senior management is responsible for forecasting. It participates actively in the discussions and facilitates communications between governance and those in charge of activities.

Strategic Protection

All the assets of an HCO are subject to known hazards. Money gets stolen; facilities get damaged; people get hurt; information gets distorted. Any kind of asset can be lost. The first line of defense is work processes designed to protect

EXHIBIT 1.13
Competitive
Tests for
Investment
Opportunities

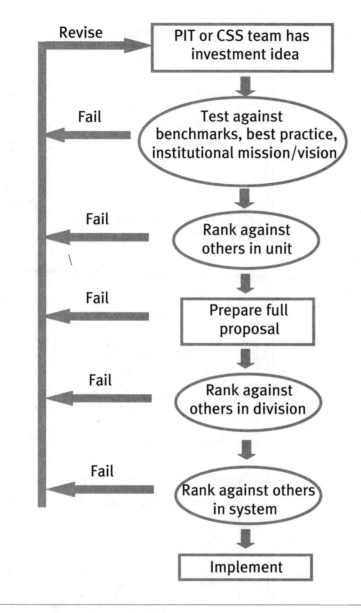

CSS: clinical support service; PIT: process improvement team

against these risks. Cash is handled in centuries-old processes that make theft and embezzlement rare. Security programs protect facilities and their people. Information handling includes careful attention to accurate inputs, safeguards for appropriate access, and backups for mechanical failure. Excellence must go beyond simply putting these processes in place. It must systematically monitor the security processes and the risks to ensure compliance. Thus, cash and cash processes are examined by external auditors; facilities and security personnel are monitored through video surveillance; data and programs are audited to verify their validity and reliability.

EXHIBIT 1.14
Strategic
Positioning
and Monitoring
Processes

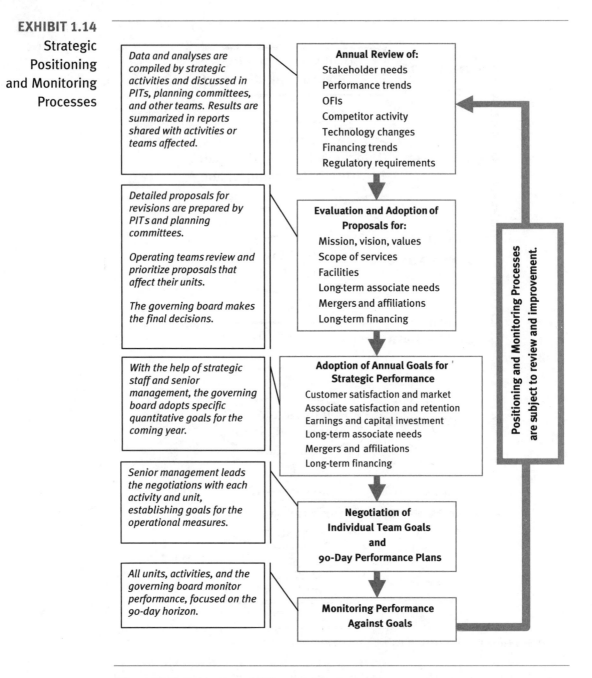

OFI: opportunity for improvement; PIT: process improvement team

A less obvious risk inherent in all organizations is the failure of an individual or a team to completely carry out its responsibilities. Individuals and teams in HCOs act as agents for patients or internal customers and must be accountable to complete their duties. Other individuals and teams must be able to trust the agents. A high level of trust is essential to sustaining the culture of excellence. As noted, agency, accountability, and trust are inherently subject to moral hazard. Any excellent organization must protect against agency failure, which can occur at all levels—from the temporary employee to the chief executive officer to the governing board chair. Excellent HCOs have learned to strengthen and protect their agency relationships through six important steps, shown in Exhibit 1.15. The first four steps are built into the culture and procedural foundations. The last two—audit and correction—require special attention.

At least three different kinds of audits go on simultaneously in an evidence-based management system and serve to strengthen accountability: *Audits*

1. *Transparent performance review.* Each level of the organization has current goals and receives performance data frequently. Excellent HCOs encourage open review of these reports, both within the units and with other units. They use 90-day plans for goal achievement, including corrective plans where necessary. The openness creates an atmosphere that makes it difficult to carry out activities that are contrary to the mission.
2. *Internal audits and reviews.* The fact that audits can be conducted at any time, by auditors deliberately isolated from the activity, on either a random or selective basis serves as a strong deterrent to misfeasance. The processes that ensure reliability of quantitative reports also discourage misrepresentation. The extensive network of listening helps ensure conformance. Reports of difficulty are carefully handled in ways that protect people who report potential problems.
3. *External reviews, audits, and oversight.* The governing board, representing the owners and stakeholders as a whole rather than the organization and its associates, is an ongoing external monitor for the organization. The services to customer stakeholders and owner stakeholders are regularly evaluated by The Joint Commission, external financial auditors, and routine financial and clinical reports. The stakeholders may pursue criminal or civil redress if they have evidence of difficulty.

		EXHIBIT 1.15
Values	Mission, vision, and values are collectively developed, prominently displayed, and frequently cited.	Foundations That
Clarity	Specific desired behaviors are advertised to potential associates and explicitly taught in orientation programs.	Reinforce Agency/
Responsiveness	The responses given by management to associate queries and requests apply the mission, vision, and values.	Accountability Relationships
Modeling	The behavior of management is consistent with mission, vision, and values.	
Audit	A system of checks and balances assists management and other associates by detecting departures from mission, vision, and values.	
Correction	When necessary, management implements a graduated corrective response that usually includes warning, retraining, second warning, and discharge.	

High-performing organizations have made the audit structure more robust. They have built reviews into the governance process so that board members evaluate each other and their performance as a team. They have voluntarily implemented the standards of the Sarbanes-Oxley Act (legislation directed at for-profit entities), calling for greater protection against fraudulent diversion of assets, fuller disclosure of actual performance, attestation to the accuracy of published results by board members and senior management, increased auditing, and avoidance of conflict of interest in all board decisions.[56]

Correction   When failures of accountability, agency, or trust occur, excellent organizations deal with them using a structured program in which managers at all levels have been trained. The program begins with a warning and discussion of causes and corrections. Subsequent failures lead to retraining and a candid discussion about the consequences of failure for the individual as well as the organization. A written record is often created. Continued failure leads to termination or reassignment. When the behavior in question is dangerous, threatening, or deliberate, discharge is often immediate. Deliberate lying, falsification of records, harassment of others, criminal behavior, and violation of community norms usually lead to immediate discharge, regardless of the rank involved.

The cultural, procedural, and strategic foundations are designed to promote excellence, and they are largely successful. When these foundations are maintained, failures of accountability and agency are rare. If they are not maintained, the entire organization is threatened and drastic reconstruction is in order. Monitoring and maintaining the foundations are strategic activities primarily of the governing board and senior management.

Additional Resources

American Hospital Association. 2014. "Hospitals in Pursuit of Excellence." [Online information; retrieved 2/3/15.] http://www.hpoe.org/.

Askin, E., and N. Moore. 2014. *The Health Care Handbook*, 2nd ed. St. Louis, MO: Washington University.

Institute for Healthcare Improvement. 2015. "Open School." [Online information; retrieved 2/3/15.] www.ihi.org/education/ihiopenschool/Pages/default.aspx.

Studer, Q. 2008. *Results That Last: Hardwiring Behaviors That Will Take Your Company to the Top*. Hoboken, NJ: Wiley.

Notes

1. Eggleston, E. M., and J. A. Finkelstein. 2014. "Finding the Role of Health Care in Population Health." *Journal of the American Medical Association* 311 (8): 797–98.

2. Shortell, S. M. 2013. "Bridging the Divide Between Health and Health Care." *Journal of the American Medical Association* 309 (11): 1121–22.

3. Hacker, K., and D. K. Walker. 2013. "Achieving Population Health in Accountable Care Organizations." *American Journal of Public Health* 13 (7): 1163–67.

4. HealthyPeople.gov. 2010. "About Healthy People: Healthy People 2020." [Online information; retrieved 7/25/14.] www.healthypeople.gov/2020/about/default. aspx.

5. Eggleston and Finkelstein (2014); Shortel (2013); Hacker and Walker (2013).

6. Burns, L., E. Bradley, and B. Weiner (eds.). 2011. "Organization Theory." In *Shortell and Kaluzny's Health Care Management: Organizational Design and Behavior*, 6th ed. Clifton Park, NY: Cengage Learning.

7. Chandler, A. D. 1977. *The Visible Hand: The Managerial Revolution in American Business.* Cambridge, MA: Belknap Press; Coase, R. 1937. "The Nature of the Firm." *Economica* 4 (16): 386–405.

8. Institute of Medicine (IOM), Committee on Quality of Health Care in America. 2001. *Crossing the Quality Chasm: A New Health System for the 21st Century,* 39. Washington, DC: National Academies Press.

9. IOM (2001).

10. Centers for Medicare & Medicaid Services. 2010. "Medicare Fee-for-Service Claims Contract Directory as of May 28, 2010." [Online information; retrieved 8/11/14.] www.cms.hhs.gov/ContractingGeneralInformation/Downloads/02_ICdirectory.pdf.

11. Iglehart, J. K. 2014. "An Uncertain Environment for US Hospitals." *Health Affairs* 33 (5): 734.

12. Kaiser Health Foundation. 2013. "Summary of the Affordable Care Act." [Online information; retrieved 7/25/14.] http://kff.org/health-reform/fact-sheet/summary-of-the-affordable-care-act/.

13. Institute for Healthcare Improvement. 2015. "Triple Aim for Populations." [Online information; retrieved 7/25/14.] www.ihi.org/Topics/TripleAim/Pages/default.aspx; Berwick, D. M., T. W. Nolan, and J. Whittington. 2008. "The Triple Aim: Care, Health, and Cost." *Health Affairs* 27 (3): 759–69.

14. Centers for Medicare & Medicaid Services. 2014. "Hospital Value-Based Purchasing." [Online information; retrieved 8/11/14.] www.cms.gov/Medicare/Quality-Initiatives-Patient-Assessment-Instruments/hospital-value-based-purchasing/index.html.

15. The Joint Commission. 2014. "Surgical Care Improvement Project." [Online information; retrieved 7/25/14.] www.jointcommission.org/surgical_care_improvement_project/.

16. Awad, S. S. 2012. "Adherence to Surgical Care Improvement Project Measures and Post-operative Surgical Site Infections." *Surgical Infections* 13 (4): 234–37.

17. Internal Revenue Service. 2014. "New Requirements for 501(c)(3) Hospitals Under the Affordable Care Act." [Online information; retrieved 7/25/14.] www.irs.gov/Charities-%26-Non-Profits/Charitable-Organizations/New-Requirements-for-501(c)(3)-Hospitals-Under-the-Affordable-Care-Act.

18. Internal Revenue Service. 2007. "Executive Summary: Hospital Compliance Project, Interim Report." [Online information; retrieved 7/26/14.] www.irs.gov/pub/irs-tege/eo_interim_hospital_report__execsummary_072007.pdf.

19. American Hospital Association (AHA). 2006. "AHA Guidance on Reporting of Community Benefit." Chicago: AHA.

20. Singer, L. E. 2008. "Leveraging Tax-Exempt Status of Hospitals." *Journal of Legal Medicine* 29 (1): 41–64.

21. Rothberg, M. B., E. Morsi, and E. M. Benjamin. 2008. "Choosing the Best Hospital: The Limitations of Public Quality Reporting." *Health Affairs* 27 (6): 1680.

22. Agency for Healthcare Research and Quality. "National Quality Measures Clearinghouse." [Online information; retrieved 8/11/14.] www.qualitymeasures.ahrq.gov.

23. Centers for Medicare & Medicaid Services. 2011. "Hospital Quality Initiative." [Online information; retrieved 8/10/14.] www.cms.gov/Medicare/Quality-Initia tives-Patient-Assessment-Instruments/HospitalQualityInits/index.html?redirect=/ HospitalQualityInits/.

24. The Joint Commission. 2014. "Facts About Accountability Measures." [Online information; retrieved 8/11/14.] www.jointcommission.org/facts_about_account ability_measures/.

25. Centers for Medicare & Medicaid Services. 2014. "National Health Expenditures; Aggregate and Per Capita Amounts, Annual Percent Change and Percent Distribution: Selected Calendar Years 1960–2012." [Online information; retrieved 9/10/14.] www.cms.gov/Research-Statistics-Data-and-Systems/Statistics-Trends-and-Reports/NationalHealthExpendData/Downloads/tables.pdf.

26. Starr, P. 1982. *The Social Transformation of American Medicine.* New York: Basic Books; Rosenberg, C. E. 1989. *The Care of Strangers: The Rise of America's Health Care System.* New York: Basic Books; Stevens, R. 1989. *In Sickness and in Wealth: American Hospitals in the Twentieth Century.* New York: Basic Books.

27. Lieberman, S. M. 2013. "Reforming Medicare Through 'Version 2.0' of Accountable Care." *Health Affairs* 32 (7): 1258–64.

28. Berry, L. L., and D. Beckham. 2014. "Team-Based Care at Mayo Clinic: A Model for ACOs." *Journal of Healthcare Management* 59 (1): 9–13.

29. Accountable Care Facts. 2014. "What Is an Accountable Care Organization (ACO)?" [Online information; retrieved 8/11/14.] www.accountablecarefacts.org/ topten/what-is-an-accountable-care-organization-aco-1.

30. Jackson, G. L., B. J. Powers, R. Chatterjee, J. P. Bettger, A. R. Kemper, V. Hasselblad, R. J. Dolor, R. J. Irvine, B. L. Heidenfelder, A. S. Kendrick, R. Gray, and J. W. Williams. 2013. "Improving Patient Care. The Patient-Centered Medical Home: A Systematic Review." *Annals of Internal Medicine* 158 (3): 169–78.

31. Institute of Medicine, Committee on Quality of Health Care in America. 2000. *To Err Is Human: Building a Safer Health System,* edited by L. T. Kohn, J. M. Corrigan, and M. S. Donaldson. Washington, DC: National Academies Press.

32. Bass, B. M., B. J. Avolio, D. I. Jung, and Y. Berson. 2003. "Predicting Unit Performance by Assessing Transformational and Transactional Leadership." *Journal of Applied Psychology* 88: 207–18.

33. Srivastava, A., K. M. Bartol, and E. A. Locke. 2006. "Empowering Leadership in Management Teams: Effects on Knowledge Sharing, Efficacy, and Performance." *Academy of Management Journal* 49 (6): 1239–51.

34. Gilmartin, M. J., and T. A. D'Aunno. 2008. "Leadership Research in Healthcare." *Academy of Management Annals* 2: 390–438.

35. Ackerman, A. L., and D. Anderson. 2001. *The Change in Leader's Roadmap: How to Navigate Your Organization's Transformation.* San Francisco: Jossey-Bass/ Pfeiffer.

36. White, K. R., and R. Dandi. 2009. "Intrasectoral Variation in Mission and Values: The Case of the Catholic Health Systems." *Health Care Management Review* 34 (1): 68–79.

37. Beauchamp, T. L., and J. F. Childress. 2012. *Principles of Biomedical Ethics,* 7th ed. New York: Oxford University Press.

38. Pfeffer, J. 1994. *Competitive Advantage Through People: Unleashing the Power of the Work Force.* Boston: Harvard Business Publishing.

39. Bronson Methodist Hospital. 2006. Malcolm Baldrige National Quality Award Application. [Online information; retrieved 9/20/08.] www.baldrige.nist.gov/ Contacts_Profiles.htm.

40. Fottler, M. D., R. C. Ford, and C. P. Heaton. 2002. *Achieving Service Excellence: Strategies for Healthcare*. Chicago: Health Administration Press.

41. Heskett, J. L., W. E. Sasser, and L. A. Schlesinger. 1997. *The Service Profit Chain: How Leading Companies Link Profit and Growth to Loyalty, Satisfaction, and Value*. New York: Free Press.

42. Griffith, J. R. 2009. "Frontiers of Hospital Management." *Journal of Healthcare Management* 54 (1): 30–44.

43. Bernd, D. L. 2008. "Executive Pay for Performance." *Trustee* 61 (2): 30–32.

44. Walshe, K., and T. G. Rundall. 2001. "Evidence-Based Management: From Theory to Practice in Health Care." *Milbank Quarterly* 79 (3): 429–57.

45. Kovner, A. R., and T. G. Rundall. 2006. "Evidence-Based Management Reconsidered." *Frontiers of Health Services Management* 22 (3): 3–22.

46. Montori, V. M., and G. H. Guyatt. 2008. "Progress in Evidence-Based Medicine." *Journal of the American Medical Association* 300: 1814–16.

47. National Guideline Clearinghouse. 2014. Home page. [Online information; retrieved 9/9/14.] www.guideline.gov.

48. Montori and Guyatt (2008).

49. Swing, S. R. 2007. "The ACGME Outcome Project: Retrospective and Prospective." *Medical Teacher* 29 (7): 648–54.

50. Pfeffer, J., and R. I. Sutton. 2006. *Hard Facts, Dangerous Half-Truths, and Total Nonsense: Profiting from Evidence-Based Management*. Boston: Harvard Business School Press.

51. Deming, W. E. 1986. *Out of the Crisis*. Cambridge, MA: Massachusetts Institute of Technology, Center for Advanced Engineering Study.

52. Griffith, J. R., and K. R. White. 2005. "The Revolution in Hospital Management." *Journal of Healthcare Management* 50 (3): 170–89.

53. Griffith (2009).

54. Kovner, A. R., D. J. Fine, and R. D'Aquila. 2009. *Evidence-Based Management in Healthcare*. Chicago: Health Administration Press.

55. For a useful summary of the issues, see Fottler, M. D., S. J. O'Connor, and M. J. Gilmartin. 2006. "Motivating People." In *Health Care Management: Organization, Design, and Behavior*, 5th ed., edited by S. M. Shortell and A. D. Kaluzny. Clifton Park, NY: Thomson Delmar Learning.

56. Sarbanes Oxley Act of 2002, P.L.107-204.

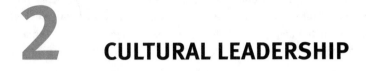

2 CULTURAL LEADERSHIP

Critical Issues in Cultural Leadership

1. *Using service excellence to create the best place to give care in order to be the best place to get care.* Listen to associates, identify what they need to fulfill the mission, and provide it.

2. *Implementing responsive leadership to build and sustain the culture.* Use training, selection, and modeling to create an environment where the values become real.

3. *Measuring and continuously improving the HCO's culture.* Use associate and customer satisfaction measures to improve relationships and communication.

4. *Establishing a program to respond to actions that undercut the HCO's values or endanger its assets.* At the senior leadership and governance levels, handle potentially divisive issues and destructive behavior.

Questions for Discussion

These questions are about applying the chapter content. It's often helpful to discuss them with classmates or mentors, gaining different perspectives on the issues.

1. Let's look closely at Exhibit 2.3. Are the responses outlined what you would have said before you read the chapter? Are they what you would have heard in your last job? Are you comfortable giving the "Negotiation Path" answers? If not, what answer would you give, and how might the associate receive it? (You could try a role-play with a classmate.)

2. Discuss the following statements. Do you believe that they are generally true, or that they don't happen in the real world? Should they be true? What competitive advantages might accrue to an HCO where these statements are true?
   a. Managers do not give orders.
   b. Managers do not make decisions.
   c. Managers spend a lot of time listening.
   d. Imagination is an important managerial skill.

3. Suppose a leader colleague at an HCO says, "I don't think our culture is where it should be." Another leader responds, "I disagree. I think our culture is fine, and we spend too much money on training and rounding." What data would you review to validate or clarify their concerns? How would you reach a consensus on defining "where it should be"? On "too much money," or, better yet, on "the right amount of money"?

4. What is the best way to answer a physician or senior employee associate who says, "We've always done it this way. I don't see why we should change"?

5. You're rounding, and associates make the following statements. How do you respond?
   a. "The toilet's broken in a patient's room. I called hours ago, but nobody's shown up."
   b. "[Name of associate] was late today and sick yesterday. Third time this month!"
   c. "[Patient]'s husband walks with a cane. She says he can't come see her because it's so far from the parking lot."

Culture establishes how an organization feels to customer and associate stakeholders. Chapter 1 notes that excellent HCOs build a transformational culture that attracts the respect and support of stakeholders using five major functions that address values, empowerment, communication, service excellence, and rewards. Leadership is critical in forming and sustaining the transformational culture. Leaders align goals with the mission, vision, and values. Leaders implement a transformational culture by listening, empowering, and teaching. Leaders explain, suggest, and remove roadblocks. Leaders inspire associates to set higher goals and reward achievement. These activities make the culture real and sustainable. The ability to perform these activities is an essential competency for leaders at all levels.

Purpose

The purpose of cultural leadership is

to implement transformational management of teams effectively from the bedside to the boardroom

and

to sustain an environment where all associates are empowered and motivated to meet their customers' needs.

Many HCOs have 100 or more work teams, including caregiving, clinical, logistic, and strategic support. All of the teams have customers. Patients are the customers of both caregiving and clinical support teams. Logistic support teams have other teams as customers, or **internal customers**. Clinical support teams and some logistic teams, such as security and patient relations, serve both patient and internal customers. All teams require support. This chapter addresses the supporting environment that encourages team members to do their best and the contribution of leaders who create and sustain that environment. Chapter 3, on operational leadership, establishes the core technology that provides effective structure, fulfilling universal team needs for people, information, supplies, and facilities.

Internal customers
Associates and teams who rely on other associates and teams within the HCO.

Functions

Excellent HCOs implement seven functions to achieve their cultural purpose. As shown in Exhibit 2.1, these seven functions are synergistic, and the whole is substantially more than the parts. Many of these functions are implemented simultaneously; for example, saying "thank you" is a communication function,

EXHIBIT 2.1

Functions
of Cultural
Leadership

Function	Intent	Implementation	Examples
Promoting shared values	Establishes a central moral focus Protects individual rights Creates an intrinsic reward	Visioning exercises Display and repetition Training Repetitive modeling Rewards	Mission/vision/ values on badges Orientation emphasis Celebration of exceptional effort
Empowering associates	Strengthens associate self-image Encourages continuous improvement Promotes responsiveness to customers	Training Manager training Repetitive modeling Rewards	Demonstrated mastery of work procedures 360-degree manager assessments Associate roles on PITs Encouragement
Communicating with associates	Identifies and responds to concerns Prevents information loss	Manager training Meeting management Display and repetition Repetitive modeling Rewards	Reports on goal achievement Rounding Blogs and e-mails PITs and group meetings
Supporting service excellence	Focuses associates on meeting customer needs	Goal setting Operational management Training Repetitive modeling Rewards	Goal negotiations Reports on goal achievement Customer relations training Service rewards and celebrations
Encouraging, rewarding, and celebrating success	Reinforces appropriate behavior Builds associate loyalty	Performance measurement Celebrations Incentive compensation	Patient satisfaction "Caught in the Act" program Bonuses
Developing and sustaining the leadership team	Ensure that the organization has adequate leaders and "bench strength"	Routine leadership assessment, individual development plans, and a leadership succession plan	High potentials program; executive coaching; leadership academies
Improving the transformational culture	Increases return from culture over time	Review of learning, perceptions, attitudes, and achievements	Better programs to assist new leaders Improvement of incentive system

PIT: process improvement team

but it is also a reward. A training session inevitably contains more messages than simply the operation lessons learned.

The culture depends on universal commitment to mission achievement and effective delivery on that commitment. Many patients require multiple care teams, and caregivers must be supported by support teams that deliver adequate supplies, staff, and facilities. Consistent results are achieved through well-planned, well-executed efforts by teams who are committed to excellence and trained to deliver on that commitment.

Leaders work daily to implement these functions. For example:

1. Leaders reinforce the mission, values, and negotiated goals by deliberate repetition and multiple displays.
2. Leaders listen to associates' concerns and respond so that barriers to achievement are promptly identified and removed.
3. Leaders model the behaviors reflected in the organization's values.
4. Leaders (and a specialist team in human resources) provide training in job processes so that the associate is not only competent but also confident.
5. Leaders train other leaders so that their actions consistently reinforce the values and the commitment to the mission. (The tools to promote culture are themselves learnable.)
6. Leaders understand that respect means acceptance of associates' viewpoints. They negotiate to reach agreement on realistic limits and points of contention.
7. Leaders reward desired behavior and goal achievement with celebrations and tangible incentives. (Positive rewards are often more effective than criticism or punishment.)

These activities are included in an integrated plan to build and sustain a culture that *delights* both associates and customers, recognizing that associates' needs must be met for them to meet customers' needs. ("Delight" is the highest possible satisfaction response.)

Promoting Shared Values

In excellent HCOs, the mission is displayed prominently and repeatedly on printed materials, on websites, and even on associates' badges. For example, the mission of SSM Health Care—"Through our exceptional health care services, we reveal the healing presence of God"—appears at the top of every page of its website (see www.ssmhc.com/internet/home/ssmcorp. nsf). SSM's values—compassion, respect, excellence, stewardship, and community—are given less display but are emphasized in other ways.

Training is a critical component in establishing a mission- and value-driven culture. Applicants are asked to read and accept the mission and values before completing an application. Orientation begins with a strong and clear commitment. Many excellent HCOs have the **chief executive officer (CEO)** or a senior leader meet all new associates to explain the mission and values and the HCO's ways of expressing its commitment to the mission and values. Training makes clear that "respect" rules out any form of harassment of customers or associates and that "stewardship" requires maintaining confidentiality of patient records and personal information. Training covers the proper forms of behavior, dress, and address, so that contacts with customers and other associates are carried out consistent to professional standards.

Leaders reinforce key messages. All leaders are trained in how to conduct personal interviews and meetings, and how to deal with recurring issues. Leaders promote shared values by asking questions: "How does this proposed action help achieve our mission?" "What services are our customers seeking?" "How can we best serve our community and patients' health needs?" Leaders "microtize" the HCO vision. In other words, they break down the overall vision to describe how it affects each work unit and individual. They ask, "What's the unit's contribution to the larger HCO mission?" They encourage each associate to think through the answer to that question, building buy-in and commitment.[1]

Empowering Associates

An empowered associate understands that she can and should change the work environment when some part of it interferes with mission achievement. Effective healthcare requires the integration and coordination of countless details. For even a moderately complex therapy, identities must be checked, diagnoses verified, treatment planned, explanation and reassurance offered, hands washed, and interventions completed correctly at the right time and recorded, and these activities must be performed many times by many associates with vastly different skill levels.

Training provides a foundation; empowerment makes it happen. Empowerment allows all associates, even those in the least-skilled positions,

to accept the professional role of agent for the patient or the customer. The leader's role is to reinforce empowerment by listening, responding, reassuring, explaining, encouraging, and rewarding. This style has been termed **servant leadership**,[2] which emphasizes the leader's obligation to be sensitive and responsive.

Empowerment and servant leadership are more than specific acts; they are learned traits. They create a culture where questions can be asked, answers sought, and changes implemented. They remove blame. They reassure associates that the HCO's commitment to its mission and values is real. They create a culture that makes teammates comrades and work intrinsically rewarding.

Communicating with Associates

Mercy Health System, a recipient of the Malcolm Baldrige National Quality Award, describes its communication program in its Baldrige application as follows:

In support of [its culture of excellence], senior leadership adopted a Servant-Leadership Philosophy. This philosophy is based on the belief that when leaders provide excellent service to partners, partners provide excellent service to customers. This approach inverts the traditional, top-down management style; thus, organizational leaders become facilitators whose role is to serve those who provide value to patients and other stakeholders. . . .

Senior leaders' personal demonstration of commitment to the organization's values is a critical element in the servant leadership approach. With this underlying philosophy, [the executive council (EC)] has adopted the following best practices:[3]

- Frequent, open, and honest communication—EC members bring issues to weekly EC meetings for full discussion, supporting integrated system strategies;
- "Cruising and connecting"—EC members perform weekly administrative rounds, connecting with partners to seek out new ways to better serve their needs; *rounding*
- Personal renewal and connections with patients and customers—EC members perform line work alongside staff annually and review patient complaints weekly; and
- Monthly luncheons—EC members conduct small group sessions [with members of their accountability hierarchy] to promote two-way communication.

The Mercy program is noteworthy for several reasons. First, it is deliberately opposite from the traditional "command and control" perspective that prevailed in many organizations until the late 1990s. That perspective is so deeply rooted in the American workplace that most associates and all leaders must be carefully taught about the new model and how to work effectively within it. Second, the Mercy program mandates frequent, direct contact between the leaders and associates and between workers and customers. Third, it includes systematic review of customer and associate complaints. Fourth, it expects the organization's senior managers to roll up their sleeves and pitch in with their teams. Fifth, it expects all leaders to model desirable behavior and to reinforce formal training.

Much of communications is about the systematic transfer of facts. It is part of the operational foundation described in chapters 1 and 3 and expanded on in Chapter 10, on knowledge management and information services. Leaders routinely participate in factual communication and accept accountability for doing it well. Cultural leadership requires more. It requires that the leader consistently reinforce the values by words, behaviors, and actions. The reinforcement is often supplied by two components of communication that have traditionally been overlooked—listening and modeling.

Listening

Transformational management depends heavily on making all communication with associates two-way. The intent is to ensure that every associate's concerns will be heard, be understood, and receive a constructive response. The emphasis on response distinguishes transformational from transactional and older management styles. It is a major factor in associate satisfaction and essential to the overall performance improvement that transformational management achieves.[4]

Listening is what makes communication two-way, and it is a skill that can be taught by example and learned by practice. Listening skill can easily be tested, by rephrasing what has been said and asking for verification: "Let me restate what I heard, and you tell me if it's right." In excellent HCOs, listening opportunities are created by planned one-to-one conversations; **rounding**, where leaders meet workers in their units; informal meetings with small groups of employees; and town-hall meetings. It includes focus groups, where small, relatively homogeneous panels are encouraged to discuss open-ended questions, and nominal group technique, where individuals and small groups pursue subjective estimates and expectations. Listening need not be face to face. It may also be done through random sampling surveys and respondent-initiated comment cards, in both paper and electronic modes.

Rounding

A planned and thoughtful practice where managers are visible on patient care units and HCO work areas to visit with associates and patients about positive experiences as well as concerns that can be addressed in real time.

Modeling

Transformational leadership relies heavily on repetition and consistency. Transformational leaders are expected to act out the HCO's values and to demonstrate how they are applied. Sharp HealthCare clearly describes the attitudes and behaviors it desires and expects from workers and leaders:[5]

12 Employee Behavior Standards
1. It's a Private Matter: Maintain Confidentiality
2. To "E" or Not to "E": Use E-mail Manners
3. Vive La Différence!: Celebrate Diversity
4. Get Smart: Increase Skills and Competence
5. Attitude is Everything: Create a Lasting Impression
6. Thank Somebody: Reward and Recognition
7. Make Words Work: Talk, Listen, and Learn
8. All For One, One For All: Teamwork
9. Make It Better: Service Recovery
10. Think Safe, Be Safe: Safety at Work
11. Look Sharp, Be Sharp: Appearance Speaks
12. Keep in Touch: Ease Waiting Times

5 "Must Haves"

1. Greet people with a smile and "hello," using their name.
2. Take people where they are going.
3. Use key words at key times: "Is there anything else I can do for you? I have the time."
4. Foster an attitude of gratitude.
5. Round with reason.

and, for all associates working with patients, an AIDET acronym:

Acknowledge: Acknowledge people with a smile and use their names.

Introduce: Introduce yourself to others politely.

Duration: Keep in touch to ease waiting times.

Explanation: Explain how procedures work and who to contact if they need assistance.

Thank You: Thank people for using Sharp HealthCare.

All leaders are expected to model this behavior. "Senior Leaders are expected to exhibit the Core Values, Behavior Standards, and Five 'Must Haves,' and serve as role models for employees, volunteers, physicians, suppliers, and partners."[6]

Supporting Service Excellence

The service excellence model diagrammed in Exhibit 2.2 is the goal of the transformational culture. It expands the concept of agency or stewardship

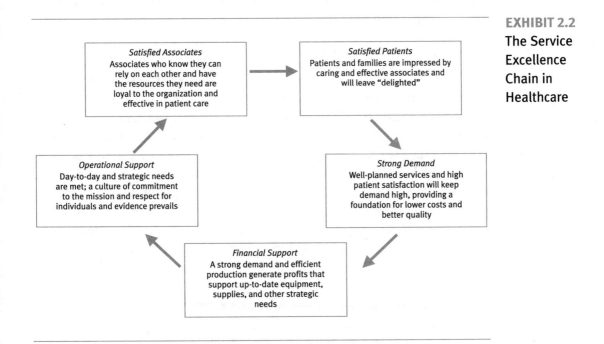

EXHIBIT 2.2

The Service Excellence Chain in Healthcare

("I am doing this *for* you") to one of shared commitment ("I am doing this *with* you"). The moral foundation of service excellence is to serve others as one wishes to be served, an important step beyond fulfilling a contract.[7] The trust implicit in agency is raised to a new level of partnership. All associates, specifically leaders, become partners in satisfying the patient as the ultimate customer. Service excellence is demonstrated rather than proven (rigorous proof is both intellectually and practically challenging), and all excellent HCOs follow the service excellence model. The model is extremely powerful financially. Small gains in the number of patients served generates big increases in profits, providing funds for the costs of the operational foundation.[8]

The new level of trust must begin with leadership. Leaders must trust associates and make that trust clear. They must also work to remove the frustrations and conflicts that associates face, freeing the energies they consumed to improve patient care. They do this by promoting shared values and empowering, communicating, and implementing the operational foundation (discussed in Chapter 3). In HCOs that are converting from transactional cultures, leaders work consistently to promote the values, increase empowerment as associates understand and accept it, and identify the most promising opportunities for improvement (OFIs). Solving all problems at once is not possible, and people learn new concepts at different rates. By identifying teams that are ready to move forward and supporting them, management demonstrates the transformational potential and gains skill in making the transition. These actions also provide compelling evidence of the strength of the organization's commitment and the power of the transformational approach. The transition snowballs. The bold volunteer, the perceptive follow, and the crowd joins in.

Negotiating

Service excellence and transformational management must deal with the realities of the world. Perfection is rarely possible. Not every problem can be addressed at once. People disagree. Some critical resources—particularly space and money—must be assigned to some and denied to others. Excellent HCOs recognize realities as part of their culture. OFIs are a measure of where realities have fallen short of desires. The leadership must resolve these realities in acceptable ways. Negotiating to find the best solutions is an ongoing process. To sustain the culture, leaders must be skilled at the process. Training, mentoring, and counseling create a culture where the following goals are universally understood and accepted and almost universally met:

1. Every position is entitled to an honest hearing.
2. The best answer is driven by two fundamental statements:
    a. Mission achievement is the basic criterion.
    b. Fact and science guide our evaluation of each decision.

3. Each decision is subject to test as it is implemented. The strategy is to measure the emerging reality, catch OFIs quickly, and correct them. Any process can be improved.
4. This decision process, while not perfect, meets every stakeholder's needs better than any alternative process does.

This set of goals is at the core of the transformational culture. Exhibit 2.3 shows some recurring sources of contention, illustrating the implications of these goals. In all cases the negotiation path is specific, honest, and factual. In most cases, it points to an underlying process, offers to explain the process, and notes how the process itself is subject to continuous improvement.

Although the solution paths in Exhibit 2.3 look like common sense, they are a major departure from traditional management styles. Weak HCOs have difficulty implementing such an approach for several reasons. First, it requires understanding that any associate is free, even encouraged, to raise any issue that concerns him or her. Second, issues like these are recurring, so they are settled by formal processes rather than by individual judgments. Third, leaders must be trained in how to respond to these concerns because they arise frequently. Good answers begin with a reassurance that the concern is legitimate; trained leaders should always assume the associate's good intentions and never place blame. They offer an explanation for how the current situation was reached and how the underlying process can be improved. The approach in itself reduces disagreement. Consistently applying it allows associates to evaluate their situation themselves, reframing concerns to suggestions that will win acceptance.

Some issues are too complex for the responses listed in Exhibit 2.3. They require detailed investigation and extensive effort to resolve. Some leaders become specialists at helping people resolve disagreement. The basic elements of this process are as follows:

1. Help the conflicting parties fully understand all aspects of their position, including the causes, implications, and alternative solutions.
2. Explore carefully for areas of agreement, and build solutions upon these.
3. Conduct the negotiations openly, and show respect for all participants and a clear commitment to the fundamentals of mission achievement and scientific evidence.

When these elements are carried out, the participants may leave thinking that they lost or that an error was made, but they concede that their case was fully and fairly heard.

Continuous Improvement

Leaders of excellent HCOs sustain a culture of continuous improvement. The culture supports a complex, ongoing improvement activity described in

EXHIBIT 2.3 Frequently Negotiated Issues and Solution Paths for Excellent HCOs

Issue	Negotiation Path	Implications
"This is an unsafe situation."	"Thank you for noticing it. Security will evaluate it and give you a report. When you get the report, let me know if you're satisfied."	Value: Safety is critical for all associates. Unsafe situations are not tolerated. Fact: A trained team evaluates risks and follows through.
"We need new equipment."	"We spend millions each year on new equipment, so we have a careful, competitive review process. Units that show how the investment will improve quality, efficiency, or customer satisfaction usually get their requests."	Value: New equipment is important to fulfilling the mission, but money does not grow on trees. Fact: New equipment is justified based on specific improvements in important operational measures.
"How many nurses (or other staff) do we have?"	"That's a good question. We have a nurse staffing system, and we monitor benchmarks and patient outcomes. If you think your floor staffing should be changed, and your coworkers agree, we'll form a performance improvement team to re-evaluate it."	Value: Providing enough nursing to ensure quality and patient satisfaction is part of our mission, but so is control of costs. Fact: Staffing is set by a specific process that includes measures of effectiveness and process improvement.
"I disagree with the protocol."	"We use caregiver panels to select our protocols, and we try to follow the evidence-based medicine rules. Would you like to meet with the chair of your panel to discuss your concerns?"	Value: Science drives the clinical practice. Fact: Any protocol is a candidate for improvement. Suggestions are welcome and are evaluated carefully.
"This patient does not fit the protocol."	"Caregivers are expected to use their professional judgment to leave the protocol when indicated. We do ask for a note in the chart, so that it reflects what is being done."	Value: Care is patient-centered. Professionals are expected to exercise judgment. Fact: Judgment must be documented for effective communication and for later review.
"My supervisor isn't fair."	"I'm sorry to hear that. Tell me more about your concerns, and we'll see how we can improve things."	Value: Associates are important stakeholders, but there are two sides to every argument. Fact: The HCO has a variety of training and counseling programs to resolve common sources of dissatisfaction, but using them requires a candid and thorough understanding of the cause.
"I want more money."	"Let's talk about that. We set our compensation carefully, and human resources can show you how we arrived at yours. We also offer bonuses, and you get a regular report on yours. One way to get more money is to win a promotion. Let's go over some steps you might take to do that."	Value: Compensation needs to be fair to all stakeholders. Associates are encouraged to improve. Fact: Compensation is based on an objective process. The HCO measures employee contribution, rewards effort, and encourages growth.

Chapter 3. Continuous improvement activities involve all leaders and many other associates, addressing all kinds of operational issues. They require a strong fact base; training in process analysis; and a formal structure usually called a performance improvement council (PIC) to select, manage, and implement improvements involving multiple work teams. Having these in place is important, but the stimulus to innovate and the implementation of improvements must come from the work teams themselves. The culture must encourage innovation. The work teams identify process-related questions. The responses to those questions should follow the initial goals of negotiation (Exhibit 2.3). When they do, their tone encourages the search for improvement. Answers that blame, are evasive, or shut off discussion cause a quick loss of team commitment.

First-line leaders can form process improvement teams (PITs) as they see fit. In excellent HCOs they are trained to do so often. They can form PITs to identify OFIs, or PITs to plan bigger PITs, or one-person PITs. The PIT is simply a device to identify improvement. As the agendas get more complex, they go to the PIC to integrate with other units. Knowledgeable superiors, internal and external consultants, and just-in-time training all support the PIT's ability to examine and improve its work processes. A key constraint—the PIT must include all who are affected by the change—is easy to learn and, when violated, easy to correct by adding the missing viewpoint to the PIT. In a transformational environment, establishing linkages to negotiate new processes, or gaining approval from the PIC, is simple.

Senior management's commitment is tested often, but is easy to sustain. Implementation is rarely uneventful, even with the best advance planning. Pilot tests are essential for complex changes. They can present extraordinary challenges for the participants, who will need extra support and encouragement. A successful transformational culture has an underlying bias toward change. This bias is expressed by being encouraging from the start, giving support during the change, and celebrating success throughout the process. Much of this is demonstrated in words, attitudes, and actions such as pitching in and getting help.

Encouraging, Celebrating, and Rewarding Success

On a day-to-day basis, all leaders must identify and encourage associate behavior that supports mission, vision, and values. Simple words of encouragement—"thanks," "good job," "that was helpful"—are the beginning, and become universal in dialogue. Celebration recognizes particularly positive examples of implementing the values. It's often exercised as informal breaks with food and public recognition before peers. Many organizations use public reporting to identify positive behavior, sometimes called "Caught in the Act." Any associate or visitor can submit a description of an act he or she thinks is exceptional. The submission identifies the associate and the act and is immediately posted to the associate's record. Weekly or monthly, a panel of associates reviews the submissions and selects the winners, who then receive recognition and prizes.

Cash bonuses often are components of best practice cultures. They are paid annually or quarterly based on achievement of goals set for unit scorecards, as depicted in Exhibit 1.10. They vary by institution, but are substantial often more than one month's pay. The operations system described in Chapter 3 and the goal-setting system described in Chapter 4 are carefully integrated. The goals are set to be meaningful improvements in mission achievement, but realistic. They are achieved more than 90 percent of the time. Some HCOs add "stretch goals," which typically see a lower success rate but come with extra rewards when achieved.

Developing and Sustaining the Leadership Team

The leadership team supports the culture and operations. High-performing HCOs systematically develop the team. They offer growth opportunities for individuals and maintain a succession plan that identifies promising candidates for every leadership position.

Assessing and Developing Leaders as Individuals

Leadership effectiveness is measured directly by **360-degree surveys** or **multi-rater reviews**. These assess leaders' skills as seen by subordinates, peers and colleagues, vendors and outside contacts, and superiors.

360-degree or *multi-rater review*
Formal evaluation of performance by subordinates, superiors, and peers of the individual or unit.

Each leader undergoes an annual 360-degree or multi-rater review to supplement the measures of unit performance. These evaluations may be supplemented with detailed competency self-assessments, such as those developed by the National Center for Healthcare Leadership and the Healthcare Leadership Alliance, which allow individuals to compare their skills with those demonstrated by successful managers.[9]

These results are then reviewed by the leader and his superior to create a professional development plan—a program that uses a mix of mentoring, special assignments, and continuing education to identify and address OFIs. For example, an early-career leader's development plan may include one or more senior mentors, an assignment to a PIT or task force in charge of an issue outside the leader's day-to-day responsibilities, and a course in process analysis such as Six Sigma. A senior leader's plan may involve a coach from outside the organization, membership on the board of a small not-for-profit, and advanced leadership education from a university.

Leaders are held accountable for their professional development plans and for assisting less experienced leaders in advancing their careers. Many organizations put a premium on diversity, seeking to advance underrepresented groups, including women, to higher management levels. The goal of this effort is to incorporate the demographic characteristics of the community into the organizational hierarchy.

Ensuring Leadership Continuity

Leadership vacancies are created through attrition, retirement, or organizational growth. They can occur suddenly, and they can seriously disrupt organizational performance. A **leadership succession plan** is a systematic process for evaluating the leadership requirements for each position, identifying potential candidates for those positions, and prompting the candidates to develop the skills necessary for being successful in

Leadership succession plan
A written plan for replacing people who depart from management positions.

higher-level roles. Its primary purpose is to fill leadership vacancies with available internal talents. The succession plan is periodically updated; at the senior levels, it is reviewed and approved by the governing board. Exhibit 2.4 shows the package of leadership function assessment, individual leadership plans, and succession plans used by high-performing HCOs to maintain and improve their leadership group.

EXHIBIT 2.4 A Comprehensive Leadership Management Program

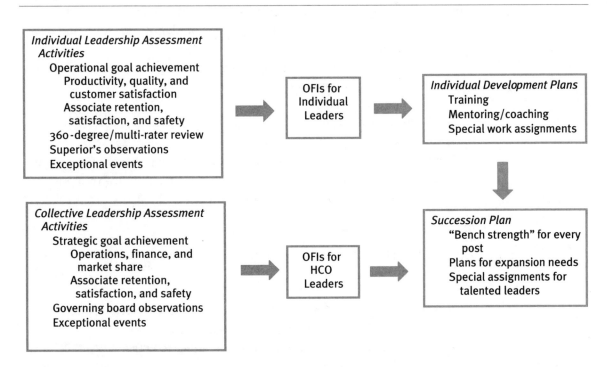

OFI: opportunity for improvement

The succession plan is relatively easy to create. Each leader identifies and rank-orders two or three candidates among her direct reports whom she deems qualified to be her successor; then, each candidate's personal development plan is reviewed and developed in preparation for the eventual opportunity. However, the process does raise some complex issues:

- The plan implies that the HCO expects its leaders to be promoted, rather than remain at one level. When a vacant position is filled, the internal candidates who are not selected may leave. The HCO will have invested in their development, but they may join a competitor.
- Associates not included on the potential candidates list may demand an explanation for why they were not chosen.

Henry Ford Health System (HFHS), a Baldrige Award recipient, maintains comprehensive leadership development and succession planning programs, termed *leadership academies*, for leaders at all levels in the organization. HFHS senior leadership identifies individual successors for the top 13 leaders in three categories: ready now, ready in two years, and ready within five years. Identified high-potential leaders work with the chief human resources officer to create individual development plans to assist them in reaching the next level. Senior leadership also selects an additional talent pool of 50 individuals who participate in the Advanced Leadership Academy to prepare for other leadership positions. Senior leaders participate in annual Talent Review sessions for the purpose of discussing progress of identified leaders and development of potential successors.[10]

The succession plan is strongly endorsed as good practice. The program has several important features:

- It tends to attract "the best and the brightest."
- It rewards learning and achievement.
- It builds a culture of "a great place to give care" that supports the retention of not only more people but also more capable people than alternative approaches, in spite of the issues mentioned in the previous list.

Improving the Transformational Culture

The culture itself, distinct from the work processes, contributes to mission achievement in several ways:

- It trains, empowers, and rewards associates, making them partners, not agents, in turning the service excellence model into a reality.
- It encourages a blame-free environment that facilitates PITs.
- It creates the "best place to give care" mind-set, which encourages associates to remain with the HCO, thus increasing the return on the ongoing training investment.

As the culture improves over time, an increasingly knowledgeable and committed associate group develops. The measures available to evaluate the culture are discussed in the Measures section of this chapter. Generally, the human resources department leads the review of the progress made, but the PIC also pays direct attention to this endeavor. Both systematic and individual OFIs can be identified and improved through the study or use of the other functions.

People

HCOs need significant numbers of leaders, from small patient care teams to CEOs. The total is on the order of 500,000 nationwide, a number similar in magnitude to the number of physicians. More than 10,000 new leaders may be needed each year to accommodate retirements. To sustain excellence, an HCO must develop a program that identifies and develops its leadership cadre.

Sources of Leaders

First-level leaders are commonly promoted from team membership, usually because they have demonstrated exceptional mastery in both the relevant knowledge and interpersonal skills. Senior leaders and division directors are often promoted from first-level leaders, but at higher ranks they may be recruited from other organizations. Executive search firms facilitate finding appropriately qualified people. In many logistic and strategic support areas, experience in other industries is relevant. While clinical leaders are often promoted from within or from similar HCOs, accounting and marketing leaders may have gained the necessary knowledge and skills in banking or retailing. Consultants often move to executive posts, and vice versa.

Senior executives of HCOs have had 10 to 20 years of experience in management and leadership with increasing accountability. For senior management, an understanding of the clinical and financial structures is essential but not easily grasped. Senior leaders usually reach their positions by following one of three routes:

1. Obtaining a graduate degree in healthcare management and moving up the organizational hierarchy from an initial administrative, support position
2. Developing an interest in management and learning its skills from being a patient care or clinical support professional; this interest then grows as the person is given broader exposure and opportunities for executive education
3. Transitioning from a strategic or logistic position into a management role through building a record of excellent performance in large HCOs or consulting companies and then pursuing graduate education in healthcare management

Many excellent senior leaders come from outside healthcare, but most have spent their careers mastering the industry and its details. Leadership development programs must recognize the differences in leaders' backgrounds and devise ways to build comprehensive skill.

Qualifications for Leaders

Leaders should be identified and promoted on the basis of their effectiveness in achieving mission-related goals. Exceptional associates may be selected to become first-level leaders, while skilled first-level leaders may become division leaders, and so on. Prior success alone is not sufficient for success after promotion. The transition is often challenging. A prominent researcher in management development notes:[11]

> [B]ecoming a manager required a profound psychological adjustment—a *transformation of professional identity*. First-time managers had to unlearn the deeply held attitudes and habits they had developed when they were responsible simply for their own performance. Prior to a managerial promotion, their contribution depended primarily on what they did personally, drawing upon their own expertise and actions. As managers, on the other hand, they had to come to see themselves as responsible for setting and implementing an agenda for a whole group. To use an orchestral analogy, new managers had to move from concentrating on one task, as an accomplished violinist does, to coordinating the efforts of many, like a conductor. To set the agenda for a whole group and to motivate and inspire others to accomplish that agenda were much more complicated than most people anticipated.

Each level of leadership presents different kinds of adjustments. Promotion generally means higher levels of abstraction, more diversity of teams, more complex problems of integration, and more challenging conflicts demanding resolution.

Leadership requirements were formerly described by global characteristics such as degrees or years of experience. The concept of **competencies**—profiles of skills, knowledge, and attributes (SKAs) that can be matched to positions and candidates—has expanded the opportunities to describe leadership requirements, evaluate candidates, and develop learning opportunities. While specific certifications remain important, particularly in medicine, nursing, and accounting, leadership position descriptions have tended to a finer-grained approach, looking for evidence of mastery of SKAs known to be associated with high performance. Gilmartin and D'Aunno, in reviewing the research in healthcare management competencies, conclude:[12]

Competency
Having requisite or adequate ability or quality that results in effective action and/or superior performance in a job.

> [A]cross the three disciplines of nursing management, public health, and health-services management, there is agreement on competencies in [seven] areas for effective leadership. These areas are (a) interpersonal relationships, (b) communication,

(c) finance and business acumen, (d) clinical knowledge, (e) collaboration and team building, (f) change management, and (g) quality improvement.

Note that three of the seven competencies listed by Gilmartin and D'Aunno are knowledge based—finance and business acumen, clinical knowledge, and quality improvement—and the other four are primarily skills. Dye and Garman identify 16 competencies that they believe distinguish great leadership from good leadership. Their list is more introspective, identifying personal values and emotional strengths.[13]

It is feasible to identify a specific leadership position—say, leader of primary care offices, or intensive care nurse leader—and describe the requirements in terms of the SKA competencies. Interviews can be conducted, references can be checked, and written documentation can be reviewed to assess each candidate's record and to compare it with the competency requirements. Of course, each candidate's profile will be different. One may have documented excellence in interpersonal skills, team building, and change management, while another may possess exceptional business acumen, clinical knowledge, and clinical quality improvement. It is unlikely that any candidate will exactly match the desired profile. Even with a specific leadership position in view, it is difficult to determine whether excellence in change management is better than excellence in clinical knowledge or whether strength in interpersonal relationships overcomes a weakness in clinical quality improvement. The task of judging is often assigned to a small search committee. Once a leader has been selected, the comparisons between desired and actual competencies are useful in planning a training program. The way the leader is supported by training and coaching may be more important than the fine details of competency or the choice between competing candidates.

Leadership Development Programs

Leadership development is a critical element of excellent HCOs. Leaders from diverse cultural and professional beginnings must collaborate effectively. All levels of leadership must reinforce empowerment, maintain the continuous improvement system, promote and implement the work of PITs, and address the identified needs of associates and customers. For long-run success, they must model the behaviors expected of associates; maintain alignment and integration between teams; and effectively use the elements of the cultural, operational, and strategic foundations. A development program with the following elements produces a leadership group with those abilities:

1. The cultural foundations are made clear to all associates and are consistently reinforced by leaders at all levels.
2. Promotion to any leadership position is based on demonstrated superiority in relevant subordinate positions and mastery of competencies required in the new position.

3. Promoted leaders receive substantial training in the cultural and operational requirements of their new position. This includes classroom education, coaching, encouragement, and modeling by superiors.
4. Every leader has a program of personal development intended to improve current performance and to prepare them for the next promotion.
5. Just-in-time training and guided experience help leaders overcome the challenges in completing their work, simultaneously broadening their skills and knowledge.
6. The organization's succession plan identifies at least one successor for every position and coordinates with the successor's development plan.
7. For individuals seeking the highest ranks of leadership, the development plan includes deliberate expansion in two directions—a graduate degree in management and experience in leading a relatively autonomous unit.

Historically, leaders have negotiated their own careers. A leadership development program brings organizational resources to help leaders in this regard. Individual skill and ambition remain critical. Management is learned by doing, and this process presents opportunities for intellectual and emotional growth:[14]

> [B]ecoming a manager was largely a process of *learning from experience*. New managers could only appreciate their new role and identity through action, not contemplation. They learned what it meant to be a manager and how to be one by facing real problems with real consequences. They grappled with four transformational tasks: (1) learning what it really means to be a manager; (2) developing interpersonal judgment; (3) gaining self-knowledge; and (4) coping with stress and emotion.
>
> . . . [M]anagers must be prepared to learn about themselves (their identities, strengths, and limitations), be willing to make necessary changes, and be able to cope with the associated stress and emotions. There is no magic or quick fix. Only with self-awareness, empathy, discipline, and practice can new managers master the human competencies.

At the same time, well-planned intervention and support are valuable. Role models, mentors, and counselors can provide material help. A supportive environment can minimize the consequences of beginners' errors. The investment pays off in two ways: (1) Supported leaders are more likely to remain with the HCO because they like the environment, and (2) supported leaders gain skill and effectiveness that help them successfully address complex issues:[15]

> [O]rganizations taking a very disciplined and rigorous approach to leadership development generally produce more leadership talent.
>
> . . . [What characterizes best practice firms] is the far greater extent to which they measure their efforts. For example, they measure the quantity of leadership

talent for specific roles. They measure the attrition rate of their leadership talent. They catalogue jobs, assignments, and bosses that are more developmental in nature. They then make strategic use of this knowledge by moving leaders into these roles and under these supervisors to ensure development.

Paths for Beginners

Transformational leadership is learned behavior. For beginners in the health-care management field, this means the following:

1. *Commitment or the will to succeed outweighs the path to success.* The evidence shows that many different paths lead to successful HCO leadership careers. Technical or professional academic credentials are relatively more important at the lower leadership levels. Even for clinical chiefs, the competency required is in leadership rather than clinical areas. The biggest barriers to advancement may be the emotional stress and new learning required, rather than any specific knowledge or skill.

2. *Practice is the foundation for mastering competencies.* Leadership is at its root a performance activity like singing, drawing, or playing soccer. As such, it can never be learned solely from printed material or classroom study; it needs to be applied in practice. Practice includes observation of other leaders. Many lessons can be learned vicariously; others' experience is a valuable guide.

3. *Guided practice—with training, coaching, and feedback—helps more leaders succeed and do so faster.* Practice without coaching and training lacks the value of history; each lesson must be learned anew through trial and error. The use of quantitative goals and routine performance measurement provides focus and identifies learning opportunities.

4. *Regular review of competencies, identification of personal OFIs, and planned actions are critical to leadership development.* As with any other kind of performance activity, leadership benefits from following a disciplined program that includes a routine review of progress.

5. *Establishing a plan or goals for the future is helpful.* A vision of what might be, a plan for realizing that vision, and a method for marking milestones reached allow leaders to get closer to their desired future.

6. *Formal education has a role in leadership development, particularly for the leader who has built the foundations of commitment and practice.* In an evidence-based environment, knowledge is steadily accumulated and codified. Formal study offers the opportunity to capture the wisdom gained from large numbers of trials.

Measures

In high-performing HCOs, culture, leadership functions, individual leadership skills, and leadership capability are all systematically measured, reported, and benchmarked. Goals are set and achieved for both the organization and the leaders.

As shown in Exhibit 2.5, culture and leadership are measured separately. Both have important direct measures. An effective culture satisfies associates, and they report their satisfaction directly on surveys. An effective culture also leads to low turnover, absenteeism, grievances, and associate injuries. All these are measured. Similarly, leadership satisfaction is measured by the same dimensions, applied to the leadership group. Leadership effectiveness is measured by the balanced scorecard, such as that in Exhibit 1.11. Effective leaders sustain an effective culture.

Managerial Issues

The transformational culture and the leadership functions described in this chapter are universal among HCOs that report high performance. No other

EXHIBIT 2.5
Measures of
Culture and
Leadership

Input Oriented	Output Oriented
Demand Counts of new hires and promotions; goal is 100% new-leader participation	**Output and productivity** Counts of program attendance and completion are routine Direct cost per leader served is a productivity measure that can be benchmarked
Cost and resources Direct costs of programs are measured and reported by human resources Total cost of leadership development is difficult to estimate because many developmental activities are integrated into other work	**Quality** Quality of training programs is assessed by survey, examination, observation, and later job performance 360-degree reviews directly measure leader capability
Human resources Leader retention is expected; each leader departure is reviewed and analyzed Leader satisfaction is assessed by survey	**Customer satisfaction** Associate satisfaction, retention, absenteeism, and work-related lost time measure the leader's effectiveness All measures of unit performance reflect on leadership

Measures of the Organization Culture
The culture of an organization can be measured directly, by survey, and indirectly, by associates' actions such as attendance at and response to training programs, absenteeism, grievances, and departures.

Measures of Leadership Effectiveness
Leadership effectiveness is measured by organization results—the balanced scorecard (see Exhibit 1.11). It can also be evaluated indirectly, using the approaches below applied to the leadership associates and the training programs specifically for leadership development.

model is documented as successful. As best can be judged, as of 2015, transformational culture is not common in American HCOs. Neither is it simple to establish or maintain. It demands a drastic shift in behavior and attitudes of some old-school managers, and a commitment to learning and change.

For HCOs today, the most critical managerial question is "What's the path from tradition to transformation?" For HCOs that have become transformational, at least three strategies may prevent an erosion of success: maintaining the ethical foundation, resolving disagreements, and protecting against destructive behavior.

Starting on the Path to a Transformational Culture

Many HCOs are "pretty good." That is, they have no crisis problems, and their associates are hardworking and committed to doing a good job. But these HCOs do not measure everything, and without measures, their goal-setting and continuous improvement efforts lag. Benchmarks, when they discover them, are eye-openers. Their culture could be described as "benign." They wouldn't disagree with Sharp's behavior standards and "Must Haves," but unlike Sharp, they don't insist upon them. They think communicating is a great idea, but unlike Bronson, they don't have a neat list of 34 specific things they do and why they do them (see Exhibit 1.8). That's where most of the known high-performing organizations started, and where most HCOs are likely to start.

How does a "pretty good" HCO move to excellence? The following strategy is a place to start:

1. They restate and recommit to their mission, vision, and values. They use the visioning process to build broad consensus on purposes. Dozens or hundreds of stakeholders participate in this process. They come to express their opinions, but they also come to understand the meaning and support behind the words themselves.[16]
2. The senior management team examines its own attitudes and behaviors and agrees unanimously to the effort.
3. The governing board adopts the concepts of the reinvigorated vision and accepts the challenge to move to excellence, recognizing that the changes will be profound. The board sets milestones and anticipated completion dates.
4. The senior leaders begin to spread the new culture by changing their behavior to reflect servant leadership.
5. As the senior leaders "cruise and connect," they seek ways to demonstrate the power of a transformational culture and look for teams to help with pilots and demonstration sites.
6. The success of pilots and demonstrations is widely celebrated and used to show the nature of the new culture and the HCO's commitment to it.
7. Mentoring, modeling, and training are used to develop managers into leaders.
8. The operational foundation and strategic protections are developed to support continuous improvement and evidence-based management.

The success of this strategy depends on two conditions. The first is that consistent commitment must be made. Many HCOs are afflicted with the flavor-of-the-month approach to improvement: This year, it is Lean, and next year, it will be servant leadership; everyone knows the year after it will be something different. Transformational management is not an annual, it's a perennial. It takes time to grow, but its rewards are continuous. Senior management's examination of its own attitudes and behaviors (step 2 above) must be diligent.

The second condition is the simultaneous move to strengthen the operational foundation and evidence-based management. It is the subject of Chapter 3. Leadership is important. Transformational culture is essential. Results require solid work processes. Even if I think my boss is great and the team is the best I have ever worked with, it is tough to improve if the staff is always shorthanded, the laundry is missing, and the medical record is unreliable. The operational foundation addresses these details.

Maintaining the Ethical Foundation

The mission, vision, and values are inherently moral statements. Patient care is recognized as a virtue by most of the world's religions. The stakeholders' commitment to mission and values is an extension of that virtue. But the day-to-day pursuit of servant leadership, continuous improvement, and stakeholder satisfaction inevitably reaches challenging ethical frontiers, causing troubling and difficult concerns for some stakeholders.

These concerns have no easy solutions: "Should our mission be community health or excellence in care?" (see Exhibit 1.7), "Is it right to pay bonuses?" and "What are patients' end-of-life rights?" Answering them requires a clear understanding of the ethical foundations underpinning not just HCOs but American culture. Senior management and governance leadership in particular need that understanding.

The ethical foundation of transformational management is rooted in a utilitarian, universalist, post-Enlightenment moral philosophy. It drives most policy in the United States and is reflected in the Declaration of Independence:

> that all men are created equal, that they are endowed by their Creator with certain unalienable rights, that among these are life, liberty and the pursuit of happiness. That to secure these rights, governments are instituted among men, deriving their just powers from the consent of the governed.

These bold assertions took centuries to implement, but we have as a nation clearly established that "men" is to be read as "persons," without regard to race or gender. Servant leadership is shorthand for "deriving their just powers from the consent of the governed." As noted in Chapter 1, the rights of life, liberty, and pursuit of happiness lead to obligations of autonomy, nonmaleficence, beneficence, and justice that underpin the ethical commitments of the caregiving professions. The Institute of Medicine reaffirmed these commitments when it established the universal goals of healthcare: safe, effective, patient centered, timely, efficient, and equitable.[17]

The ethical foundations are supported by laws and regulations that reflect formal stakeholder consensus. Various laws and regulations speak to obligations, conflict of interest, and transparency of information (e.g., federal acts covering employment practices, emergency care, confidentiality, compensation, and accounting practices). Professional HCO leaders, like professional caregivers, are expected to adhere to professional codes of conduct, such as the American College of Healthcare Executives *Code of Ethics*.[18] The commitment to empiricism also stems from Enlightenment Era thought. Evidence-based medicine and evidence-based management are simply recent adaptations of the scientific method that arose in the seventeenth century. It means that the search for facts drives all analytic and improvement activity.

Excellent HCO cultures systematically help their associates follow these codes by developing and implementing policies and procedures that promote ethical decision making. Their training programs reflect both the spirit and the letter of regulation. Their policies are carefully checked for compliance. Many have compliance officers who are assigned full time to that task. Their servant leadership structure offers ready assistance when ethical questions arise, as they frequently do in healthcare.

Consistent support of these values is essential. Leaders are required to model ethical behavior. Sharp's insistence on its associates' adherence to standard behaviors reflects the importance of consistency. Associates are entitled to wonder if the organization is sincere; if leaders do not follow through consistently, a climate of doubt develops and the culture deteriorates. Reinforcing the desired behavior is also important, and opportunities to do so arise frequently. Team leaders can reassure and comfort caregivers who have faced particularly demanding situations. Extra efforts can be reported by anybody, using "Caught in the Act" cards.

Organizational **ethics committees**, which began as support for clinicians facing difficult issues related to individual patients, have expanded their role to advise on broader ethical issues. In HCOs undertaking research, the ethics committee is complemented by an institutional review board, which

Ethics committee
A standing multidisciplinary committee that is concerned with biomedical ethical issues and decision-making processes, formulation of policies, and review and consultation of medical ethical issues.

monitors ethical issues in research and approves research protocols for involving patients or associates. The ethics committee strives for membership that reflects stakeholder concerns, often drawing on ethicists, leaders, clinicians, patient representatives, and local religious leaders. Ethical decision-making tools identify and involve all stakeholders of an ethical conflict in determining root causes and implementing approaches that reduce their occurrence and associated costs. Some evidence suggests that having an ethics committee is highly cost-effective because an unresolved ethical concern reduces the effectiveness and efficiency of the treatment process.[19]

The ethical foundation is especially sensitive to, and must be protected from, unethical behavior. "Everybody does it" is an easy excuse for all kinds of unacceptable activity. It must be countered promptly with "but not around here." Senior management commitment to enforcement is essential. Enforcement of ethical rules is deliberately divorced from training programs and consultation opportunities. Instead, it is carried out as part of the strategic protection audit activities, although compliance officers have dual roles of consultation and enforcement. Excellent HCOs view violations of individual rights and the regulations established to protect them as extremely serious. Deliberate violation is often grounds for immediate discharge.

Resolving Conflicts

The transformational culture emphasizes negotiations to allow stakeholders to seek the solutions best for all. The program of negotiation, described earlier, is deliberately designed to identify and resolve differences of opinion as quickly as is consistent with stakeholder rights. Negotiating in this manner is effective; it not only resolves many concerns and disputes, but it reassures associates that independent thought is desirable behavior, and if it leads to dispute the path to resolution is reasonable. Many common disagreements are ironed out at the level closest to the source of the conflict. Some issues, however, are deeply imbedded and thus require more attention; these are usually addressed by senior management and governing board members.

What might be called the *appeals process* is driven by a set of the following agreed-upon principles:

1. *Evidence drives the decisions.* Objective measurement trumps tradition, status, and opinion. What is best for the patient is what is scientifically determined to be best. What is realistic for the associate is the best the associate can expect elsewhere.

2. *Negotiation is improved by patience, listening, and imagination.* Many apparent conflicts are actually misunderstandings. Careful listening expands understanding and reveals consensus opportunities. Imagination—thinking outside the box—identifies new opportunities to resolve apparently conflicting needs.

3. *Equity, not equality, drives the organization's ultimate position.* Under an equity concept, each stakeholder is treated fairly in terms of his or her contribution. Under an equality concept, each is treated equally.[20] While the definition of contribution is never easy, the concept forces participants to recognize realistic differences in influence.

4. *Stakeholders and associates are free to terminate their relationship with the organization; conversely, the group can terminate its relationship with any stakeholder.* The usual goal for everyone is to retain and strengthen relationships, but it is occasionally necessary for some people to seek separate paths.

5. *The governing board's calendar ultimately forces a decision.* The calendar itself is set for the good of the whole, and it is always subject to negotiation and amendment. Again, for the good of the whole, the organization must appropriately, as Hamlet says, "take arms against a sea of troubles, and thus opposing, end them."[21]

Additional Resources

Burns, L. R., E. H. Bradley, and B. J. Weiner. 2011. *Shortell and Kaluzny's Health Care Management: Organization Design and Behavior,* 6th ed. Clifton Park, NY: Cengage Learning.

Collins, J. C. 2001. *Good to Great: Why Some Companies Make the Leap . . . and Others Don't.* New York: HarperBusiness.

Dye, C. F., and A. N. Garman. 2014. *Exceptional Leadership: 16 Critical Competencies for Healthcare Executives,* 2nd ed. Chicago: Health Administration Press.

Filerman, G. L., A. E. Mills, and P. M. Schyve. 2013. *Managerial Ethics in Healthcare: A New Perspective.* Chicago: Health Administration Press.

Kouzes, J. M., and B. Z. Posner. 2012. *The Leadership Challenge,* 5th ed. San Francisco: Jossey-Bass.

Mosser, G., and J. W. Begun. 2014. *Understanding Teamwork in Health Care.* New York: McGraw-Hill.

White, K. R., and J. S. Lindsey. 2015. *Take Charge of Your Healthcare Management Career: 50 Lessons That Drive Success.* Chicago: Health Administration Press.

Notes

1. Kouzes, J. M., and B. Z. Posner. 2012. *The Leadership Challenge,* 5th ed. San Francisco: Jossey-Bass.

2. Greenleaf, R. K. 2002. *Servant Leadership: A Journey into the Nature of Legitimate Power and Greatness,* edited by L. C. Spears. New York: Paulist Press.

3. Mercy Health System's application to the Malcolm Baldrige National Quality Award. 2007. [Online information; retrieved 3/25/14.] www.baldrige.nist.gov/Contacts_Profiles.htm.

4. Gilmartin, M. J., and T. A. D'Aunno. 2007. "Leadership Research in Healthcare." *Academy of Management Annals* 2: 394–96.

5. Sharp HealthCare's application to the Malcolm Baldrige National Quality Award. 2007. [Online information; retrieved 3/25/14.] www.baldrige.nist.gov/Contacts_Profiles.htm.

6. *Ibid.,* p. 1.

7. The precept is fundamental in most religions, in most moral philosophy (including Immanuel Kant and John Rawls), and in most judicial systems.

8. Raman, A. 2013. "Healthcare's Service Fanatics." *Harvard Business Review.* [Online article; retrieved 2/4/15.] https://hbr.org/2013/05/health-cares-service-fanatics.

9. National Center for Healthcare Leadership. 2014. "NCHL Leadership Competency Model." [Online information; retrieved 3/25/14.] www.nchl.org/static.asp?path=2852,3238; Healthcare Leadership Alliance. "About the HLA Competency Directory." 2013. [Online information; retrieved 3/25/14.]. www.healthcareleadershipalliance.org/directory.htm.

10. Henry Ford Health System's application to the Malcolm Baldrige National Quality Award. 2011. [Online information; retrieved 3/25/14.] www.baldrige.nist.gov/Contacts_Profiles.htm.

11. Hill, L. A. 2004. "New Manager Development for the 21st Century." *Academy of Management Executive* 18 (3): 121–26 [124].

12. Gilmartin, M. J., and T. A. D'Aunno. 2008. "Leadership Research in Healthcare." *Academy of Management Annals* 2: 397.

13. Dye, C. F., and A. N. Garman. 2014. *Exceptional Leadership: 16 Critical Competencies for Healthcare Executives,* 2nd ed. Chicago: Health Administration Press.

14. Hill, L. A. 2004. "New Manager Development for the 21st Century." *Academy of Management Executives* 18 (3): 121–26.

15. Conger, J. A. 2004. "Developing Leadership Capability: What's Inside the Black Box?" *Academy of Management Executive* 18 (3): 136–41.

16. Ryan, M. J. 2004. "Achieving and Sustaining Quality in Healthcare." *Frontiers of Health Services Management* 20 (3): 3–11.

17. Institute of Medicine, Committee on Quality Health Care in America. 2001. *Crossing the Quality Chasm: A New Health System for the 21st Century,* 39. Washington, DC: National Academies Press.

18. American College of Healthcare Executives. 2011. "ACHE *Code of Ethics.*" [Online information; retrieved 3/25/14.] www.ache.org/ABT_ACHE/code.cfm.

19. Nelson, W. A., W. B. Weeks, and J. M. Campfield. 2008. "The Organizational Costs of Ethical Conflicts." *Journal of Healthcare Management* 53 (1): 41–53.

20. Phillips, R. 2003. *Stakeholder Theory and Organizational Ethics,* 85–118. San Francisco: Berrett-Koehler.

21. Shakespeare, W. *Hamlet,* Act 3, Scene 1.

3 OPERATIONAL LEADERSHIP

1. *Maintaining contact with all stakeholder groups.* Conduct surveys, listen, and hold formal meetings to ensure a balanced, timely flow of information from external to internal stakeholders.

2. *Sizing the organization and its components.* Use the epidemiologic planning model to size clinical and other units to meet clinical needs.

3. *Measuring and improving performance.* Maintain a system of complete, timely performance measures, goals, and benchmarks. Identify OFIs, support PITs, and negotiate and achieve improvement goals.

4. *Supporting a learning organization.* Maintain information, consultation, and training services to meet all performance improvement needs.

5. *Resolving issues in a timely manner, and adhering to an annual calendar.* Use the board's authority to limit negotiations and prevent unnecessary delay.

Questions for Discussion

These questions are about applying the chapter content. It's often helpful to discuss them with classmates or mentors, gaining different perspectives on the issues.

1. What do first-line leaders need to understand about how the HCO implements the functions of operational leadership? If you were helping a newly appointed first-line leader (for example, a head nurse or a food service supervisor), what would you say to her about each of the functions:
   a. Boundary spanning: how this HCO relates to its community
   b. Forecasting: how the HCO prepares for patients in each service line
   c. Knowledge management: what kinds of knowledge resources are available to her
   d. Accountability and corporate design: who owns the HCO, and how the owners retain control of patient care
   e. Continuous improvement: how she can identify OFIs and then change processes to improve
   f. Improving the operational structure: how the HCO applies the continuous improvement process to all its components, even the governing board

2. The new leader is likely to be concerned about how the goal-setting, accountability, and continuous improvement functions play out for her unit. How would you reassure her that she can succeed in her new role?

3. Senior leadership forms a PIT to be sure annual and long-term forecasting are as good as they can be. What data should the PIT review? With whom should it confer? What questions should the PIT ask to identify important OFIs in the forecasting process?

4. Consider Exhibit 1.2, the scope of comprehensive personal health services. Stakeholders need, and your HCO can offer, service lines in each of the care levels—primary, acute, rehabilitation, continuing, and palliative. What are the critical questions to be asked about the HCO's actual plan? That is, how does the HCO determine that it should offer, or not offer, a given service line?

5. The planning committee of the governing board believes that the HCO's goal-setting efforts, the process shown in Exhibit 3.6, might be improved. It will establish a PIT of trustees, senior leaders, and others to investigate. What data should the PIT review? With whom should it confer?

Chapter 1 describes the excellent HCO as an array of teams empowered, assisted, and rewarded for seeking excellence in their activity. The teams must be aligned and integrated; the whole must be as effective as the parts. Alignment and integration demand a common culture (Chapter 2), a common infrastructure of processes, and rules that facilitate the solutions to complex problems. The infrastructure (or operational foundation) is essential to strategic scorecard success. It keeps the HCO and its mission consistent with stakeholder needs. It ensures that every team receives support services. It generates a consistent approach, deployed across many different teams, that allows the teams to learn, improve, and collaborate in producing a superior overall product. The infrastructure is systematically sustained by specific actions of senior leadership. This chapter describes those actions. Like other components of the HCO, the infrastructure itself is measured and improved.

Purpose

The purpose of operational leadership is

> **to sustain an infrastructure to ensure that the HCO's array of services is effectively designed, aligned, integrated, and continuously improved.**

Effective design emphasizes having all the services the market needs, but not those the organization cannot properly support. Effective alignment rests on a uniform approach to culture, training, and communication. Effective integration requires shared information and collective goal setting. Continuous improvement requires a common mission, capital allocation, and a reward system.

Achievement of the purpose is measured by the improvement of the strategic scorecard (see Exhibit 1.11). Operational leadership complements and is equally essential to cultural leadership and transformational management (see Chapter 2).

The operational infrastructure is a large and expensive component of most HCOs. It includes all the logistic and strategic support activities described in chapters 10 through 15. It is managed by senior leadership, which establishes the direction, importance, and implementation of these activities. Senior leadership stimulates the widespread use of these activities and aggregates the information into an ongoing strategic process, fitting the HCO to its environment.

Functions

To implement the operational infrastructure, senior management returns conceptually to the basic contribution of the organization—fulfilling needs that the stakeholders cannot fulfill by themselves—and improves the processes for reaching decisions rather than focusing on the decisions themselves. When these processes are aligned, the chances of correct decisions—those that optimize the long-run contribution to the mission—are maximized. The functions shown in Exhibit 3.1 ensure that alignment is reached between the HCO and its stakeholders.

Boundary Spanning

Long-term survival requires ongoing adaptation to changes in the environment. Boundary spanning is a deliberate, ongoing surveillance that identifies the changes that arise and the opportunities for improvement (OFIs) those changes generate. Effective boundary spanning identifies the strategic opportunities (Chapter 15). Operational leadership evaluates those opportunities and uses them to create a specific plan for every existing and proposed unit of the HCO and for all critical resources, including funds, caregivers, facilities, and information. These plans must stretch several years into the future, far enough to allow orderly adaptation to change.

Technology, population changes, prevailing attitudes in society, caregiver shortages, financing mechanisms, and regulations drive change in healthcare. Processes that worked well last year will require a redesign to work next year. HCOs that fail to adapt to changing needs fade and disappear, sometimes with surprising speed. The increased importance of population health expands the need for diligent boundary spanning. The HCO should participate in community-related discussions about issues such as income, education, health, safety, and needs of the disadvantaged.

HCO stakeholders expect progress, but also continuity and stability. More than other service industries, the community HCO is expected to keep pace with changes in the environment rather than to be replaced by a new model. This emphasis on long-term survival is promoted by the not-for-profit corporate structure, which is more difficult to dismantle than stock corporations or partnerships, and by tax exemptions that give not-for-profit HCOs a competitive advantage. HCOs' actual life spans reflect this. Many U.S. hospitals have century-long or longer histories, much longer than public stock corporations.

Identifying and rank-ordering the OFIs that arise from external change require an ongoing system of listening to and negotiating with all stakeholders (see Exhibit 1.3). Members of the governing board (see Chapter 4) are selected, in part, to be aware of many stakeholder constituencies. Its members and senior management are expected to keep current on state and national developments that might affect the HCO. Associates are encouraged to participate and assume leadership roles in community activities beyond healthcare. Marketing surveys and customer-listening activities cover a broad spectrum of current and potential customers and target specific groups with unique needs. Senior management meets often with community groups and managers of other services. Much time is spent exploring what stakeholders like and do not

EXHIBIT 3.1 Functions That Sustain Operational Infrastructure

Function	Intent	Implementation	Examples
Boundary spanning	Monitor all external stakeholder groups to identify changes in their needs/desires.	Governing board members, senior executives, and other managers solicit stakeholder perspectives and describe HCO opportunities.	Board members selected for prior community service. Senior managers participate in community services for education, housing, etc.; monitor state and national developments potentially affecting the HCO.
Forecasting	Forecast patient needs to plan staffing and facilities.	Ongoing market analysis identifies trends in patient and associate needs. Epidemiologic planning model sizes all clinical units.	Quantified plans for services, facilities, and personnel reflect trends in community need.
Knowledge management	Provide prompt, complete, reliable information for any associate's or team's purpose.	Strong clinical and business information systems, widespread access, and a culture of communication. Training for repetitive tasks, just-in-time training for arising tasks.	Automated patient record and access to clinical information. E-mail and an internal website. "Data warehouse" with operational measures, goals, benchmarks, and current achievements. Access to public information sources like Medline and Guidelines.gov.
Accountability, integration, and corporate design	Establish explicit expectations of every team. Provide an integrated array that optimally meets community needs.	Expectations and accountability are established and integrated in the annual goal-setting process. Corporate structures such as subsidiaries, joint ventures, and strategic partnerships support a broad scope of healthcare activities, including primary, acute, and post-acute care.	Ninety-day plans used to reach agreed-upon goals. HCO includes primary and continuing care services, forms joint ventures with medical staff, merges with another HCO. HCO organizes caregiving teams into service lines and ensures that effective clinical support services are available.
Continuous improvement	Improve measured performance. Reach decisions in a timely and coordinated fashion.	PITs develop improved processes, guided by a PIC, which coordinates and integrates improvements. PITs and goal-setting process follow a quarterly and annual calendar.	The annual goal-setting and budgeting activities proceed according to a prearranged timetable initiated and finished by governing board action. PITs are scheduled to complete their work in time to coordinate with budget deadlines.
Improving the operational infrastructure	Improve the operational and strategic foundations.	Educational sessions of the governing board and senior management meetings are devoted to review of infrastructure effectiveness measures, identification of OFIs, and development of improvements.	Annual goal-setting process improved, additional performance measures installed and benchmarked. Strategic protection is expanded. Analytic and training support for PITs are expanded.

OFI: opportunity for improvement; PIC: performance improvement council; PIT: process improvement team like, how deep their concerns are, and which alternatives are attractive. This knowledge allows process improvement teams (PITs) and planning teams to formulate proposals that meet a broader spectrum of stakeholder needs. The inputs from systematic listening often form the difference between a successful proposal and a contentious negotiation.

The program that helps Sharp HealthCare relate to the San Diego community is one example. Sharp, a recipient of the Malcolm Baldrige National Quality Award, claims its "involvement in San Diego's well-being is comprehensive":[1]

- When key community health issues or new health threats are identified, Sharp collaborates with appropriate public officials for a safe, evidence-based, patient-centered, timely, efficient, and equitable resolution.
- Sharp's leaders serve as board members on many community organizations.
- Sharp's comprehensive environmental, health, and safety management program, including emergency/disaster management, ensures a safe and secure environment for customers/partners.
- Staff and leaders present a strong showing of support and participation each year in community fundraisers.
- Sharp hosts many free community preventive health offerings, such as flu shots, lectures, and screenings.
- Sharp offers the Weight Management Health Education program, providing health maintenance to employers and employees and free, weekly programs to the community.
- Managers are encouraged to donate a minimum of 22,000 collective hours annually to community service.

Effective boundary spanning, as shown in Exhibit 3.2, has four requirements:

1. A network of listening activities must be established so that the HCO has entrance into and recognition with specific stakeholder groups.
2. Trust must be established and common values recognized so that the stakeholders are candid and comfortable with discussing complex topics.
3. Associates must be trained to hear accurately what the stakeholders are saying and to represent the HCO's perspective.
4. The knowledge gained from dozens of individual contacts must be systematically assembled, analyzed, and integrated.

Excellent HCOs achieve these components by consistently pursuing listening opportunities, repeatedly demonstrating their commitment to values, training their associates, and systematically assembling and reviewing notes from contacts. The results serve as a rich source of OFIs and a valuable background for improving all kinds of internal processes.

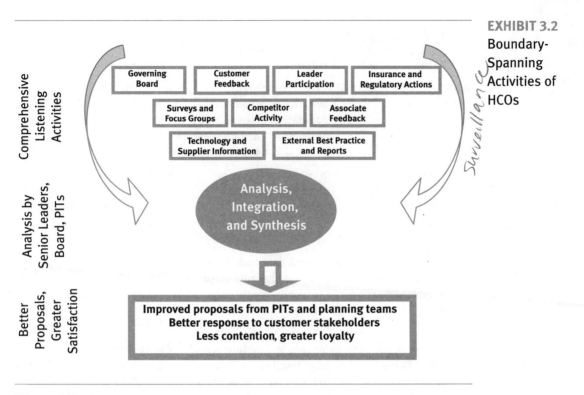

EXHIBIT 3.2
Boundary-
Spanning
Activities of
HCOs

PIT: process improvement team

Forecasting Need and Demand to Plan Services

All healthcare services are ultimately delivered by specialized teams and facilities. The success of the HCO depends on the correct sizing of those teams and facilities. Each service offered must be large enough to meet needs and operate effectively, but no larger. The array of services must meet community needs without exceeding the available funds. It must be carefully based on population, market trends, and competitor behavior. Each service must be evaluated against available funds, performance benchmarks, and alternative investments. Some services will be referred to distant HCOs, as the local community does not generate enough demand to support them. Some will be implemented in competition with others; some will be offered in partnerships with others. These plans require years to implement; decisions must be made months or years in advance. An **epidemiologic planning model** generates the most reliable forecast for the number of patients who require a specific service. Most HCOs purchase access to a sophisticated computerized model that combines population forecasts and usage data from a variety of national sources to identify factors affecting the incidence and prevalence of specific conditions and to forecast demand on a community level. Its elements are shown in Exhibit 3.3.

Epidemiologic planning model
A statistical analysis and forecast of the health needs of the community served.

EXHIBIT 3.3
Elements of the
Epidemiologic
Planning Model

For any specific clinical service

Question	Solution	Example
What population will use the service?	People live in small geographic areas. The population of these areas is measured and forecast by the U.S. Census Bureau.	Births for Ann Arbor, Michigan, and surrounding areas
What part of that population is at risk for needing the service?	The risk of a disease is dependent on age, genetics, income, and lifestyle. These factors are used to forecast demand.	Births are a function of the number of females by age and certain socioeconomic characteristics.
What part of the population at risk will select our service?	Historical data and surveys estimate the fraction of those with the disease who seek care from our team (market share).	Women in and around Ann Arbor choose between two obstetrics services. Home deliveries and travel to other services are rare.
How many specialized people will we need to meet this demand?	Protocols and historical and benchmark data show the number of patients an individual provider can successfully treat.	Each of the obstetrics services must establish the numbers of obstetricians, family practitioners, midwives, registered nurses, and other caregivers required.
How big a facility will we need to meet this demand?	History, benchmarks, and simulation models show how many rooms and specialized facilities will be required.	The 2012 University of Michigan obstetrics delivery service will have "50 single room maternity care beds in the Birth Center."*

*Information from the University of Michigan Health System, C. S. Mott Hospital. 2008. [Online information; retrieved 4/21/09.] www.med.umich.edu/mott/touch/new_facts.html.

The epidemiologic planning model draws on five major sources of data to produce forecasts of the proper size and staffing for a specific service:

1. *Population.* Unbiased population forecasts for states are prepared by the U.S. Census Bureau. These forecasts must be translated to small areas, minor civil divisions, or postal codes. Most HCOs draw patients from a few dozen small areas and heavily from only a few. Both the counts and the characteristics of the small-area population must be forecast at least a decade into the future.

2. *Disease risk.* This is estimated based on population characteristics. Large databases of hospital admissions, specific treatments, drug usage, and other indicators are used to identify the risk of occurrence of specific medical needs, which are measured by the following:

- Incidence: the number of new cases in the population in a given period
- Prevalence: the number of cases at a point in time
- Demand: the number of cases that actually sought service

By dividing the population into small, homogeneous groups (e.g., white males, aged 40–65 years, earning between $50,000 and $75,000 per year, with post–high school education) and analyzing patterns of incidence of common diseases for these groups, precise estimates of incidence, prevalence, and demand can be made.

3. *Market share.* This is the fraction of the total demand from care-seeking activity at a specific HCO. Patients have choices for most services, such as selecting a local competitor, traveling to a larger HCO, or deferring care. Surveys and historic usage data are used to estimate market share. Market share is forecast subjectively, on the basis of the HCO's ability to retain or increase its attractiveness to patients.

4. *Staff requirements.* These are estimated on the basis of the capacity of each skill level required. Capacity is measured by history, survey, and benchmark. Requirements for physicians by specialty, registered nurses, other nursing personnel, and total personnel are forecast for each service. These are compared against intentions of current staff to identify recruitment needs.

5. *Facility requirements.* These are estimated on the basis of the numbers of patients expected and the length of time they will require service plus allowances for idle time. Allowances are as small as feasible, given the need to not turn patients away and to meet patient and associate schedules. Allowances differ by service, and they significantly increase the physical capacity required. Some services, such as newborn delivery and emergency cardiac catheterization, cannot be delayed. Allowance must be made to meet the peak, rather than the average, demand. For less pressing care, neither patients nor associates like night or weekend service. Allowances are forecast using protocols, history, and benchmarks. Facility requirements are often calculated by simulation models or by comparison to best practices.

The basic estimating equations are as follows:

$$\{\text{Demand}\} = \left\{\begin{array}{c}\text{Population}\\\text{served}\end{array}\right\} \times \left\{\begin{array}{c}\text{Risk of}\\\text{need of}\\\text{service}\end{array}\right\} \times \left\{\begin{array}{c}\text{Market}\\\text{share}\end{array}\right\}$$

$$\left\{\begin{array}{c}\text{Total}\\\text{personnel}\\\text{required}\end{array}\right\} = \left\{\begin{array}{c}\text{Demand}\\\text{per work}\\\text{period}\end{array}\right\} \div \left\{\begin{array}{c}\text{Service}\\\text{per}\\\text{provider}\end{array}\right\}$$

$$\left\{\begin{array}{c}\text{Facility}\\\text{required}\end{array}\right\} = \left\{\begin{array}{c}\text{Maximum}\\\text{or average}\\\text{demand per}\\\text{work period}\end{array}\right\} \times \left\{\begin{array}{c}\text{Time}\\\text{required}\\\text{per service}\end{array}\right\} \div \{\text{Allowance}\} \div \left\{\begin{array}{c}\text{Time of}\\\text{facility}\\\text{availability}\end{array}\right\}$$

Calculations for a scheduled service (e.g., primary care office visit) are relatively straightforward. The epidemiologic planning model forecasts the demand, aggregating the incidence of all causes for office visits. Market share is established by a planning committee, considering relevant prior experience. The HCO forecasts the expected output of each caregiver. If the demand is 300 visits per week, the anticipated market share is one-third, and the office teams (one physician, one registered nurse, and one clerical associate) can see 15 visits per shift for 10 shifts, then

$$\left\{\begin{array}{l} \text{Teams} \\ \text{required} \end{array}\right\} = \left\{\begin{array}{l} 30 \text{ visits} \\ \text{per shift} \end{array}\right\} \div \left\{\begin{array}{l} 15 \text{ visits} \\ \text{per shift} \end{array}\right\} = 2$$

If each visit requires 30 minutes per examining room, and cleanup sometimes delays room readiness, only 90 percent of capacity can be used:

$$\left\{\begin{array}{l} \text{Number} \\ \text{of rooms} \end{array}\right\} = \left\{\begin{array}{l} 30 \text{ visits} \\ \text{per shift} \end{array}\right\} \times \left\{\begin{array}{l} 30 \text{ minutes} \\ \text{per visit} \end{array}\right\} \div \{0.9 \text{ allowance}\}$$

$$\div \left\{\begin{array}{l} 240 \text{ minutes} \\ \text{per room} \end{array}\right\} = 4.17 \text{ rooms}$$

The planning committee must address the question of four rooms, with delays and overtime as factors about one day a week, or five rooms. Given customer and caregiver satisfaction issues, the committee will probably decide on five rooms, but this decision will increase project cost. The resulting projections are translated to actual personnel and facility forecasts by internal or external consultants, negotiating the personnel and facilities parameters with local associates. The size of many support services, such as parking and human resources, is driven by the aggregate forecast of clinical services; this process is described further in chapters 14 and 15. The epidemiologic planning model is essential to virtually every service and is referenced in all the following chapters. The governing board has the final decision on the size of clinical services. Senior management is responsible for negotiating a recommendation that is acceptable to the board and the associates involved in the service.

Knowledge Management

Knowledge—evidence—is at the core of high-performing HCOs and the theory of evidence-based management. Poudre Valley Health System (PVHS), a Baldrige Award recipient, explains what is involved in knowledge management:[2]

> PVHS' ability to meet and exceed the expectations of quality care, prompt service, and friendly staff is dependent upon the timely availability of information

for the workforce, suppliers, partners, collaborators, patients, and the community. To optimize the flow of accurate, real-time information, PVHS has established a secure, user-friendly network that is appropriately accessible to all stakeholders, regardless of geography or time of day. In this network, the central repository [has] associated content-specific functions such as:

- Clinical Information. Electronic health records, Picture Archive and Communication System (PACS), lab results, poison control, [automated pharmaceutical dispensing, and medication reconciliation].
- Physician Information Center (Provider LINK). Clinical information (see above); subscription-based online resources, such as MD Consult, CINAHL, and online medical journals.
- Decision Support. "Key Performance Indicator" reports; electronic data interchanges (automatic supply tracking, ordering, and billing with nearly 100 percent of PVHS vendors); Information Center (service utilization, patient demographics, market trends).
- Financial Information. Patient billing, payroll, accounts receivable, revenue cycle management.
- Employee Information Center. Patient census (by unit or outpatient department); bed management (number of patients by unit/facility and admission/discharge projections); time clock; due dates for mandatory annual learning test, tuberculosis testing, performance reviews, time clock entries, pay stub, and benefits; performance reviews; balanced scorecard and quality data; patient satisfaction data; Medline; policies/procedures; forms; calendars; job postings; directories.
- Patient Information Center. GetWell Network, educational materials, gift shop, newborn photo gallery, and health resources, such as a diabetes management tool and a database for identifying potential drug interactions.

This array of information is increasingly web-based and supported by a substantial infrastructure that maintains electronic access and helps associates find and use all the information appropriately (further described in chapters 10 and 14). The knowledge infrastructure implements the following criteria:

1. *Access.* The user gets the screens or documents needed with minimal delay.
2. *Protection.* Access is limited to appropriate users and protected against loss, service interruption, or deliberate distortion.
3. *Accuracy.* The information is valid and reliable.
4. *Completeness.* The user gets all the information needed.

These criteria are achieved by systematic processes that support the library of work processes, protocols, and measures; training; and the communications network.

High-performing HCOs deliberately pursue a broad access strategy. Personal information about patients and associates must be protected by law. A small set of strategic information, largely relating to work in process, must be protected to allow orderly decision making. Beyond that, the strategy is to make information available. Access is made faster by electronic records and search engines. PVHS notes that it also communicates "through newsletters, reports, bulletin boards, posters, mailings, media, and [other] approaches."[3] Open access enhances empowerment, speeds communication, and reduces errors. Under this strategy, much information becomes public, or nearly so. The dangers cited against broad access (competitors, lawsuits, misinterpretations) have not proven to be significant.

Protection is achieved by providing each user with an identification and a password, organizing the users in groups and the knowledge in sets, and allowing groups access to specific sets of information. Protection also requires safeguarding not just the records but also the communications network. (This is handled by specific information services functions described in Chapter 10.)

Accuracy of information is critical. Modern information management uses three approaches to improve the accuracy of information (they are expanded on in Chapter 10):

1. *Screens and information input design.* Well-designed screens (and paper forms) discourage errors and encourage completeness. Electronic entry adds edit and audit protections that increase accuracy and completeness. Procedures can follow an outline or a template that helps make them complete and easier to comprehend. Tags allow cross-referencing and retrieval.

2. *Standardization of performance measures.* Performance measures have become increasingly complex. Ideally, users should be assured that (a) each measure reflects the process it purports to measure (validity); (b) variation from prior values, goals, or benchmarks is meaningful (reliability); and (c) the cause of the variation is reasonably under the users' control. High-performing HCOs rely on a measurement review committee to assist in developing and testing measures. The committee emphasizes nationally defined measures as a priority for two reasons: These definitions are rigorously developed and tested, and national standardization is essential for benchmarking. When unique measures must be created or national measures adjusted for local conditions, the committee also provides expert guidance.

   Many measures are obtained by survey. The design and administration of surveys are a science, and commercial companies provide standardized packages for various purposes. Such a package ensures the consistent application of surveys and provides automatic benchmarking and analysis of statistical sensitivity.

3. *Audits.* High-performing HCOs have extended the internal audit activity to all dimensions of the operational and strategic scorecards.[4] Critical and other measures may be audited routinely to check their accuracy.

The goal of these efforts is to make transparent the measures used to evaluate performance, identify OFIs, and analyze alternative processes. The measures are valid and reliable, and they are accepted as reliable by the participants in PITs and planning sessions.

Completeness as a criterion means that the library is constantly expanding. Processes get extended, additional measures and adjustments get approved, and histories get longer. Modern knowledge management depends on computer technology. High-performing HCOs expect to expand applications, usage, and storage.

Training

High-performing HCOs are distinguished by their commitment to training, providing 80 to more than 100 hours a year per full-time associate, about twice the average HCO investment.[5] Training takes two forms: scheduled and just in time. Scheduled training prepares associates for recurring needs. It is used for orientation, preparation for promotion, standardization of work methods, and implementation of ongoing values such as the Health Insurance Portability and Accountability Act enforcement and harassment prevention. It can be offered in a variety of modes, including online courses and on-site exercises. Just-in-time training is offered when the skill involved is used less frequently. With access to the library, it is often self-training. Looking up clinical evidence and verifying a procedure on the Internet are just-in-time training topics. Coaching a new manager and helping a PIT chairperson manage a meeting are other examples.

Communications Network

A great deal of the knowledge necessary for HCOs is ephemeral. It is essential in framing short-term responses to patient and other needs and must be communicated quickly and accurately. E-mail, which is documented and does not require simultaneous participation, has proven to be a major advancement, as are electronic records where current observations and requests can be entered. Broad access to communication is encouraged, as in other knowledge management activities. Accuracy and completeness are improved by multiple users; erroneous material is questioned and corrected or abandoned. Protection has not proven to be a serious issue. E-mail and web access are certainly misused, but the key to control is passive rather than active. Policies are in place to forbid spamming, deliberate distortion, and other improper messaging. They are supported by the recorded identity of senders and investigated when complaints are received.[6]

The culture is an important factor in making communications networks effective. PVHS and other high-performing HCOs make clear that communication must be responsive. Failing to answer completely and constructively is not acceptable.

Accountability and Corporate Design

Accountability

Much has been written about how to design organizations in general[7] and for HCOs specifically.[8] The traditional starting point is the accountability hierarchy, a reporting path that allows each team to communicate its needs to the larger organization and to assure the governing board of negotiated acceptance of goals. The hierarchy groups teams with closely related interests into a single division, divisions into departments, and so forth. It establishes managerial rank and titles, with work teams reporting directly to "managers," who report to "division directors" or similar titled leaders, who report in turn to senior management. (Titles differ, but they should be consistent within a single HCO.) The hierarchy is reflected in the traditional pyramid table of organization (see Exhibit 3.4).

Excellent HCOs that operate under evidence-based management have moved substantially beyond the hierarchy concepts. They retain an accountability hierarchy, because it is essential in negotiating goals and monitoring performance, but they emphasize multiple lines of communication as shown in the lower section of Exhibit 3.4. Direct communication between teams is encouraged. Support teams are encouraged to think of serving other teams as internal customers. PITs deliberately seek representatives of all affected teams. Management listening activities and surveys are avenues for less structured discussion. Unlike the classical bureaucratic organization where the hierarchy connoted power and authority, the hierarchy in the modern HCO connotes resources and support. Power accrues from facts, ideas, vision, and goals; authority is a last resort in conflict resolution.

Senior management maintains the hierarchy. Most hierarchies organize patient care around service lines and clinical support around groups of related services. Service lines group similar patients together, allowing teams to specialize and supporting clinical protocols and work processes built around the patients' needs. Service lines allow HCOs to manage very different patient needs effectively, ranging from preventive care through ambulatory services of various kinds to inpatient acute care, rehabilitation, chronic inpatient care, and end-of-life care. The HCO's logistic support services—functions such as knowledge management, human resources management, and financial management—are organized around their professional skills. Specifics differ with size and system structure. For example, a small unit of a multisite system might rely on nearby referral centers for several service lines and the corporate offices for logistic systems.

The levels of Exhibit 3.4 identified as "leadership" constitute the HCO's leadership team. The higher levels carry broader and more diffuse responsibilities.

Managers at every level of the hierarchy are expected to do the following:

Leadership Level	Common Names	Goal Setting and Monitoring Function
Governance	Governing board, board of trustees	Set corporate goals, monitor progress and strategic protection, make strategic decisions
Senior leadership	Senior leadership, senior management, or senior vice presidents	Provide fact base for all goal-setting activities, assist all units in goal achievement
Intermediate leadership	Division directors	Translate corporate goals to individual teams, assist teams in coordinating with other teams, assist teams in goal achievement
Team leadership	Managers, head nurses, chiefs	Negotiate team goals, maintain coordination with supporting teams, assist team in goal achievement
Work team	Named by function	Participate in goal setting, monitor team performance, report OFIs, participate in PITs
Associate	Employees, partners, volunteers	Participate in goal setting, monitor personal performance, report OFIs, participate in PITs

EXHIBIT 3.4

Leadership Structure, Communications, and Accountability

Traditional Table of Organization

The traditional pyramidal Table of Organization is created by identifying a line of formal communication from the governing board to the associates such that each associate has a single point of contact to a team leader and each team leader has a single point of contact to a superior:

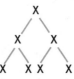

While the line of formal communication is still important, Tables of Organization themselves seriously understate the communications possibilities and are now infrequently used.

Modern Communications Network

Each team is engaged in multiple ongoing relationships, and the same is true of all its partners.

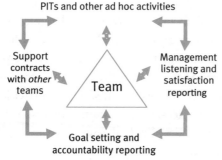

OFI: opportunity for improvement; PIT: process improvement team

- Listen continuously to the units, individuals, and patients in their assigned area.
- Achieve agreed-on goals for service, and resolve all issues that threaten goal achievement, either by direct action or by seeking assistance outside their area.
- Initiate requests for assistance from other areas, and respond to requests from other areas.
- Convey the organization's global needs, and negotiate realistic improvement goals in their assigned area.
- Participate in PITs and other continuous improvement activities.

These obligations ensure that each team has a prescribed purpose, a guideline for size, an operating location, a formal contact for communicating unmet needs, and a path for negotiating goals for operational measures. These elements both support the individual teams and coordinate their contribution to the organization as a whole.

At higher levels, the expectations of leaders are more complex. By definition, senior management is accountable not only for large groups of services but also for the support activities (including measurement) that underpin the HCO's performance. To be successful, accountability must pass three tests:

1. *Control.* Operational scorecard performance should equal or exceed negotiated goals. In units large enough to have strategic scorecards, senior leaders are collectively accountable for strategic performance.
2. *Comparability.* The organization's scorecard values should be less than the values in alternative sources for the product or service, and they should be acceptably close to benchmark or values that support best practices.
3. *Profitability.* At the level of aggregation at which revenue is received, expenditures should equal the amount paid minus an allowance for funding the long-run strategic goals of the organization. (Very few accountability centers actually receive revenue. With insurance payments increasingly "bundled" around a care episode, only service lines and hospitals receive revenue and can assess profitability. Certain services may be deliberately subsidized; this amounts to a negative allowance.)

Corporate Design

The corporate design of an HCO consists of charters, bylaws, and long-term contracts that establish the HCO's legal entities and link together its major units. Historically, American healthcare has been fragmented into a large number of separate vendors. The traditional provider groups—such as community hospitals, medical practices, and specialty providers—each provided a small fraction of the care needed to sustain individual or community health. Care was so fragmented and individual units were so small that healthcare was frequently called a "cottage industry."

Healthcare reform has increased pressure for both *vertical* integration (across service lines) and *horizontal* integration (uniting similar service lines). Advantages of scale—such as the ability to gain debt financing or the ability to support advanced knowledge management systems—drive both horizontal and vertical integration. Most not-for-profit hospitals are now in systems, albeit mostly small, single-community systems. There are many large and growing not-for-profit multistate systems, supporting a wide variety of service lines. National companies dominate for-profit hospital systems. National for-profit companies have acquired large market shares in nursing home care, dialysis, and pharmacies. Medical practices have moved toward large groups, many of which have formal employment arrangements with the health systems in which they practice.[9]

The high-performing HCOs presented in this book often operate multisite, multipurpose systems. They are acquiring or joint venturing with medical practices and nonacute services. Many with population health missions have extended their influence through a variety of collaborative efforts, forming consortia, joint ventures, and partnerships with private, charitable, and government organizations.[10,11] Also, many include their own health insurance or healthcare financing mechanisms.

The emerging corporate design includes a parent corporation, wholly owned subsidiaries, partially owned joint ventures, and long-term strategic partnership contracts without ownership. Increasingly, it is both vertically and horizontally integrated. The levels of corporate design are shown in Exhibit 3.5. The exact form varies, but the purpose of affiliations is to use advantages of scale to increase mission achievement. As indicated in Exhibit 3.5, central corporate offices typically establish a shared mission, vision, and set of values; rules for doing business such as timetables and approvals required for the annual cycle of improvement; and long-term corporate finance. HCO subsidiaries are empowered under these rules, and they support hospitals and similar groups of service lines. The service lines focus on their clinical specialty.

The growth of healthcare systems has helped overcome the cottage industry identity problem, but the overall performance remains well below benchmark on quality and related indicators.[12]

Senior management and governance at the HCO level must define the service line structures and revise them as local conditions change. Both tax-exempt and taxable structures are used. Specific rules in the Internal Revenue Code define permissible relationships between entities. Tax exemption generally requires community control and pursuit of a purpose consistent with congressional intentions for exemption.[13] All corporate design decisions are ultimately made by the governing board as part of its strategy function (see Chapter 4) or by the corporate office. Empowerment requires senior managers to work closely with the associates directly involved in the activity under study.

EXHIBIT 3.5 Organization Structures for Hospitals and Healthcare Systems

Organization	Trends
Corporate Office	Large, multistate HCO systems have grown rapidly by acquiring community HCOs and aggregating systems. Many pursue a deliberately broad scope of service lines in response to healthcare reform. They use the tools of empowerment and continuous improvement to support their subsidiaries.
Examples Intermountain Health Care, Ascension Health, HCA, Veterans Health Administration *Focus:* • Mission, vision, and values • Long-term finance • "Reserved powers," e.g., – acquisition of local sites – approval of annual plans – appointment of governing board members and chief executives – review of annual audit • Support for regional HCOs	
Community HCOs	Community HCOs historically were small and independently owned. Many of these have merged, usually around the not-for-profit community hospital. The merged organization can better support integrated, efficient care.
Examples: local hospitals, surgical centers, nursing homes, physicians' offices *Focus:* • Annual plan (balanced scorecard, Exhibit 1.11) • Operation of one or more service lines • On-site support to service lines and logistic services	
Service Line	Service lines are built around caregivers with training to care for similar patients. A service line may have several teams, at several locations.
Examples: primary care, mental health care, women's health, surgery, cardiovascular care, rehabilitation, end-of-life care *Focus:* • Clinical protocols • Annual plan (unit scorecard, Exhibit 1.10) • Operations	

Continuous Improvement

The management approach used in *The Well-Managed Healthcare Organization* has four characteristics of evidence-based medicine and evidence-based management that make it successful:

1. It strengthens the physician's role as selector of protocol (diagnostician) and monitor of protocol, with the obligation to depart from the usual path when it is failing the patient.
2. It empowers nurses and other caregivers both to provide physician-ordered services and to identify and meet additional patient needs so that the care supports maximal recovery.

3. It stresses measured, audited, benchmarked performance in all components of care, enabling the results to be shared with the governing board and the stakeholders.
4. It approaches benchmark performance through continuous improvement.

The HCOs that have followed the approach and documented their achievement have annual expenses that range from $500 million to several billion dollars and offer a relatively broad scope of services in several geographic locations. They have religious and secular not-for-profit owners. It appears likely that government and for-profit HCOs can also benefit from the evidence-based transformational model, although thus far no such example has been reported. Small corporate structures will continue to be important as joint venture partners and affiliates of large organizations.

The system for continuous improvement must imbed the cycle of identify/analyze/test/evaluate into the routine of the organization. The search for OFIs must be ongoing, PITs must make steady progress, PIT findings must be implemented, and expected results must be included in next year's goals. The operational foundation for continuous improvement has three major parts: an annual planning calendar, an internal consulting resource, and a process for conflict resolution.

Calendar for Annual Planning

All business organizations must have a system for timely planning that adheres to a calendar. Whether the HCO is a 20-bed **critical access hospital** with three or four physicians and 50 nursing personnel or a healthcare system like Kaiser Permanente with 150,000 associates in eight states, the

Critical access hospitals
Rural community hospitals that receive cost-based reimbursement.

outside world does not wait for the HCO. Excellent organizations maintain their timeliness with an explicit calendar that tracks the fiscal year. Adhering to the calendar is the responsibility of senior leadership. Following are the main steps of the annual planning process followed by Mercy Health System (see Exhibit 3.6):

- *Step 1.* The process starts at the governing board retreat with the board's thorough review of data and information gathered from boundary spanning, responsive communication, and performance measurement. The board refines long-range plans into short-term goals for all dimensions of the strategic performance measures (see Exhibit 1.11). The board's task is to balance customer and associate needs, establishing organization-wide goals that sustain excellence but are still realistic.
- *Steps 2, 3, and 4.* The senior management team begins the translation to operational goals for every unit. With advice from the team, the board's finance committee establishes the amount of funds available for capital replacement and expansion. The team begins dialogue and negotiations with division leaders, who in turn work with unit managers.

EXHIBIT 3.6 Mercy Health System's Annual Planning Calendar

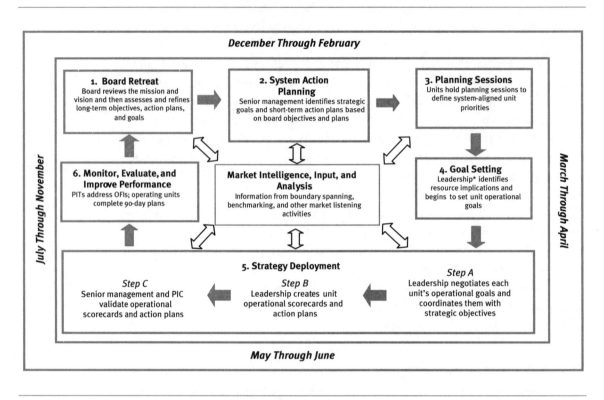

OFI: opportunity for improvement; PIT: process improvement team
*Leadership is composed of all management associates.
Note: Market intelligence activity occurs throughout the year, but it is emphasized at the board's annual retreat. The activity is described in Chapter 15.
Source: Adapted from Mercy Health's Malcolm Baldrige National Quality Award application, p. 7.

- *Step 5a.* All work groups set operational goals using the strategic goals as a guide along with OFIs. The division and senior leadership must integrate the operational goals to meet the strategic goals through negotiation. This is a complex process that is central to empowerment.
- *Step 5b.* Consensus is reached on the goals at all levels and then summarized in dashboards or scorecards.
- *Step 5c.* Negotiations conclude, and explicit operational goals for every group in the accountability hierarchy are established. These operational goals are aggregated to the board's strategic goals.

  The process through Step 5c takes six or seven months, leaving five or six months for Step 6.

- *Step 6.* PITs design new processes to address OFIs. These improvements allow the board to raise the strategic goals in the next annual planning round, driving continuous improvement. The improvements anticipated by the PITs must be implemented and included in goal negotiations. Every PIT project managed by the performance improvement council (PIC) is monitored on an implementation queue, and appropriate changes in unit goals are built into the next budget cycle. The implementation is achieved by 90-day interim goals. The 90-day goals are usually achieved, but a recovery process is in place should plans not work out as expected.

The relentlessly forward-looking characteristic is a major source of strength for an HCO. The boundary-spanning, communication, PIT, planning, and 90-day implementation activities seek, find, and celebrate better performance. The negotiated goals are realistic, the improvements to support them have been tested, and the unit teams have accepted them. Thus, almost all operational goals in high-performing HCOs are achieved. There is little to fix because the planning activities anticipate the problems and prevent them.

Managing Process Improvement

The larger PITs and the PIC follow formal processes as well. Each PIT, large or small, has a charge, a specified membership, and a timetable. Larger PITs usually have two kinds of technical assistance—meeting management and systems analysis. Members of the PIT have ongoing responsibilities, and their time must be used efficiently. PIT meetings must be well managed, and information must be prepared in advance, agendas defined, debate appropriately moderated, and minutes kept. The PIT chair is trained to lead meetings and is assisted by a meeting manager, who handles the details.

Fact-finding and analyses must be assigned to personnel who have the time, skills, and resources to do them. A number of formal approaches are popular, including Lean and Six Sigma. These approaches provide rigor, objectivity, and thoroughness, and they require trained leaders. Tasks such as implementing the epidemiologic planning model or designing a staffing system demand experience and skills and take substantial time. To support their continuous improvement efforts, large HCOs rely on in-house consultants, while small HCOs hire external consultants. The roles that consultants fill are detailed in chapters 14 and 15.

Process for Conflict Resolution

Change frequently requires substantial relearning and occasionally painful adjustment. Conflicts, defensiveness, and denial can be anticipated in the PIT process. These are best handled in private sessions where emotions as well as facts can be explored, alternatives investigated, and accommodations made. The process of conflict resolution discussed in Chapter 2 is a negotiation activity that supports the culture. The annual planning calendar is an essential part of conflict resolution because it establishes a deadline for resolution. Many serious conflicts will test that deadline, and it is the governing board's job to hold to this date judiciously. That action rules out foot-dragging, red herrings, and obfuscation as strategies to protect limited interests. It does not rule out legitimate concerns expressed by any associate. The culture reinforces the board's action. Listening has occurred, facts have been gathered and tested, and the opinion of colleagues has been established. The case is won or lost, and continued objection is fruitless.

Sustaining and Improving the Operational Structure

The senior leadership team leads the PIC and assists the work teams and accountability groups in carrying out continuous improvement. The team must also apply this process to the cultural and operational infrastructure. This is done by evaluating both quantitative and qualitative evidence about the improvement processes themselves. Quantitative measures begin with the balanced scorecard. A number of supplementary measurements are suggested in Exhibit 3.8, later in the chapter.

Many qualitative indicators arise from various listening activities and unexpected events; examples are shown in Exhibit 3.7. These are the "ear to the ground" activities that identify social trends, competitor plans, and similar matters of great interest. They are an important part of boundary spanning and the annual strategic review.

Systematic listening, suggested several times in Exhibit 3.7, includes generating logs or written reports of noteworthy findings. Logs and reports must be aggregated, summarized, and critically reviewed. Aggregation and summary are assigned to an appropriate internal consulting unit. The OFIs can then be rank-ordered by importance and feasibility. Members of the PIC can individually identify and rank-order OFIs. Their written reports can be aggregated and consensus can be reached using nominal group technique.[14] Using several perspectives generates a more objective and thorough evaluation.

Many of the questions that arise in evaluating the infrastructure revolve around "How do we fall short on our values and vision?" Those questions are challenging to answer. Inherent biases cause disabling blindness. Cultural competency is an important example. It is not uncommon to overlook some population sectors, leaving them to feel ignored. The first step toward overcoming these weaknesses is for the senior leadership team to reflect on the question. The second is to form review teams who are sensitive to the issues. These teams can pursue several possibilities to identify OFIs, such as comparing the HCO's boundary spanning with best practices in other communities and those reported in the literature or conferring with leaders of cultural groups.

People

HCO leadership requires an extensive and challenging set of operational competencies. These competencies are typically supplied to first-line leaders by

EXHIBIT 3.7
Qualitative
Indicators of
OFIs for
Maintaining the
Cultural and
Operational
Infrastructure

Function	Qualitative Indicators	Sources
Boundary spanning	Stated satisfaction of major customer stakeholders Competitor activities Activities of excellent HCOs in other communities Changes in healthcare financing Changes in healthcare technology Changes in local employment, attitudes, or civic commitments	Systematic listening and comments of customer stakeholder leadership Published and suspected actions of competitors Published reports and awards Consultants' reports Government legislation and regulation Reports from literature, trade, and professional associations
Organization design	Requests for service expansion Effectiveness of PITs Customer and associate complaints or service concerns Effective adoption of new technology	Systematic listening and comments of associate stakeholders Logs and reports of unexpected events Consultants' advice and record of other HCOs
Responsive communication	Associate complaints or concerns Unionization efforts Success of new hires and promotions Terminal interview comments	Systematic listening and comments of associate stakeholders Individual interviews and personal evaluations
Continuous improvement	Difficulty in negotiating goals Complaints about PITs or timetable	Minutes and observations of PIT participants

OFI: opportunity for improvement; PIT: process improvement team

in-house training and coaching. The program of preparation for senior leadership usually includes formal education, planned experience, and mentoring. (See Chapter 2 for an expanded discussion of these concepts.)

Measures

Evidence-based management assumes that objective measurement is the best source for all judgments and evaluations. The strategic and operational performance measures assess inputs (demand and quantity, cost, and quality of resources) and outputs (production, efficiency, quality, unit cost, and customer satisfaction). This approach does not translate easily to the infrastructure. The infrastructure does not create a tangible product, and much of the resource used to maintain it is blended into other activities. It is still necessary to measure the infrastructure as objectively as possible to keep it sound and identify its OFIs.

The quantitative measures available for assessing the infrastructure are shown in Exhibit 3.8. These measures indicate how well a specific part of each function has been addressed.

They are often difficult to benchmark and complicated to interpret. For example, "board self-evaluation" and "ad hoc surveys of other stakeholders" cannot reasonably be compared across different communities. Community health measures can be compared and benchmarked, but the HCO is only one of many factors that affect the statistics. As a result of these complexities, interpreting these numbers is not as straightforward as it is for operational and strategic measures. Qualitative information is relatively more important. The full array of opportunities must be carefully explored to establish the right goals.

The issues involved in evaluating local market information provide an illustration. Much about the local market can be measured, such as the percentage of patients leaving the community and their reasons, the shares of local competitors and their trends, the number and size of competitors, and the per capita cost of care for the community. For many of these measures, even the proper goal is debatable. The desirable level of patients leaving the community is different for different locations. Two communities—one 40 miles outside Phoenix and the other 40 miles outside Minneapolis, for example—are not likely to accept the same levels as goals. The number of competitors is likely to be a historic accident, and one cannot say that two competitors are better than four or that Community A is better than Community B because it has more HCOs per 100,000 people.

While the per capita cost of care can be benchmarked, community income and education are important contributors. An HCO in a community with high unemployment and low post–high school education should not be directly compared with an HCO in a suburban community filled with professional families. Both HCOs can lower the per capita cost in their communities, but they cannot overcome the social and economic differences.

The process for evaluating OFIs and establishing goals should give primacy to objective measures, but it should never ignore qualitative information. When judging the measures of infrastructure, the balance shifts toward qualitative information. The key questions for evaluation are as follows:

1. Is the HCO moving in the correct long-term direction? Has the overall progress been sufficient?
2. Is progress uniformly deployed across the HCO?
3. What are the most important OFIs and improvement goals?

Because of the complexity and importance of the task, the evaluation is usually carried out by both the governing board and senior leadership. They

EXHIBIT 3.8 Performance Measures for Infrastructure Functions

Function	Infrastructure Concept	Measures	Sources	Examples
Boundary spanning	Maximizing external stakeholder satisfaction	Trends and variations in satisfaction surveys Counts of unexpected events Financial performance Quality-of-care measures Community health measures	Ongoing patient surveys Ad hoc surveys of other stakeholders Records of complaints and incidents Financial reports Medical records Community health surveys	Surveys of employers and potential patients Profit and funds available for investment Bond rating Global patient satisfaction scores Adverse patient care events Percent of community immunized Percent of community with premature loss of life or function
Corporate design	Uniformity of performance Extent of service Competitor relations	Market share Efficiency of care Per capita cost of care Variation in internal performance improvement Unmet or delayed demand	Surveys of market share Cost per case and length of stay Analysis of trends, variation and percent of benchmark for operational and strategic measures	Patients leaving area for care Case-mix adjusted cost per case Dartmouth Atlas* cost and use per capita Unit(s) not progressing toward benchmark Undersized unit with service delays Oversized unit with excess capacity Competitor growth
Responsive communication	Associate satisfaction, retention, and complaints	Satisfaction surveys Retention, absenteeism, and vacancy measures Number of issues raised	Routine surveys and human resources statistics Summaries of rounding and other listening activities	Tenure of associates Percent of "loyal" associates Percent of RN positions vacant Number of food service complaints
Timekeeping	On-time planning	Delays in annual planning process PITs completing on time	Annual planning activity Minutes and records of PIC	Budget delivered on time Percent of PITs completing charge without time extension
Sustaining and improving	Continuous improvement	Board scores Outside audits	Board self-evaluation Auditor reports	Percent of board stating "complete satisfaction" Joint Commission deficiencies

PIC: performance improvement council; PIT: process improvement team; RN: registered nurse
*Information from the Dartmouth Atlas of Hospital Use, a web-based, small-area reporting system. The site provides estimates of cost per capita and hospital days per capita from Medicare data. See www.dartmouthatlas.org.

meet at a retreat to allow time for thorough discussion of carefully analyzed quantitative and qualitative data. The consensus reached establishes the priorities for strategic OFIs and shapes the future position of the HCO.

Managerial Issues

The transformational and evidence-based approach described in chapters 1, 2, and 3 is an unchallenged best practice for managing community-oriented HCOs. The measures and benchmarks that document excellence are themselves a major step toward evidence-based management. The case for transformational management is strongly supported by the general management literature and by its documented HCO applications.

The fact that this model for high performance is relatively rare as of 2014 suggests that the most critical managerial issues are starting and sustaining the transition. The case studies discussed in this text developed the cultural and operational elements in parallel. It is likely that pursuing the cultural transition creates demands for knowledge that are supported by the evidence-based approach, and efforts to use the knowledge are successful in a culture of empowerment. The Managerial Issues section of Chapter 2 pursues these questions for the transformational culture. This chapter discusses the issues that arise in evidence-based management.

Starting on the Path to Evidence-Based Management

Assuming that your HCO is "pretty good," how does it strengthen the operational foundation? The path is clear enough.

1. *Senior leadership must assemble the available strategic measures.* High-performing HCOs use about 30 strategic performance measures (see Chapter 1, Exhibit 1.11, and Chapter 4, Exhibit 4.3), many of which are commonly available and benchmarked. The Centers for Medicare & Medicaid Services maintains deliberately public records on all participating hospitals, accountable care organizations, and long-term care facilities. Private organizations support websites like WhyNotTheBest.org and Leapfrog.org for easy retrieval of these data. For most HCOs, the news on initial review of these indicators will be grim. Even the best HCOs have numerous failures in safety and quality.[15] A similar variation exists in the community cost of care.[16] Data on quality of care suggest modest improvement at best.[17] Based on these measures, most HCOs have substantial OFIs. The quality improvement potential is measured in tens of thousands of lives and the cost improvement in hundreds of billions of dollars.

2. *The governing board must renew its commitment to a community mission.* The board must accept the opportunity to improve and the reality of that task. Although it would seem automatic that members of the governing board of an HCO would be committed to achieving a mission of excellent care or health

for their community, it is not. A for-profit HCO must put emphasis on return to shareholders ahead of all other concerns. Board members of a not-for-profit HCO may have several personal goals that conflict with the HCO's mission, such as using the membership as a tool for social or business gain or viewing the membership as an honorific role rather than as a community obligation. These are forms of agency or accountability failures—that is, the board members are failing to act as agents for the community as a whole. Defenses against such failures lie in board leadership process and selection (described in Chapter 4). Leadership, selection, and process are particularly powerful. Board officers can focus attention on the mission. They can insist on boundary spanning and order a visioning exercise. They can use the agenda to ensure that OFIs are not forgotten and calendar deadlines are met. They can identify and elect new members from the community who can commit to the HCO's mission and are skilled in transformational and evidence-based management.

3. *The governing board must understand the opportunity to improve and be motivated to pursue improvement.* Board members are selected for their community commitment and demonstrated skill. They arrive with little knowledge of HCO management and often strong emotions remaining from personal and family healthcare. High-performing HCOs educate them specifically about their board roles. New board members in the best HCOs receive several days of initial training,[18] and a portion of each meeting is devoted to continuing education. The education clarifies the commitment to transformational and evidence-based management so that each trustee understands how the OFIs are addressed and what the board's responsibility is. Members learn that the board must complete six functions (listed in Chapter 4) for the HCO to reach excellence. They learn to expect measured performance and continuous improvement on the strategic scorecard and to work with management and clinical leadership to attain the goals.

4. *Senior leadership must embrace the model.* The initiative and the work to achieve excellence must come principally from senior management. While the effort is not overwhelming, it is probably harder than sustaining mediocre performance. The first step—leaving the front office and starting to listen sincerely to associates and patients—is not dangerous, but senior managers must have the skill to solve at least a few of the problems presented, the vision to understand what is being built, and the personal leadership skills to explain and convince. The skills necessary for these tasks are not difficult to acquire (they are discussed in Chapter 2). Developing measures and continuous improvement should be done sequentially, beginning with the strategic scorecard and continuing unit by unit as time and funds permit. A number of consultants offer assistance on both the transformational and evidence-based aspects. The Baldrige process and its state analogues offer an inexpensive method of learning that is strongly endorsed by award recipients.[19,20] Unfortunately, if senior leaders do not understand the opportunity to improve, it is not likely that the governing board will correct them, and no public agency or market device exists that stimulates interest and learning.

The last three elements—board commitment, board knowledge, and senior leadership capability—appear to explain why progress is so halting. The lack of a public agency that insists on improvement makes it easy for HCOs to remain "pretty good." Two elements frequently cited as requirements for the transition are, in fact, not.

First, the transition is not capital intensive. The HCO does not need a substantial financial reserve to start or sustain the transition. The underlying dynamic of the approach, that better-supported associates do a better job—suggests that listening and measuring are critical starting points. Both activities are self-sustaining, and a small initial investment in each is likely to identify a number of relatively easy-to-solve OFIs. These generate efficiencies that lead to cash surpluses and quality improvements that improve both patient and caregiver satisfaction. Material improvement can be seen in the second year, and major shifts are possible in three years.[21,22]

Second, although the traditional management model divides the HCO into domains of authority (e.g., "the doctors," "the board," "the nurses"), these groups have good reason to support rather than oppose a convincing plan for an evidence-based approach because they (and other associates) will find the work more satisfying. When incentive compensation is added to the plan, few caregivers will argue for the old ways. For the governing board, improvement in the strategic measures, which reflects mission achievement, is a compelling argument. There are undoubtedly transition failures, although none are documented in published reports. The cause of failure is more likely related to a breakdown in trust and systematically meeting associates' needs than to resistance to change.

Understanding the Risk Factors of the Model

So far, none of the documented implementations has reported difficulties that caused the Baldrige award–winning HCOs to question the model; in fact, these HCOs are strongly committed to pursuing it further.[23] Therefore, a review of the weak links or risk factors is hypothetical. The following factors deserve careful consideration:

1. *Good physician and nurse relations are crucial to the culture and to overall success.* Physicians and nurses are the people who actually deliver care and relate most closely to patients and families. Any successful improvement program requires their active support. Evidence suggests that many caregivers in traditional settings are less than satisfied.[24] High-performing HCOs have recognized the primacy of these two groups, building extra listening mechanisms, investing in expanded training for supervisors of caregiving teams, working through leaders recognized by their peers, and celebrating gains. Their record shows that the startup interval—when OFIs vastly exceed improvements—is manageable. Obviously, not every OFI can be pursued and fixed in the short run. Evidence that

progress can be made and that the support is genuine is sufficient to increase caregiver satisfaction and win caregiver support. The cultural change that results from the initial efforts helps PITs address more complicated problems. Caregiver support, satisfaction, and performance improvement should continue to grow as the transition matures.

2. *Changes in the payment system have made the model much more important.* The evidence suggests that high-performing HCOs can thrive under prevailing reimbursement schemes. All high-performing HCOs report adequate earnings and cash flow for their operations, usually surpassing comparable institutions. Improvements in clinical and logistic processes eliminate waste. The savings pay for the extra costs associated with the model—chiefly a vastly expanded investment in education, added costs for managing the measurement system, and incentive payments. Note, however, that some HCOs receive substantially less income than others, even though they deliver as much or more care. They are in highly disadvantaged economic areas, with large numbers of uninsured and persons covered under Medicaid. It is not clear that these HCOs can overcome their disadvantages of location and limited finance and sustain the model in the same form as it is described here.

    High-performing HCOs are better equipped to respond to changes in reimbursement. Recent changes—elimination of readmission payments, incentives for higher quality—and proposed changes to global episodes of care reward HCOs whose care is safe, effective, timely, and efficient. The revised reward structure supports a mission of excellence in care and a mission of population health.

3. *Unrealistic governing board demands could threaten the model.* To preserve a culture of trust and respect, the negotiations between stakeholders must be perceived as fair. An effort by some stakeholder groups to exploit others is likely to destabilize the model and potentially destroy it. The governing board has sufficient power to do this by demanding more for customer stakeholders than the current processes can support. This situation can occur in several ways. First, the board can set unrealistic goals at the outset of the annual budgeting process. Second, the board can insist on substandard wages or benefits, creating shortages of critical personnel. Third, the board can accept unrealistic demands from a specific stakeholder group, leading to imbalances and destroying trust. To avoid all this, the board's membership must reflect the entire community, with a clear customer majority. Board discussions must not only strive for equal representation but also be conveyed to all stakeholders. In other words, fairness and transparency of board discussions and actions can strengthen the model.

4. *Operations management failure could threaten the model.* Empowerment demands servant leadership, an effective response to an honest, mission-related concern. If an associate points out that a process is failing, the HCO must redesign that process to prevent further failures. If a measure is incorrect and misleading, it needs to be fixed. A responsive attitude is important to sustain the culture; a responsive organization is important to sustain the operations.

Consequently, certain logistic and strategic components must grow in size and effectiveness. Training expands and recruitment shrinks, diminished by the high retention rate. Counseling and mentoring must grow. In-house consultation must grow. Audit activities must grow. Information processing must grow to support the library and communications network. Marketing must grow to support more refined boundary spanning.

Measuring and benchmarking these services are challenging. It is easy to undersize them because the effects are deferred and widely dispersed. The successful approach is to use demand and customer satisfaction measures as a guide to find the appropriate size. The customers are all internal, and they demand prompt, effective service. Delays can be measured. The quality of service can be assessed by auditing the work product. Cost and productivity can be benchmarked against other programs of similar capability. Large systems have some advantages. They can centralize some services, standardize others, and analyze details of comparable programs. Small systems, on the other hand, may be well advised to meet customer needs as their dominant goal, only secondarily working to improve cost and productivity.

5. *Lack of sincere commitment could threaten the model.* The model succeeds because it gains greater support and loyalty from stakeholders than competing approaches. The gravest danger is to lose that support, and the greatest threat is the presence of unfair advantage. Free riders are inherently destructive; they destroy the dynamic of working together for rewards and replace it with self-serving agendas and hypocrisy. The seriousness of this risk is what makes strategic protection and the vigorous correction of fraud and malfeasance necessary. No high-performing HCOs brag about their protection system, but that system is present as a silent portion of the culture. The continued record of the reported organizations suggests that it is effective.

The evidence-based model, which has led a growing number of HCOs to success, is not simple. With its cultural, operational, and strategic foundations and its leadership functions, the approach demands ongoing effort from a large number of well-trained people. But the training can be easily mastered, and the effort itself is more effective and more rewarding. The overview of the model presented in this chapter sets the stage for the specific actions discussed in the following chapters.

Additional Resources

Collins, J. C. 2001. *Good to Great: Why Some Companies Make the Leap . . . and Others Don't* New York: HarperBusiness.

———. 2009. *How the Mighty Fall . . . and Why Some Companies Never Give In.* New York: HarperCollins.

Fine, D. J., R. D'Aquila, and A. R. Kovner. 2009. *Evidence-Based Management in Healthcare.* Chicago: Health Administration Press.

Baldrige Performance Excellence Program. Updated annually. "Health Care Criteria for Performance Excellence." [Online information; retrieved 4/20/14.] www.nist. gov/baldrige/publications/hc_criteria.cfm.

Notes

1. Sharp HealthCare's application to the Malcolm Baldrige National Quality Award. 2007. "Preface," p. vi. [Online information; retrieved 4/20/14.] www.baldrige. nist.gov/PDF_files/2007_Sharp_Application_Summary.pdf.

2. Poudre Valley Health System's application to the Malcolm Baldrige National Quality Award. 2008. "Summary," pp. 17–18. [Online information; retrieved 4/20/14.] www.baldrige.nist.gov/PDF_files/2008_Poudre_Valley_Application_ Summary.pdf.

3. *Ibid.*, p. 18.

4. Griffith, J. R., and K. R. White. 2003. *Thinking Forward: Six Strategies for Highly Successful Organizations.* Chicago: Health Administration Press.

5. Griffith, J. R. 2009. "Finding the Frontier of Hospital Management." *Journal of Healthcare Management* 54 (1): 59–72.

6. American Health Lawyers Association. 2003. "Sample E-Mail Usage Policy for Healthcare Organizations." *Journal of Health Law* 36 (2): 365–76.

7. Daft, R. L. 2012. *Organization Theory and Design,* 11th ed. Clifton Park, NY: Cengage Learning.

8. Leatt, P., G. R. Baker, and J. Kimberly. 2011. "Organization Design." In *Shortell and Kaluzny's Health Care Management: Organizational Design and Behavior,* 6th ed., edited by L. Burns, E. Bradley, and B. Weiner. Clifton Park, NY: Cengage Learning.

9. Corrigan, J. M., and D. MacNeil. 2009. "Building Organizational Capacity: A Cornerstone of Health System Reform." *Health Affairs* 28 (2): w205–w215.

10. Griffith, J. R., and K. R. White. 2005. "The Revolution in Hospital Management." *Journal of Healthcare Management* 50 (3): 170–89.

11. Gurewich, D., J. Prottas, and W. Leutz. 2003. "The Effect of Hospital Ownership Conversions on Nonacute Care Providers." *Milbank Quarterly* 81 (4): 543–65.

12. Hines, S., and M. S. Joshi. 2008. "Variation in Quality of Care Within Health Systems." *Joint Commission Journal on Quality and Patient Safety* 34 (6): 324–32; Griffith, J. R. 2014. "Understanding High-Reliability Organizations: Are Baldrige Recipients Models?" *Journal of Healthcare Management* 60 (1): 44–61.

13. Internal Revenue Service. 2006. "Application for Recognition of Exemption Under Section 501(c)(3) of the Internal Revenue Code, Instructions for Form 1023." [Online information; retrieved 4/20/14.] www.irs.gov/pub/irs-pdf/i1023.pdf.

14. Tague, N. R. 2005. *The Quality Toolbox,* 2nd ed. Milwaukee, WI: ASQ Press.

15. Chassin, M., and J. M. Loeb. 2013. "High-Reliability Health Care: Getting There from Here." *Milbank Quarterly* 91 (3): 459–90.

16. Griffith, J. R., J. A. Alexander, and D. A. Foster. 2006. "Is Anybody Managing the Store? National Trends in Hospital Performance." *Journal of Healthcare Management* 51 (6): 392–406.

17. Dartmouth Atlas of Health Care. 2012. "Total Medicare Reimbursements per Enrollee, by Adjustment Type." [Online information; retrieved 4/20/14.] www. dartmouthatlas.org/data/topic/topic.aspx?cat=21.

18. Leapfrog Group. 2013. "Hospital Errors Are the Third Leading Cause of Death in U.S., and New Hospital Safety Scores Show Improvements Are Too

Slow." [Online information; retrieved 4/20/14.] www.leapfroggroup.org/policy_leadership/leapfrog_news/5123987.

19. Griffith and White (2003, 35–40).

20. Calhoun, G. S., J. R. Griffith, and M. E. Sinioris. 2008. "The Foundation of Leadership in Baldrige Winning Organizations." *Modern Healthcare* (Suppl.): 9–20.

21. Bea, J. 2009. "Practitioner Application." *Journal of Healthcare Management* 54 (1): 45.

22. Griffith and White (2003); North Mississippi Medical Center's Baldrige application.

23. North Mississippi Medical Center's Baldrige application.

24. Calhoun, Griffith, and Sinioris (2008).

25. Weinstein, L., and H. M. Wolfe. 2007. "The Downward Spiral of Physician Satisfaction: An Attempt to Avert a Crisis Within the Medical Profession." *Obstetrics & Gynecology* 109 (5): 1181–83; Ruggiero, J. S. 2005. "Health, Work Variables, and Job Satisfaction Among Nurses." *Journal of Nursing Administration* 35 (5): 254–63.

4 GOVERNANCE

Critical Issues in Governance

1. *Establishing and sustaining a mission of clinical excellence and a culture of respect, honesty, and service:*
   - Work with the chief executive officer (CEO), the clinical staff, and senior leadership.
   - Maintain governance processes that implement the HCO's mission, vision, and values.

2. *Integrating boundary spanning and forecasting to create a strategic plan for mission achievement:*
   - Listen to stakeholder voices, and fairly balance stakeholder needs.
   - Translate the mission to a strategy implementing an effective long-range financial plan.
   - Establish annual improvement goals and monitor the strategic scorecard.

3. *Working with physicians and other caregivers to improve quality and efficiency of care:*
   - Support and encourage caregiver efforts to achieve safe, effective, patient-centered, timely, efficient, and equitable care.
   - Maintain a mutually rewarding partnership with physicians and caregivers.

4. *Monitoring the overall performance of the HCO using the strategic scorecard and qualitative feedback.*

5. *Improving the board's ability to identify and meet stakeholder needs:*
   - Ensure that the board maintains an understanding of stakeholder needs.
   - Monitor and improve the board's performance.

Questions for Discussion

These questions are about applying the chapter content. It's often helpful to discuss them with classmates or mentors, gaining different perspectives on the issues.

1. Should every community have its own HCO, with its own governing board and its own mission? Or should hospitals be like CHE Trinity Health, where the mission is nationwide? If there is a virtue to a local community mission, what is it, and how will a local governing board achieve that virtue? If a national mission is appropriate, what is the role of a local governing board? Could a single corporate board and central office carry out the remaining functions better than a local governing board?

2. Consider board decisions like the mission, scope of services, corporate structure, and annual operating goals. What does the CEO contribute to those discussions? How does the board evaluate the CEO's contribution? What makes the relationship effective, and what erodes the relationship?

3. Should every HCO become a "high-reliability organization," putting outcomes quality and patient safety first and foremost in operational goals? If the question was raised by a governing board member, how should the CEO respond?

4. Review Saint Luke's Hospital's strategic scorecard (Exhibit 4.3) and Exhibit 1.11. What are the important differences?
   - Might the Saint Luke's board change some measures next year? Why would they do that?
   - If a change is proposed, what should senior management do to facilitate the board's decision?
   - If a new board member asks why the HCO needs so many measures, how should senior leadership respond?
   - What happens if the board sets a goal that's too challenging? What happens if a measure is below benchmark and goal, and not improving?

5. Why should the governing board evaluate its own performance? How does a board build in evaluation so that it is not overlooked? Why should a board use both the balanced scorecard and the "ten measures" process (see Exhibit 4.4) to evaluate its work?

Purpose

The purpose of the governing board of a well-managed HCO is

to create and maintain a foundation for relationships among the stakeholders that identifies and implements their wishes as effectively as possible.

This purpose has always been challenging, and the twenty-first century brings a new level of accountability. Customer stakeholders demand improvements in patient safety, more rigorous cost control, greater scrutiny of community benefit, and the transparency of managerial practices. Provider stakeholders expect strong support and a congenial culture. Stakeholders' decisions to participate are based on their perceptions of the HCO's ability to fulfill their needs, and their needs conflict. The board's central purpose is to resolve the conflicts in a way that maximizes the total benefit.

This purpose, called the *corporate* or *managerial perspective* of governance, is deceptively complex and not universally understood;[1] it is contrasted with and often confused with two other purposes that have been proposed for not-for-profit governance. The *resource distribution* perspective views the organization as a source of largesse and the governing board as a body to distribute resources. Such a purpose is sometimes called "political" because the role of legislative bodies and politics, in general, is to distribute resources.[2] The HCO's expenditures are income to various stakeholders and an important economic resource. The HCO is among the largest employers in any community, and a large share of its income comes from outside that community. Under this perspective, physicians, suppliers, and employees gain importance, compared to patients and families. Distributional equity is a matter of constant concern.[3] The focus on distribution distracts from improvement opportunities that often benefit all.

The *resource contribution* perspective is less common but is still used. It views board members as contributors of resources to the organization. This model emphasizes the funds or services board members may donate or the influence they can bring to bear on critical external relations. Naming a member of the richest family in town or appointing the mayor to the HCO board are examples.

The HCO ownership can complicate the board's purpose. In the for-profit tradition, the focus is on maximizing profit. Stockholders—the owners—are the dominant stakeholders, and success is measured by profitability. Board members—usually called *directors*—are compensated for their efforts and are typically given strong incentives to achieve financial goals. In the not-for-profit tradition, the owners are the members of the community served. This community ownership concept arises from legislation and the courts and is less precise than the stockholder ownership concept. The original concept of a charitable organization was to make no profit and disburse assets,[4] but in recent decades HCO boards have accepted the need to ensure continued, and even expanding, mission achievement. That need requires a profit and its reinvestment for the community's benefit.[5]

Trustees

Members of the governing board of not-for-profit HCOs who volunteer their time to the organization; their only compensation is the satisfaction they achieve from their work. The title reflects their acceptance of the assets in trust for the community; also may be called *directors*.

The Well-Managed Healthcare Organization focuses on nonprofit governing boards. Board members are commonly called **trustees**, rather than directors, reflecting their acceptance of the assets in trust for the community. By tradition, and reinforced by tax law, their decisions should be based on what will best fulfill community needs. Trustees are rarely compensated, except for out-of-pocket expenses.

Important legal barriers exist to the board's ability to liquidate or transfer the assets of the HCO outside the owning community. The equity of a not-for-profit HCO cannot be distributed to any individual. So-called community benefit provisions of the Affordable Care Act now also require boards to review community needs and report the value of contributions such as charitable care, education of caregivers, and losses on government-supported insurance to the Internal Revenue Service (IRS). The report, IRS Form 990 Schedule H, also requires reporting of senior leader compensation. The IRS requires that such compensation be "reasonable."[6]

Excellent organizations emphasize the *managerial perspective*.[7,8] Evidence shows that not-for-profit HCOs that have adopted the managerial perspective achieve better organizational performance.[9]

Functions

The functions that HCO boards must complete to achieve excellence are described in Exhibit 4.1. They describe the governance activities of any economic organization, although in smaller organizations they are required of the owners directly rather than trustee representatives.

Maintaining Management Capability

Typical trustees have full-time occupations, volunteer their services, and have only limited time for the HCO. They may serve only a few years and will be replaced by others. Board decisions require careful factual study, or due diligence. They are made by committee but must be implemented by individuals. All of these factors—competing obligations, diligence, lack of continuity, and implementation—limit what a board can accomplish on its own. Thus, the first function of governance is to assemble an executive team. Typically, this is done by hiring a CEO, establishing a rewarding relationship, and assisting that individual in building and supporting an effective team.

EXHIBIT 4.1 Functions of the Governing Board

Function	Intent	Implementation	Examples
Maintaining management capability	Establish a professional capability to • provide the board with timely, thorough, relevant, and accurate information and • implement the board's decisions	Recruit a CEO and review her/his contribution to the HCO Establish policies for recruiting, developing, and compensating other managers Maintain a plan for management succession	Select a CEO Evaluate executive performance Establish senior management compensation Review compensation and bonus program for all managers
Establishing the mission, vision, and values	Agree on common goals and core values of the organization Articulate the goals as a guiding concept	Undertake a visioning exercise Maintain ongoing communication with stakeholder representatives Conduct an annual review	Revise mission/vision/ values Meet with medical staff leadership Hold a retreat for annual environmental assessment
Approving the corporate strategy and annual implementation	Establish the scope and organization of services, and set strategic annual improvement goals	Balance the vision against current realities Establish plans for expansion and renewal Maintain competitive plant and equipment	Approve plans for implementation Set annual strategic goals Approve capital and new programs budget
Ensuring quality of clinical care	Maintain a central commitment to quality patient care Attract and retain the most competent physicians, nurses, and other caregivers	Approve the strategic goals for quality improvement Approve the privileges of attending staff Approve compensation programs for caregivers	Encourage PITs to address important quality-of- care OFIs Approve clinical staff bylaws Approve quality-related incentives
Monitoring performance against plans and budgets	Ensure implementation of annual goals	Review reports of strategic performance Monitor progress of long-term projects	Review quarterly reports of strategic scorecard Review progress reports of search activities and construction
Improving board performance	Ensure that the governance function remains competitive	Annually review individual and collective performance	Conduct confidential survey of member perspectives

PIT: process improvement team; OFI: opportunity for improvement

CEO Selection and Support

The CEO selects and/or ensures accountability of all other employees of the organization, coordinates the design and operation of the HCO, and represents the board and the owners internally and externally. CEOs act for the board in all emergencies and in rounding and listening activities, where they must infer and interpret the board's desires. The CEO controls much of the due diligence, influencing the facts brought to the board's attention. The CEO is critical to building an ongoing board education and improvement program, timely sharing of relevant and accurate information, and a relationship that actively advises and challenges management.[10]

The CEO and the senior management team are often the only people in the community who are professionally trained in healthcare management. That training covers technical questions of need, demand, finance, quality, efficiency, law, and government regulation that are not included in the training of doctors, lawyers, or businesspersons. With the training comes a professional obligation similar to that of physicians and lawyers.

Many say that selecting the CEO is the most important decision a board will make because of the impact the CEO has on other board decisions. The decision is also exceptionally difficult. It involves judging the future skills of individuals. It is made without the assistance of a CEO, whereas other decisions have the benefit of the CEO's counsel. It is made infrequently, and the people who make it may never have selected a CEO before.

How does a board make such a difficult decision? The best way is to follow with extra thoroughness and care the rules that improve all high-level personnel decisions. A description of duties and responsibilities should be in place. The job description is translated into selection criteria that identify the desired competencies, skills, and attributes of the individual. The priority or importance of these criteria and the ways in which these skills will be measured in specific applicants should be specified. A national search for candidates is usually appropriate. For most U.S. organizations, the law requires not only equal opportunity on the basis of race, age, sex, and disability but also affirmative action in seeking candidates who are disadvantaged on those grounds. The backgrounds of qualified individuals must be carefully verified. Executive search firms provide assistance with each of these steps; they contribute by having broad relevant experience and by developing a pool of potential candidates.

The selection process is only the beginning of a relationship. Sustaining the CEO–board relationship over time allows both the organization and the executive to grow. Four major elements are the focus of ongoing review in addition to a formal annual process:

1. *Develop a mutual understanding of the employment contract.* Formal, written contracts are now the rule, but much of the relationship depends on an

underlying relationship of trust and communication.[11] The contract specifies the duties of the CEO, the mechanisms for review of performance, and the approach to compensation. It also states the procedures for terminating the relationship, including appropriate protection for both the organization and the CEO. Properly performed, the CEO's job is now—and always has been—high risk. Thus, even handshake agreements should include appropriate protection if the CEO must leave the institution.

2. *Agree on short-term (usually one year) personal goals.* The CEO is expected to achieve the goals reflected on the balanced scorecard. In well-run organizations, all managers have explicit personal goals as well. The CEO's personal goals are established by discussion with the governing board.

3. *Establish the base compensation.* Compensation includes salary, employment benefits offered to all employees, unique benefits offered to the CEO, terms for bonuses and merit increases, an agreement on the disposition of any incidental income the CEO might earn as a result of related professional activity, and an agreement on both voluntary and involuntary termination compensation. The compensation should comply with IRS regulations. Review by legal counsel is essential.

    The only enduring guideline for designing a compensation package is the marketplace—that is, what the institution pays a specifically prepared person and what that person could earn in a similar employment situation elsewhere. For all large HCOs, and for increasing numbers of small ones, the marketplace constitutes the national market for people trained and experienced in healthcare management.

4. *Establish incentives for goal achievement.* Incentive compensation is increasingly common, although the evidence is mixed on the organizational outcomes that influence CEO compensation.[12] The incentive should be based on the overall achievement of the organization and is determined either by a prospectively agreed-on formula or by retrospective evaluation against previously agreed-on criteria. Incentive payments can be quite large—on the order of 50 percent of total compensation. Incentive-based compensation motivates the executive, documents that community needs are being met, and may be more palatable to the general public than a high CEO salary.

Management Development and Succession

The board is responsible for a management succession plan and a program to develop managers.[13] The plan and the program are designed by the CEO and senior management and approved by the board with at least an annual review (see Chapter 11). The plan identifies specific internal candidates to replace key executives, including the CEO. The management development program includes a review of management compensation and incentives, evaluation of the competencies of all managers, identification of individual improvement opportunities and plans for enhancing skills, and an assessment of preparation for promotion.[14] Many leading HCOs pay particular attention to issues of diversity in management, seeking not only equal opportunity for women and members of disadvantaged groups but also a diverse managerial workforce that mirrors the characteristics of the population served and the employee workforce.[15]

Establishing the Mission, Vision, and Values

The governing board establishes the mission, vision, and values. It manages the extensive stakeholder discussions that support both the statements and their acceptance throughout the organization (see Chapter 1; examples of missions are shown in Exhibit 1.7). The board's role is to monitor the realism and effectiveness of the mission in light of evolving stakeholder needs. It implements this function through its annual environmental assessment and goal-setting activities. It sets aside time to periodically revisit the mission, vision, and values in terms of how the organization sees itself in the future, not so much to change these core commitments as to refresh stakeholder understanding. The board approves all the formal statements about mission, vision, and values. It must uphold the statements in its actions, modeling the behavior it expects from employed leaders. Consistently doing this is a major element of sustaining the HCO's transformational culture.

Approving the Corporate Strategy and Annual Implementation

As the board and the HCO progress through the annual calendar (see Chapter 3, Exhibit 3.6), the board makes the final decisions in shaping both short- and long-term performance. These are resource allocation decisions, distinguished from the mission and vision by the commitment to expend resources in certain directions. They progress from corporate strategies to long-term plans, financial plans, and annual goals. In all cases, management proposes the action and its justification. The board reviews the proposal for consistency with stakeholder needs, the mission, and prior actions, and in most cases the board approves the management proposal.

Setting Corporate Strategies

The initiative for identifying strategic opportunities comes from the HCO's environmental assessment processes (see chapters 3, 14, and 15). A successful assessment generates dozens, even hundreds, of new business opportunities and ways of meeting old goals. The most realistic of these should be developed and evaluated through the use of scenario building. **Scenarios** often begin with sketches of various outcomes for the community; several common topics for these scenarios are shown in Exhibit 4.2. The initial scenarios can be quite abstract and ambiguous. They evaluate alternative **strategic opportunities** and must eventually be refined

Scenarios
Alternative approaches to improving the profile of opportunities reflected in the environmental assessment.

Issue	Strategic Response	Questions
Expansion/ closure	Expand existing services Add new services Close or reduce services	Demand trends, financing Cost and quality of service Ability to support high-tech specialties Impact on other services
Local affiliations	Specific affiliation opportunities	Expansion, closure Existing affiliations Size and strength of competitors Antitrust considerations Regional affiliation opportunities
Regional affiliations	Specific affiliation opportunities	Expansion, closure Impact on local market share Costs and benefits foreseen Local political issues
Relation to insurers	Contract acceptance Cash flow reduction Joint venture	Market response Profit and cash flow implications Variety of plans available to local buyers
Relation to physicians	Contracts Joint ventures	Primary care physician preferences Specialist preferences Existing physician organization
Relation to employees	Shortages Surpluses Workforce skills	Projected supply and demand for workers by specialty Programs for associate development Programs for associate satisfaction, commitment

EXHIBIT 4.2

Strategic Scenario Questions for Healthcare Organizations

[handwritten: Approving the Corporate Strategy & Annual Implem..]

into specific **business plans** that shape the HCO's directions. Business plans often involve seemingly quantum shifts in facilities, service capabilities, or market share and may include mergers, acquisitions, joint ventures, or large-scale capital investments. Strategic opportunities are sometimes triggered by external events and require rapid decisions. The governing board of the well-run HCO quietly but thoroughly evaluates the more probable strategic scenarios in advance and is therefore prepared for prompt action when required.[16]

Strategic opportunities
Opportunities that, when narrowed for use in business plans, involve quantum shifts in service capabilities or market share, usually by interaction with competitors, large-scale capital investments, and revisions to several line activities.

Business plan
A model of a specific strategy or function that guides design, operations, and goal setting.

Long-Term Planning

Once the strategies and priorities are established, management develops specific plans for facilities, personnel, marketing, and operations (see chapters 14 and 15). These are often multiyear plans with specific implications for the annual plans. The board enters the decision process at critical stages, usually when resources are about to be committed. It ratifies or selects among the final proposals. The board's earliest decisions—establishing the strategic direction and outlining the specific goals to be met—are the most critical, but the board's continued surveillance keeps projects focused on mission.

Long-Range Financial Plans

A crucial test of the strategic and long-range planning activities comes when the financial impact is assessed. This involves realistic assumptions about future market share, prices, and costs that are used to build a **long-range financial plan (LRFP)**, which shows earnings, debt, and capitalization for at least the next seven years. The plan is actually a sophisticated financial model that integrates forecasts from the epidemiologic planning model and changing insurance payment structures to reflect the implications of major decisions.

Long-range financial plan (LRFP)
An ongoing projection of financial position showing earnings, debt, and capitalization for at least the next seven years.

The plan integrates the strategic business plans and tests their realism. It accepts estimates of the demand, revenue, and cost for various strategic opportunities and shows the impact on profit and debt structure under varying market and price assumptions. The alternatives that generate the most favorable combination of customers served and capital structure can be identified. All the elements are interrelated. A new service affects market share, prices, cost, and profits. It may be redesigned several times to fit the LRFP. The process—generally undertaken by management and reported to the board when an ideal fit has been reached—is a critical step in ensuring that productive plans are realized.

The LRFP is also used to identify immediate financial needs. The survival of any enterprise, for-profit or not-for-profit, requires ongoing cash flow. Long-term obligations such as construction contracts or bond debts must be met along with current price needs. Equipment and facilities must be replaced. Most HCOs operate in a relatively fixed price environment. Medicare and other government programs establish revenue; the HCO has little chance to negotiate the amounts. The LRFP generates a cash need for each year. Forecasts of costs come from the internal goal-setting process described in Chapter 3 in the Continuous Improvement section. The two must be resolved. The governing board initiates this process by setting financial goals from analysis of the LRFP.

Annual Goals

Boards of high-performing HCOs set goals for all of the balanced scorecard strategic measures. The process, originally limited to financial goals, is still called *budgeting* in many HCOs. *Goal setting* is a more accurate term.

A mock-up of the summary report of a strategic scorecard for Saint Luke's Hospital, a recipient of the Malcolm Baldrige National Quality Award in Health Care, is shown in Exhibit 4.3. Expanding on Exhibit 1.11, Saint Luke's used five financial goals; seven customer satisfaction goals; five "development" or marketing goals; eight "clinical and administrative quality goals," six of which were indexes reflecting composites of more detailed dimensions; and six "people" goals. In the goal-setting process, the governing board negotiates the performance expected for each measure. Saint Luke's has expanded the concept of goal achievement to stretch goals—those that might be achieved with luck and effort. It has also established a target—the benchmark for the measure. The color-coded system reports progress toward each goal. (The green, yellow, and red zones are represented in shades of gray in the printed text.)

The specific measures used in the strategic goals can be changed from year to year as part of the goal-setting process. Strategic goals are the basis for senior management to negotiate the operational goals used by the smaller units of the organization.

The governing board participates in goal setting at three critical points—establishing the dimensions to be included, setting budget guidelines, and approving the final budget proposal. In addition to the dimensions shown in Exhibit 4.3, the board establishes a target for programmatic capital expenditures each year. The amount sets the stage for competitive review of capital and new program requests (see Chapter 14).

Referents for Goal Setting

The boards of high-performing HCOs use four conceptual referents to evaluate current performance and the opportunity to improve (some referents may be unavailable for specific measures):

1. *Trends.* Last year's value, or a time series of several years, provides an initial baseline and allows judgment on the direction of the measure.
2. *Competitor and industry comparisons.* What other similar organizations are achieving provides crude guidelines, even if the available information is not strictly from competitors.
3. *Benchmarks.* The benchmark value may be from a non-HCO—for example, the standards for financial ratios that are driven by the total bond market, not simply healthcare bonds, or the healthcare cost levels of a country with a different system.
4. *Values.* The benchmark for some measures (e.g., worker injuries, patient safety violations, infant deaths) is not good enough. The proper goal for these measures is zero. Focusing on the zero goal is often a powerful motivator, producing major gains and falling benchmarks.

The board's emphasis on these referents is an important reinforcement for evidence-based management.

EXHIBIT 4.3 Saint Luke's Hospital Strategic Scorecard

Scoring Criteria 2010

	Key Measures	Bench-mark	Adj. Score	+4 / 9	+3 / 8	+2 / 7	+1 / 6	Goal / 5	-1 / 4	-2 / 3	-3 / 2	-4 / 1	Raw Score
PEOPLE	Retention												
	RN Vacancy Rate												
	Employee Satisfaction**												
	Diversity												
CLINICAL & ADMINISTRATIVE QUALITY	Inpatient Clinical Care Index												
	Appropriate Care Measure (ACM) Index												
	Order Set Utilization Index												
	eICU Index												
	Outpatient Clinical Care Index												
	Patient Safety Index												
	Operational Index												
	Infection Control Index												
	Medical Staff Clinical Indicator Index												
CUSTOMER SATISFACTION	Would Recommend (HCAHPS)												
	Patient Loyalty - SLHS "Would Recommend" 5's only												
	Timeliness of Care and Service												
	Responsiveness to Patient Needs												
	Aver ER Wait time - Home Disposition (Tracking BRD)												
	Student Education Index												
GROWTH & DEVELOPMENT	Eligible IP Market Share (Primary/Secondary)												
	Eligible IP Market Share - Strategic Product Lines												
	Profitable Eligible IP Market Share (Primary Only)												
	OP Surgeries - Count												
	Unsuccessful ER to ER Transfers Not Meeting Criteria												
	Days to Budget												
	Research Index												
FINANCIAL	Operating Margin												
	Operating Cash Flow												
	Days Cash on Hand												
	Net Days in Accounts Receivable (IP/OP)												
	Patient Volume (revenue % to budget)												
	Realization Rate vs Budget												

Scores at this level will be flagged blue. (column +4 / 9)
Scores at this level will be flagged in green. (column Goal / 5)
Scores at this level will be flagged in yellow. (column -3 / 2)
Scores at this level will be flagged in blue. (column -4 / 1)

** Indicates annual measure.

Exceeding Goal	
Goal	
Moderate	
Risk	

		1 Qtr	2 Qtr	3 Qtr	4 Qtr
2010 Overall Score					

Overall Score	
Goal	
Stretch	

For current performance to be scored greater than Level 1, the current performance value must meet or exceed the scoring criteria within a Level.

For FINANCIAL: Scoring ranges based on agency ratings

Note: The scoring criteria was modified in 2006: The scoring range changed from a 10-tier range to a 9-tier range, and the color coding for meeting goal was expanded to accommodate common cause variation.

Source: Reprinted with permission from Saint Luke's Hospital.

solid processes to id OFIs a address them Thru protocol changes?, implement changes via training?/incentives? leadership

High-reliability organizations make safety and effectiveness their preeminent concerns.[17] While no HCOs have achieved near zero defects,[18] scattered evidence suggests that high reliability is consistent with overall high mission achievement—reduced cost per case and improved patient and associate satisfaction.[19] The path to high reliability is consistent with the approach used by Baldrige-recipient HCOs and documented in *The Well-Managed Healthcare Organization.*

The goal-setting process is a detailed, complicated construction that involves almost the entire organization and requires several months to complete. (Goal setting is discussed in many chapters in this book: Chapter 10 expands the measurement concepts; the contributions of management support services to the goals are described in chapters 11 through 15.) The final goal set is a book-length document for larger HCOs, containing the expectations for each work group. The financial expectations—the traditional budget—are major works in themselves, with several parts (see Chapter 13). The final capital budget lists the approved projects in priority order and is supported with detailed descriptions and timetables for each project. In general, the final review is a fine-tuning exercise within the original guidelines. Final approval should be anticlimactic; a well-managed goal-setting process uses the referents, conforms to the guidelines, and settles most questions before it is submitted for approval.

Approval of Annual Goals

Ensuring Quality of Clinical Care

The fourth essential function of the governing board is unique to HCOs. The governing board is legally responsible for ensuring the quality of clinical care. Despite this, some HCO boards do not identify quality as a top priority, and a small minority of board chairs report that they routinely receive training in quality of care. High-performing HCO boards, however, regularly review quality dashboards.[20]

The HCO board is responsible for exercising the duty of care on behalf of the patients and the community and on behalf of physicians who desire to participate, and the organization as a whole is liable for damages should they fail. In addition to these legal requirements, The Joint Commission has specified many of the structures by which the board and the hospital clinical staff discharge this duty. The growth of quality measurement, service lines, and evidence-based protocols has simplified the issues involved. The Joint Commission and the Centers for Medicare & Medicaid Services (CMS) require the measurement and improvement of outcomes of care as published in the common measure specifications documentation known as the *Specifications Manual for National Hospital Inpatient Quality Measures.*[21] CMS is now compensating hospitals directly for achieving quality goals.[22]

In addition to approving explicit annual quality goals, the board has the following five obligations related to ensuring the quality of clinical care:

1. Approve the **clinical staff bylaws**. (Clinical staff includes the clinical associates who are legally and contractually permitted to make a medical diagnosis and, in some cases, undertake specific treatments such as surgery or obstetrical delivery. They include physicians, who are by far the most numerous, and licensed independent practitioners (LIPs), such as physician assistants, nurse practitioners, psychologists, and others.
2. Appoint clinical staff executives at all levels.
3. Approve the plan for clinical staff recruitment and development.
4. Approve appointments and reappointments of individual physicians.
5. Approve contracts with physicians and physician organizations.

Some basic facts heighten the importance of the board's quality-of-care activities. First, the HCO is an expensive capital resource made available to the doctors by the owners in return for either profit or community health-care delivery. The board has an obligation to see that the owners receive fair value for the use of the resource. The courts have interpreted that obligation to include limiting privileges to the competence and proficiency of each physician or other affiliate of the clinical staff (i.e., allied health professionals not employed by the HCO requesting privileges). Second, physicians are a uniquely expensive and critical resource for the community. A shortage of physicians in a community is a serious threat to the quality of care and indirectly limits growth of the workforce. A surplus may encourage marginally necessary treatment that is both costly and dangerous. If community demand is low relative to the supply, costs will mount drastically, and lack of practice may impair quality. Third, most practitioners would find their income severely reduced without participation in an HCO. Clinical practitioners deserve fair treatment and equitable opportunities to participate. The process of peer review can be subverted for the personal gain of some members;[23] the board's responsibility is to see that this does not occur. In short, the issues involve a sensitive balance of community and professional needs on both quality and economic dimensions.[24]

Most of the activity is carried out by management and the medical staff. The details of the processes involved are addressed in Chapter 6. The core concept is one of **peer review**—the care of all patients is subject to review by a group of similarly trained and experienced professionals. Peer reviewers work within the bylaws, and the **clinical staff organization** and the senior management team provide appeal and mediation opportunities that keep the review process fair. The board's role is usually limited to oversight and final approval. The board also serves as a final arbiter in case of disputes, but these should be rare.

Monitoring Performance Against Plans and Budgets

Well-managed organizations work on a no-surprises assumption through care-fully negotiated plans. The board's trust obligation requires it to <u>monitor performance</u>. Recent law and social action in the United States have empha-sized the duty of governance to control compliance with ethical and legal standards, including such issues as accurate information, protection of assets, protection of confidentiality and other individual rights, and conformance to laws governing contracts. While much of the legal obligation to control is established only for publicly listed for-profit corporations,[25] the trend has widespread support both in society at large[26] and among healthcare influ-entials.[27] Board review builds a culture where noncompliance is never a reasonable path to follow.

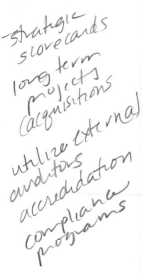

strategic scorecards
long term projects
(acquisitions
utilize external auditors
accredidation
compliance programs

The board performs three monitoring functions that promote both excellence and compliance.

Routine Surveillance of Performance Data

The strategic measures established in the goal-setting process are monitored by the board monthly or quarterly on a scorecard like Saint Luke's (Exhibit 4.3). The expectation is for no surprises. Most values will be in the green or blue zones, exceeding the minimum goal and moving toward benchmark. Values in the yellow zone are a signal to management rather than the board. Values in the red zone—that is, below the minimum goal—are rare but seri-ous. For yellow and red values, management is expected to prepare and implement a 90-day plan for recovery.

Acceptance of Reports from External Agencies

Any data-intensive system is at risk for fraudulent or accidental errors. The audit system (chapters 3 and 13) minimizes the risk. Good practice now requires that the auditors report directly to the governing board so that they are insulated from threats and conflicting interests. The result is not only reduced fraud; greater accuracy promotes greater trust in the numbers throughout the organization.

Several outside agencies monitor performance from a public perspec-tive and report directly to the board. The no-surprises assumption applies: Clean reports are expected, and exceptions, though rare, get immediate and unpleas-ant readjustment.

The **external auditor** is selected by and accountable to the board, usually through an audit

External auditor

A certified public accounting firm that attests that the accounting practices followed by the organization are sound and that the financial reports fairly represent the state of the business.

committee. The audit attests that the accounting practices followed by the organization are sound and that the financial reports fairly represent the state of the business. A **management letter** points out real or potential problems that might impair either of these two statements in the future. The management letter is, in effect, an audit of the internal auditor. It is the board's ultimate protection against misrepresentation, fraud, or misappropriation of funds.

Management letter
Comments of external auditors to the governing board that accompany their audited financial report.

CMS requires HCOs to achieve *deemed status* to receive payment from Medicare and Medicaid.[28] CMS has authorized eight accrediting organizations as deemed-status designees and can also grant it directly. Accrediting organizations typically make their decisions public and, in some cases, publish additional performance data. Although other organizations are prominent in specific service lines, The Joint Commission is by far the largest accrediting agency.

Accreditation standards increasingly rely on measured outcomes and quality and patient satisfaction data from both the strategic scorecard and the service line scorecards. They offer procedural guidelines and standards that promote high reliability. Excellent hospitals generally exceed accreditation standards; serious or repeated difficulty meeting them suggests major weaknesses in the organization. The HCO governing board receives all reports from accrediting agencies.

Various laws now govern specific activities such as patient record confidentiality, rights of employees and physicians, management of environmental hazards, and compliance with accounting regulations. **Compliance programs** are procedures designed to ensure compliance with specific regulation, such as the Civil Rights Act, the Health Insurance Portability and Accountability Act, and the Medicare Fraud and Abuse Act. Compliance is the responsibility of the executive office, but governing board oversight is required. Bond-rating agencies investigate all outstanding judicial or regulatory issues; their reports are a useful summary for the board. In 2002, Congress passed the Sarbanes-Oxley Act to impose numerous requirements on corporations regarding their governance and internal control arrangements.[29] Although Sarbanes-Oxley does not apply to not-for-profit corporations, the mandates from the legislation have been widely accepted by leading HCOs.[30] If a committee of the board receives and acts on a thorough annual report of compliance and any interim reports of serious difficulties, the organization is protected from the more severe penalties of these laws.[31]

Compliance programs
Programs designed to meet statutory and regulatory requirements; may be based on legislation or voluntary efforts such as accreditation.

Approval of Major Contracts and Transactions

In addition to approval of medical and LIP contracts, the governing board routinely approves real estate transactions, acquisitions, mergers, joint ventures, and contracts involving large sums of money. The review includes compliance with legal requirements, and the existence of the review protects stakeholders against unexpected major changes in direction. In well-managed HCOs, these transactions arise from strategic opportunities that the board has previously discussed.

Improving Board Performance

An effective board must be thorough in its environmental assessment, imaginative in its search for solutions, and deliberate in its eventual actions. It must also be timely—responding to issues promptly—and efficient—not wasting the time of its members and other participants in the decision process. Well-managed organizations meet these criteria by using a triple strategy of disciplined operation that emphasizes preparation and delegation; educational programs for board members; and the use of systematic board performance review.[32]

The board monitors and improves its own performance through an annual self-assessment that is usually led by a committee of the most senior members, a group that often also serves as the nominations committee. The committee surveys individual members' opinions of how well the board has completed the five functions and what opportunities for improvement OFIs should be pursued. The members are often asked to assess their personal contribution, an approach that helps identify new leadership and discourage "deadwood." The committee compiles these comments and its own observations and leads a discussion of how board processes can be improved. Regular executive sessions, where only nonmanagement board members remain, allow outside members complete freedom to discuss the performance of the CEO or of senior leadership or other issues. Such discussions help patient and community stakeholders identify important interests and reach consensus on them.

The essential question in assessing the board's performance is whether stakeholder wants have been satisfied as well as realistic alternatives would permit. The board's performance is the HCO's performance, as reflected in the strategic scorecard and as compared to competitors and benchmarks. In addition to the strategic scorecard measures, boards can use checklists of recommended practice to assess their performance; Bryant and Jacobson (2005) have proposed the ten measures shown in Exhibit 4.4. This checklist of good practices helps the board carry out its trust obligations. It complements, but does not replace, the balanced scorecard. A successful board should comply with all ten measures, but it should also have a near-benchmark scorecard. The American Hospital Association's (AHA) Center for Healthcare Governance offers the Government Assessment Process, which can be used as a self-survey or with consultants recommended by the Center. Its survey pursues more detailed processes than the Bryant and Jacobson model does. The Center has developed specific surveys for standing committees and one for individual board members. [33]

1. Meeting legal requirements	Bond-rating agencies include a due diligence review of the organization's compliance with all outstanding legal obligations. The board, at a minimum, should always require that one of its committees have access to all such due diligence reports and any responses from senior management.
2. Compliance orientation	Corporate compliance is a process of honest self-scrutiny, often involving objective third-party evaluators. When done properly, it produces an attorney–client privileged report that the board of directors or an appropriate board committee can study in depth and monitor steps taken in response. Boards should insist that senior management develop a corporate compliance mentality, in which legal shortcomings are routinely defined, identified, analyzed, and corrected. A formal compliance program reduces legal risks and constitutes another best practice of good governance.
3. Continuing governance education (CGE)	The board chair, the CEO, and the governance committee chair should together take the lead in ensuring meaningful CGE for the entire board and not just its new members. Every board should have its formal and informal CGE calendar for each year, supplemented by having individual board members lead the discussions after their attendance at CGE events.
4. Use of dashboards	Dashboards (e.g., Exhibit 4.3) help boards realize that policy decisions should result in performance improvements. Appropriate and regular use of dashboards will build governance confidence and will easily distinguish those boards from the ones not using such governance best practices.
5. Agenda practice	Some form of board self-evaluation and executive sessions should occur at *each* board meeting. Good practice encourages questions, seeks balanced presentations, and makes a deliberate effort not to disparage any good-faith question.
6. Conflicts of interest*	Conflicts of interest should be announced at every meeting. "If board members will just remember three simple rules about conflicts of interest, they will generally want to do the right things. a. Undisclosed conflicts are, by definition, not 'in good faith,' which has the legal effect of nullifying all the directors' statutory immunities. b. Undisclosed conflicts can, since 1996, produce substantial federal excise taxes on affected individuals who are corporate insiders and who obtain excess benefits from their organizations. c. An apparent, but not real, conflict can cause almost as much trouble as a real one in terms of public embarrassment for individuals and [not-for-profit] boards."
7. Corporate governance committee	The committee should meet regularly throughout the year; seek and nominate appropriate new members; review all outside reports and board effectiveness materials, plans, and continuing education; propose new measures, procedures, and bylaws as indicated; and investigate violations of confidentiality and conflict-of-interest policies.

EXHIBIT 4.4
Ten Measures
of Board
Effectiveness
(continued)

8. Voluntary Sarbanes-Oxley compliance	The landmark Sarbanes-Oxley Act does not apply to not-for-profit organizations except to provide whistle-blower protection. But its rationales *do* apply. Governance committees should study the act and recommend such easily identifiable steps as CEO and CFO certification of financial statements and clarification of who should and should not serve on the board and various committees.
9. CEO evaluation	CEO evaluation is best coordinated through a board committee, but all members of the board should be invited expressly to participate. The evaluation should relate to board-established objectives and include an opportunity for open-ended comments as well as ones responsive to specific questions. The evaluation should directly affect a year-end bonus or the next year's base compensation. The board chair should share the evaluation with the CEO in a personal meeting. The process should include both the CEO's self-evaluation and the CEO's reaction to the board's evaluation.
10. Board planning and evaluation	Each of the foregoing nine areas of conduct includes some form of planning for the institution, but no single one of them "asks whether the full board is invested in helping to plan the overall future of the organization. Board self-analysis should include what *all* directors/trustees think about: a. their collective tackling of the foregoing nine measurable elements in the last year, b. the organization's prospects for the future, and c. their individual contributions and/or misgivings about what each has done or not done for the organization."

*Conflicts of interest: real or potential personal financial benefit that may accrue from a given board decision.

Source: Used with permission from the National Center for Healthcare Leadership. Bryant, L. E., Jr., and P. D. Jacobson. 2006. "Practices for Measuring the Effectiveness of Ten Best of Nonprofit Healthcare Boards." *Modern Healthcare* Supplement, December.

In short, these are valuable tools to assess board processes. They do not replace the balanced scorecard, which is the ultimate measure of HCO and board performance. Ultimately, a successful board is one with a near-benchmark scorecard.

People

Board Membership

Society has established, through law and tradition, two minimum criteria for the actions of governing boards. The first is that the actions are measured in terms of their *prudence* and reasonableness, rather than being well intentioned (a looser standard) or successful (a stronger standard). Board members should be careful, thoughtful, and judicious in decision making; they need not always be right. The second is that the board members hold a position of *trust* for the owners. They must not take unfair advantage of their membership and must, to the best of their ability, direct their actions to the benefit of the whole ownership. Board members must avoid situations that give some owners special advantage.

Excellent boards seek members who are committed to the criteria of prudence and trust. They select their members through a continuing search, and they support their members with ongoing programs to help them make the biggest possible contribution. This section discusses board selection criteria, processes, compensation, education, and support. It also addresses two special issues of membership: (1) conflicts of interest for board members and (2) roles for physicians and CEOs on boards.

Membership Qualifications

Skill and Character Criteria

Board members should be able to make the challenging and sophisticated decisions required in the five managerial functions. Members should bring to each meeting good judgment based on an acute sense of the best interest of the owners as a whole. In not-for-profit HCOs, board members must recognize the community as the owner. What characteristics predict these critical skills?

- *Familiarity with the community.* The raison d'être of community boards is their ability to relate healthcare decisions to local conditions. This means insight into how much money the community should pay for care, how to recruit professionals to the community, how to attract volunteers and donations, how to make community members feel comfortable as patients and associates, and how to influence local opinion and leadership. Different groups in the community will have different views on these questions. The board should have members who represent the diversity of the community but whose understanding transcends their own sex, race, and social group.
- *Familiarity with business decisions.* Most board decisions involve multimillion-dollar commitments. They are measured and described in the languages of accounting, business law, finance, and marketing. The HCO boardroom is a place where technical language is frequently used to communicate complex concepts. There is also an emotional component to multimillion-dollar decisions. Although individuals from all walks of life can make excellent board members, moving from hundred-dollar decisions to million-dollar decisions takes some practice. Previous experience at decision making is important for board members to gain the necessary familiarity with the language and as psychological preparation.
- *Available time.* Board service on even a medium-sized community hospital requires a substantial time commitment—one day per month at a minimum; more for officers and committee chairs. People who do not have the time to master

the information and participate actively in debate are unlikely to guide the organization effectively.

- *A record of success.* The best predictor, more important than general experience or formal education, is how well the person has performed on similar assignments. This indicator is important after the individual has joined the board as well. Effective members should be promoted to higher board offices. Reliance on achievement is a way of overcoming biases in selecting board officers. Objective criteria open opportunities for members of disadvantaged groups.

- *Reputation.* The general reputation or character of an individual is important in two senses. First, like the record of success, it is an indication of what the individual will do in the future. Second, it serves to enhance the credibility of the individual. Persons with reputations for probity frequently gain influence because of that reputation. Boards have a legal obligation for prudence. The appointment of people whose reputation is suspect could be construed as imprudent.

Representation Criteria

Representation criteria are related to the resource distribution functions of the board. Many people support the argument that only a member of a certain constituency can truly understand how the organization treats that group. They believe a good board should have representation from women, the poor, ethnic groups, labor, and so forth. The concept of representation can be extended to include employees, physicians, nurses, religious bodies involved in ownership, and other groups. Stakeholder constituencies are usually pleased by recognition at the board level.

Several caveats must be attached to representation criteria. First, and most important, representatives who lack the necessary skills and reputation are unlikely to help either their constituency or the community at large. Second, excellent boards act by consensus for the community as a whole. The concept of resource distribution tends to foster adversarial positions, compromise instead of consensus, and division instead of enhancement of resources. Third is the problem of tokenism. A seat on a board, particularly a single seat, does not necessarily mean influence in the decisions. Finally, the appointment itself changes the individual. The lessons of the boardroom are not available to their constituents, and over a period of time, the board members are co-opted from the view for which they were selected. Tokenism and co-optation can be deliberate adversarial strategies to diminish a group's influence.

Affirmative action to ensure that competent individuals are not excluded from board membership is encouraged under the law and is likely to make organizations more successful. High-performing organizations understand that a diverse board may be more likely to make improved decisions, due to the diversity of perspective. To that end, they seek out board members who are patients and family members, women, and from a variety of racial and ethnic backgrounds. A balance can be best struck if two points are kept in mind:

1. *Board members are appointed as individuals, not as representatives.* They should be competent to serve in their own right, regardless of their position in the community.
2. *Board members act on behalf of the community as a whole.* This does not rule out special considerations of groups with unusual needs, but it places those considerations in a context—they are appropriate to the extent that they improve the community as a whole.

Board Selection

Selecting board members involves issues of eligibility, terms, offices, committees, and the size of the board as well as the actual choice of individuals. Officers and committee chairs have more power than individual members, so their selection is especially important. A 2012 review of the literature concludes:[34]

> Recent empirical studies linking board composition and processes with patient outcomes have found clear differences between high- and low-performing hospitals, highlighting the importance of strong and committed leadership that prioritizes quality and safety and sets clear and measurable goals for improvement. Effective oversight is also associated with well-informed and skilled board members. (p. 738)

Appointment to Membership and Office

Most HCOs have self-perpetuating boards—the board itself selects new members and successors. Other methods include election by stockholders—the prescribed procedure in stock corporations—and election by members of the corporation who sometimes are simply interested members of the community. Boards of government institutions are frequently appointed by supporting jurisdictions or, rarely, through popular vote. In multicorporate systems the parent corporation appoints subsidiary boards, usually from local nominations. Boards generally elect their own officers. In addition to the officers, a number of committee members and chairs must be appointed, a job usually left to the chair but appropriately subject to discussion or approval.

Role of the Nominating Committee

The nominating committee is responsible for nominating both board members and board officers. As Exhibit 4.4 notes, the committee also manages the board's self-evaluation and resolves issues of conflict of interest. It is usually a standing committee with membership determined by the bylaws. It is common to put former officers on the nominating committee; such a strategy emphasizes continuation of the status quo in the organization. Thus, organizations wishing for fresh ideas broaden nominating committee membership and charge the committee with searching more widely for nominees. It is typically in the confidential discussions of the nominating committee that individuals are suggested or overlooked, interviewed, compared against criteria, and accepted or rejected. This makes the nominating committee one of the most powerful groups in the organization.

Board nominees are usually asked beforehand if they will serve, and the best candidates frequently must be convinced. Truly contested elections and overt campaigning are rare. Many organizations nominate only one slate for boards and board offices. Formal provisions for write-in candidates and nominations from the floor are safeguards that are rarely used. In the normal course of events, selection occurs in the nominating committee. The committee often proposes not only board members but also corporate and board officers and chairs of standing committees.

Size, Eligibility, and Length of Terms

The number of nominations to be made each year is a function of the number of board members and the length of their terms. Board sizes range from a handful to a hundred, although between 10 and 20 members is most common. Terms are generally three or four years, and the number of terms that can be served successively is usually limited. Lengthy terms or unlimited renewal of terms can lead to stagnation; it is difficult for the nominating committee to pass over a faithful member who wants to serve another term unless the rules forbid it. Too-short terms reduce the experience of officers as well as members.

Board size, terms, and limits are related. If there are 15 members, three-year terms, and a two-term limit, there will be five nominations each year, but only two or three new people will be added in most years. The median experience of board members will be about three years. Similarly, 16 members, four-year terms, and a two-term limit will add two new people yearly, and the median experience will be nearly four years.

In addition to length of service, many organizations have eligibility clauses related to the owning corporation. For-profit boards can require stock ownership. Church-sponsored organizations, even when they are operated as secular community institutions, can require that board members be from the religious group. Some government and voluntary not-for-profit institutions require residence in the political jurisdiction for board membership. Other eligibility clauses include phrases like *good moral character*, although so much judgment is implied that they are more selection than eligibility criteria.

Compensation

The rewards for board service are complex. They include the satisfaction of a desire to help others, pride in professional achievement, public recognition, association with community leaders, and sometimes commercial opportunities that relate indirectly to recognition and association. In not-for-profit HCOs, they do not include significant direct financial reward; board members are rarely compensated. The Volunteer Protection Act of 1997 affords greater protection against personal liability for trustees who are not compensated.[35] Some evidence suggests that noncompensated boards have equal or superior performance.[36]

CEO Membership

The CEO is an active participant in board deliberations. Because his or her principal livelihood is from employment at the organization, the CEO has fundamental conflicts of interest, particularly when possibilities arise for consolidation or conversion and when other employees or doctors present grievances against the CEO. Although less obvious, CEOs can influence the board by controlling the information it receives and the board meeting agenda. Despite the conflict, most hospital boards make the CEO an ex officio member. CEOs sometimes hold offices, such as chair of the executive committee or president of the corporation. The justification lies in the same rule governing other conflicts—that the community's potential benefit exceeds its potential loss.[37]

Physician Membership

Physicians who practice at the HCO also have clear conflicts of interest. The national consensus, however, is even clearer for physicians than for CEO board membership; in fact, The Joint Commission recommends physician representation on HCO boards. Empirical evidence indicates that hospitals with physicians in board roles have better mortality and morbidity[38] and financial[39] performance. Physician representation improves overall success: The board needs to hear the viewpoints of doctors, and doctors need to know their views are being received.[40] Many HCOs set aside seats for doctors and solicit nominations from the clinical staff. It is not uncommon for the clinical staff to elect its representatives to a minority of the board. Physician representation can approach 50 percent, but such large fractions in not-for-profit corporations raise questions of inurement, tax exemption, and antitrust. The IRS relies on explicit rules for not-for-profits to avoid inurement and retain tax exemption.[41] Antitrust considerations forbid physicians (or other vendors) from collusion in restraint of trade.

Appointment of a few physicians to the board is not a panacea, however. They are added to the board as community members, not representatives of the medical profession. Conflict-of-interest rules can silence a physician when his or her viewpoint is most critical. HCOs use a variety of other mechanisms to emphasize each physician's participation in the decisions most immediate to his or her practice (see Chapter 6).

Board Organization

Committees

Board committees weigh the importance of various issues, evaluate differing perspectives, identify interrelationships and opportunities to combine or separate issues, and resolve issues that do not require full board attention. They analyze facts and educate members. They develop expertise in a given area, such as finance. They often expand representation, including others beside board members. Finally, they can take on especially sensitive issues, such as compensation, nomination, auditing, and clinical staff membership, in more discreet settings.

Well-managed boards delegate routinely to **standing committees**—permanent units of the board, established in the bylaws of the corporation. As shown in Exhibit 4.5, finance, compensation, audit, and nominating committees are almost universal. The majority of HCO governing boards have a quality committee to review processes of care, mortality, dashboard indicators for clinical quality, patient safety, and patient satisfaction.[42]

> *Standing committee*
> A permanent committee established in the bylaws of the corporation or similar basic documents.

Each standing committee should have a clear, recurring agenda that cannot be handled well by other structures. The use of an executive committee appears to be diminishing among small boards, where routine use is unnecessary. The overall tendency is toward a small, active board with a few important standing committees.

Beyond the few standing committees, well-managed boards of all sizes use **ad hoc committees**, formed as appropriate to the issue at hand for a specified time period. An organization often has several ad hoc committees working simultaneously and reporting to the board or its standing committees. Ad hoc committees bring the most knowledgeable members into each decision. They open opportunities for conflict resolution and promote understanding and consensus. Even if a minority is opposed to the final outcome, the members understand the logic that determined it and are convinced that the process was appropriate.

> *Ad hoc committee*
> A committee formed to address a specific purpose for a specified time period.

The rules for operation of the board are recorded in **governance bylaws**. These specify quorums, requirements for passage of specific items, duties of committees and officers, and procedures for the conduct of business. Matters such as the use of a consent agenda or the board's calendar are usually covered in procedural memoranda that supplement the bylaws.

> *Governance bylaws*
> A corporate document that specifies quorum rules of order, duties of standing committees and officers, and other procedures for the conduct of business.

Multicorporate Governance Structures

Health systems with multiple operating units may establish governance functions for each of the affiliates, setting up boards that report to other boards.

EXHIBIT 4.5
Typical
Standing
Committees of
the Governing
Board

Committee	Function	Membership
Executive	Act on behalf of full board in emergencies Less commonly, assume governance functions, making the full board advisory or honorific	Officers (chair, vice chair, secretary, treasurer), standing committee chairs, CEO and CFO
Quality	Develop strategic goals for quality improvement and safety Set the quality agenda Receive and recommend approval of quality and safety reports Review physician appointment and reappointment and results of focused quality studies	Board chair, COO, CMO, CNO, chair of the quality improvement council, clinical and nonclinical members
Finance	Establish long-range financial plan, debt structure, and initial budget guidelines Monitor budget performance	Treasurer, CFO, potential future chairs
Compensation	Review executive performance Award increases and bonuses Link senior executives' compensation to quality and patient safety indicators Ensure compliance with IRS, GAO, and Sarbanes-Oxley	Officers, former officers, legal counsel
Audit	Review financial audit, Joint Commission reports	Officers, former officers
Nominating	Nominate new board members and board officers Review board performance and individual contribution Annually evaluate individual conflicts of interest Suggest improved processes	Senior board officers

CFO: chief financial officer; CMO: chief medical officer; CNO: chief nursing officer; COO: chief operating officer; GAO: Government Accountability Office; IRS: Internal Revenue Service

For example, an HCO that operates two hospitals, a medical group practice, a home care business, and a hospice as subsidiaries needs at least one board, but it might have as many as five—one for each entity. (Technically, any separately incorporated unit must have a board, but the requirement can be met by a small group of employed officers. The discussion here is of boards that include other stakeholder representation.)

Subsidiary boards make four contributions that have made them popular in larger HCOs:

1. They expand representation, allowing local leaders to retain a sense of influence over their institution and local preferences to be reflected in operating decisions. This is particularly important when the subsidiaries operate in different markets; as a result, most multistate systems have local subsidiary boards.
2. They allow board specialization. The home care and hospice board would allow input from stakeholders with expertise and interest in these services, for example.
3. They permit joint ventures with other corporations and partnerships with the clinical staff. Various service lines can be separately incorporated with different groups of physicians who serve on the boards.
4. They allow identification of taxable endeavors and protect the exemption of activities that qualify under the Internal Revenue Code.

Subsidiary boards operate under the concept of **reserved powers**. Reserved powers are held permanently by the corporate board. Their purpose is to make sure the subsidiary continues to follow the central mission and vision and to resolve conflicts between subsidiaries.

Reserved powers
Decisions permanently vested in the central corporation of a multicorporate system.

Within the limits imposed by reserved powers, subsidiary boards tend to work as corporate boards do. They carry out the managerial and resource-related functions for their organization, making recommendations to the parent board on the reserved matters.

Exhibit 4.6 shows the board structure of Henry Ford Health System, a $3.4 billion–a-year HCO that serves about 20 percent of the metropolitan Detroit market of 4.5 million people. The system has 12 subsidiary boards that involve 150 members and report to a system board of 44 members. The 12 boards allow almost 200 people to participate in the activity of the corporation. It is sufficiently flexible to allow the system to run a successful insurance company, participate in a variety of partnership activities with several other large healthcare providers and insurers in the area, and operate HCOs oriented to specific local communities and that reflect their histories and preferences. About a dozen other corporate entities exist but are managed by internal directors. With the exception of the 1,000-member Henry Ford Medical Group, which is accountable to the system board through the regional units, these entities are mainly special-purpose organizations that handle insurance and real estate activities.

Joint Venture Boards

Much acute care is now delivered in service lines that focus on a specific clinical area such as women's health. It is common to establish the service line as an explicit collaboration between the HCO and a group of its physicians. It is often desirable to incorporate the service line separately and to share its governance with the participating physicians. The arrangements can either be contractual or made by establishing jointly owned corporate subsidiaries, commonly called *joint ventures*.

EXHIBIT 4.6 Henry Ford Health System Governance Structure

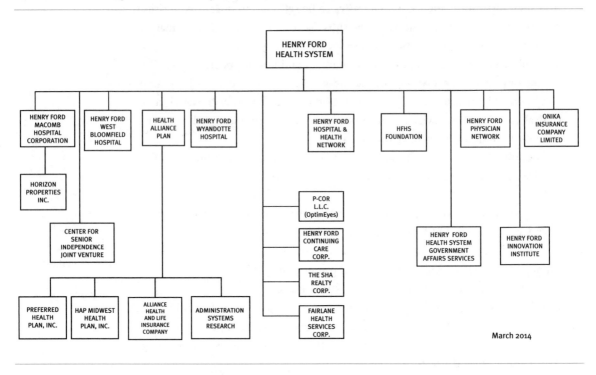

Source: Reprinted with permission from Henry Ford Health System.

Joint ventures normally have boards that represent the participating groups. They can be either for-profit or not-for-profit. They are often designed to require approval of parent corporate boards or supermajorities on matters such as major expansion, change in direction, or dissolution. The joint venture structure is flexible and convenient to allow physician ownership and shared financial rewards. The actual models in place are not automatically effective, however. A review of literature concludes, "The evidence base for the impact of many models of economic integration is either weak or nonexistent, with only a few models of economic integration having robust effects."[43]

Joint ventures need not be limited to service lines. Understanding the competition, even in hotly contested local markets, is a form of cooperation. For healthcare, competition is regulated by federal and state law, which generally encourages rivalry to win customers under specified conditions such as licensure, fair advertising, and avoidance of collusion or discrimination. The law permits various kinds of collaboration. HCOs are learning to exploit both aspects of regulated markets. Thus, they can, and do, compete and collaborate with each other simultaneously. In Kansas City, Missouri, Saint Luke's Health System and the local unit of HCA, a national for-profit hospital system, collaborate to run a cancer center.[44] In Iowa, two Catholic systems collaborate to provide referral care and telemedicine to a larger rural area.[45] Arrangements like these are formed because they offer routes to market advantages that are more practical than other available alternatives.

Education and Information Support for Board Members

Evidence from California voluntary hospital boards shows that educated boards achieve greater financial success.[46] New members need education in several unique aspects of healthcare management. There are also issues unique to the particular institution. While new members should bring fresh perspectives, they should not operate in ignorance of history. New-member orientation programs include tours, introductions to key personnel, conveyance of written documents and texts, and planned conversations and presentations. A typical list of subjects is shown in Exhibit 4.7. Catholic Health Initiatives, a successful HCO system operating in 20 states, mandates a three-day, off-site training program for each new trustee in its member HCOs.[47]

Ongoing board education is accomplished by special programs—time set aside from business to explore new ideas and best practices—often using consultants. To be effective, formal programs for board members should follow certain rules. Brevity is essential. Small segments should be scheduled for each specific topic. Most important, members should be active participants. Questions should be encouraged, the style should be conversational, and the

---

Mission, Role, and History of HCOs

What healthcare organizations give to the community

Difference between for-profit, not-for-profit, and government ownership

How HCOs Are Financed

Operating funds
Private insurance
Government insurance
Uninsured patients
Sources and uses of capital funds

How HCOs Strive for Excellence

Quality and safety agenda
Service lines
Empowerment and transformational management culture
Performance measurement
Continuous improvement

HCO–Physician Relations

Nature of contract between doctors and healthcare organizations
Concept of peer review
Trustee responsibilities for the medical staff

Functions of the Governing Board

Maintain management capability
Establish the mission, vision, and values
Approve the corporate strategy and annual implementation
Ensure quality and appropriate medical care
Monitor organizational performance
Continuously improve board performance

Duties of Trustees

Duty of loyalty (conflict of interest)
Duty of care
Fiduciary and compliance duties
Trustee liability
Confidentiality

EXHIBIT 4.7
Board Member Orientation Subjects

discussion should be extended over several sessions. After orientation, most board members' learning is informal and on the job. Well-organized boards make committee appointments carefully, allowing new members to become acquainted with the organization in less demanding assignments. They fill chairs with experienced members; they use chairs and organization executives to help members learn as they serve.

In addition to on-the-job learning, high-performing HCOs now include educational programs in their agenda. These serve to clarify specific situations, keep the board current with national and regional trends, and provide background on complex issues. Many disagreements between stakeholders stem from avoidable misunderstandings and ambiguities of positions. Thus, the "backgrounding" helps the board make clearer, less controversial decisions.

Measures

Board performance is measured primarily by the HCO's strategic scorecard. Values on the scorecard should be improving and approaching benchmark. If they are stagnant or declining, the board must negotiate more aggressive goals and explore with management or outside consultants how to achieve them. Specific OFIs for the board arise from the measures proposed by Bryant and Jacobson (see Exhibit 4.4). Many OFIs emerge from qualitative comments; the board's nominating committee identifies and prioritizes them in its review processes of individual board members and the board as a whole.

Managerial Issues

The board's continuous improvement function, structure, and educational program described in this chapter are all designed to increase board and HCO effectiveness. They have all been used effectively by high-performing HCOs— that is, those that are near benchmark on strategic performance measures. They help many boards overcome the pitfalls of governance: incomplete information, inability to reach decisions, and unbalanced response to stakeholder needs. Even with them, boards and senior management must be vigilant to help the board make the best decisions. The available evidence, although limited, suggests that governance is a major differentiator for high performance.[48]

Unfortunately, few HCOs achieve best practices in governance. A 2011 survey by the AHA reports many deficiencies. While three-fourths of surveyed hospitals report having quantitative quality-of-care goals, 90 percent rate finance and patient satisfaction as more important measures of performance. Only a third have a succession plan for the CEO. Only half review community health needs annually. Ninety percent of board members are white, and 75 percent are men.[49] The survey was offered to all AHA members, with about a third (1,520) responding. While the respondents were similar to the total hospital population, it is reasonable to assume that data from nonrespondents would not improve the results. Interestingly, two-thirds of the responses were by CEOs only. For the third where both CEO and board chair responded, significant differences appeared in the responses. The difference suggests problems with the first governance function, CEO selection and support. A survey of large healthcare systems raises similar concerns.[50]

Operating Discipline

Operating discipline keeps track of the agenda so that no item is lost and all items receive a timely decision. The board's operating discipline is critical, because it maximizes the value of the board's time. It is provided by the CEO and supported by board leadership. The board's six functions are driven by the HCO's annual planning calendar (see Exhibit 3.7). They provide a check-list for what must be done each month. If the board falls behind in its duties, the rest of the organization is stymied.

Maintaining timeliness is often challenging. Most board actions are by consensus—unanimous agreement—rather than by a majority vote. This gives minority positions substantial power. A committed minority can successfully stall a position valuable to the whole. In the worst case, when several stakeholder groups take advantage of this possibility, the board becomes a deliberate weapon to avoid change. Operating discipline brings to the board items that can be handled without acrimonious dissent. Preparation, agenda management, use of committees and subcommittees, and deliberate negotiation all have a role. Board leadership and senior management use these tools to identify and resolve differences, building both the proposal details and the consensus in a stepwise progression.

Preparation

CEOs and their staffs are responsible for preparing appropriate factual documentation for every agenda item. They are responsible for conducting the environmental surveillance, identifying issues, analyzing and developing proposals, and understanding the needs of the community. Staff is used extensively to gather and disseminate facts and to identify potential conflicts. Establishing the fact base is a major justification for the strategic support activities described in Chapters 10 through 15. Not only does it provide the due diligence that foresees and avoids implementation problems, but it also identifies potential conflicts and opens alternatives for negotiated solutions.

The other aspect to preparation is general rather than specific to the issues at hand. Most issues take meaning from context; the better the environment and the decision-making processes are understood, the better the specific decision is likely to be.

Focused Agendas

The board's agenda management falls heavily on the board chair, the committee chairs, and the CEO. A discussion may have any of several outcomes in view: general education and backgrounding, exploration of controversial or complex topics, plan to develop a proposal through committees, or action on specific proposals. Both the outcome and time allotment are made clear to the board at the start of the discussion. A major issue may come before the board for each of these outcomes as it evolves, is understood, and is finally resolved.

Successful boards tend to focus on major issues one at a time, attempting to comprehend all aspects of the single issue and reach a consensus understanding of it. Meetings feature a few issues or a single issue in depth, rather than a superficial review of several topics. Ongoing information not related to the priority issues is often consolidated into a **consent agenda**—a group of reports passed without discussion. Members may request to remove a matter from the consent agenda if they have a specific concern. Such requests are rare and are usually granted by the chair or by motion of the board.

Consent agenda
A group of agenda items passed without discussion unless a member requests a review; used to focus attention on priority matters.

Retreats are effective as devices to focus board attention. They can be held in comfortable off-site settings, emphasizing the departure from usual practice. Longer sessions allow fuller presentation of issues and background. Additional representatives of the clinical staff and management can be invited, facilitating understanding, acceptance, and implementation of the final decision. Consultants and guests from the community can be used to expand knowledge of factual and political issues.

Use of Committees and Subcommittees

A consequence of the focused agenda is extensive use of committees. Issues are referred to standing or ad hoc committees and subcommittees for less formal and more extensive discussion. Moving the issue away from the boardroom allows more voices to be heard, more alternatives to explore, and more candid expressions of viewpoint.

Senior management plays a critical role in this process. It identifies stakeholders with interests and brings them to the committees. It seeks best practices that demonstrate the ways others have solved the issues. It painstakingly explores positions, developing the understanding that is the first stage of negotiating solutions. Data from an AHA survey in 2011 suggest that many HCO boards do not use committees effectively.[51] Fewer than two-thirds have a governance or nominating committee, and only 80 percent have a finance committee.[52]

Negotiation

Progress usually involves designing proposals that meet most or all stakeholder needs and do not impair the special needs of any one group. Proposals that might generate powerful resistance are avoided. Compromise is the rule; radical reform is rare. Although this reality slows progress, it is inherent in the culture of respect. The fact that high-performing HCOs use this model shows that there are avenues where material progress can be made. Extensive negotiation is often necessary to find them. Negotiation takes place at all levels, from individual meetings to major committees, but rarely in the board meeting itself. Senior managers often negotiate directly to shape proposals that will gain consensus. Their skill at shaping consensus proposals and then implementing them "as advertised" is a major factor in maintaining stakeholder loyalty.

Board Membership

Selection

Weak boards fail to generate turnover and do not develop members for leadership roles. They sometimes have large memberships, diluting each individual's sense of obligation or opportunity. Conversely, they are sometimes too small to fully represent stakeholders. Ironically, they can be both—large, with disinterested members and a small cabal dominating decisions. Size limits, term limits, and member development go together in building board strength.

Legal and Ethical Issues

Three areas of legal and ethical concern are known to create governance difficulties:

1. *Conflict or duality of interest,* where a board member has a personal financial gain or risk in the decision at hand. The duty of loyalty holds that members of governing boards not serve when their personal financial interests conflict with those of the owners. Conceptually, this is clear enough. In practice, it is hard to find people who meet the criteria for board membership but who have not also become involved in activities that eventually will conflict. Conflict of interest is inherent in any democratic structure, and it cannot be permanently resolved. Each member annually declares in writing his or her major activities and holdings. Individuals are expected to disqualify themselves from discussion and voting on an issue whenever appropriate, but they may be asked to do so by the chair or another member. Good practice calls for an announcement of conflicts at each board meeting, with attention to the specific agenda. It is generally agreed that the external auditor and the legal counsel should not serve as board members.
2. *Inurement,* where a board member improperly receives financial gain from the assets of a corporation. Actions by trustees that lead to their personal financial gain can be inurement. Inurement often means compensation in excess of the market value provided. The IRS monitors executive and other high-level salaries and can deny tax-exempt status to an organization that allows inurement.[53]

3. *Conversions,* where the assets of a not-for-profit corporation are transferred to a for-profit corporation at less than their true value. Conversion (when not-for-profit assets are converted to for-profit ownership) and consolidation (when one corporation merges with another, regardless of tax structure) raise important questions of fairness to the owners. Because of this, they place trustees and directors at unusual risk. Boards usually hire special legal counsel skilled in these transactions. Large-scale conversions and consolidations often require regulatory or judicial review.

Lawsuits over these matters serve to reinforce the ethical duties. Board members can be sued as individuals, although such suits are rare. Lawsuits must demonstrate a trustee's failure in one or more of the three duties of loyalty, care, and disclosure, such as failing to take due care, deliberate self-serving, or unnecessarily risky behavior. The board's legal counsel should guard against individual liability as well as guide the board as a whole. Directors' and officers' liability insurance provides legal and financial assistance against suits that might be placed.

Additional Resources

Alliance for Advancing Nonprofit Health Care. 2009. "Advancing the Public Accountability of Nonprofit Health Care Organizations: Guidelines on Governance Practices." www.nonprofithealthcare.org.

American College of Healthcare Executives. 2010. *Contracts for Healthcare Executives,* 5th ed. Chicago: Health Administration Press.

Biggs, E. 2011. *Healthcare Governance: A Guide for Effective Boards,* 2nd ed. Chicago: Health Administration Press.

Conger, J. A. (ed.). 2009. *Boardroom Realities: Building Leaders Across Your Board.* San Francisco: Jossey-Bass.

Joshi, M. S., and B. J. Horak. 2009. *Healthcare Transformation: A Guide for the Hospital Board Member.* Chicago: American Hospital Association.

McGinn, P. 2009. *Partnership of Equals: Practical Strategies for Healthcare CEOs and Their Boards.* Chicago: Health Administration Press.

Prybil, L., S. Levey, R. Killian, D. Fardo, R. Chait, D. Bardach, and W. Roach. 2012. *Governance in Large Nonprofit Health Systems: Current Profile and Emerging Patterns.* Lexington, KY: Commonwealth Center for Governance Studies.

Showalter, J. S. 2014. *The Law of Healthcare Administration,* 7th ed. Chicago: Health Administration Press.

Notes

1. Kane, N. M., J. R. Clark, and H. L. Rivenson. 2009. "The Internal Processes and Behavioral Dynamics of Hospital Boards: An Exploration of Differences Between High- and Low-Performing Hospitals." *Health Care Management Review* 34 (1): 80–91.

2. Alexander, J. A. 1990. "Governance for Whom? The Dilemmas of Change and Effectiveness in Hospital Boards." *Frontiers of Health Services Management* 6 (3): 39.

3. Ehrenreich, B., and J. Ehrenreich. 1970. *The American Health Empire: Power, Profits, and Politics*. New York: Random House.

4. Rosenberg, C. E. 1987. *The Care of Strangers: The Rise of America's Hospital System*. New York: Basic Books.

5. Seay, J. D., and B. C. Vladeck. 1988. "Mission Matters." In *In Sickness and in Health: The Mission of Voluntary Health Care Institutions*, edited by J. D. Seay and B. C. Vladeck, 1–34. New York: McGraw-Hill.

6. Young, G. J., C. H. Chou, J. Alexander, S. Y. Lee, and E. Raver. 2013. "Provision of Community Benefits by Tax-Exempt U.S Hospitals." *New England Journal of Medicine* 368 (16): 1519–27; Song, P. H., S. Y. Lee, J. A. Alexander, and E. E. Seiber. 2013. "Hospital Ownership and Community Benefit: Looking Beyond Uncompensated Care." *Journal of Healthcare Management* 58 (2): 126–42.

7. Collins, J. 2001. *Good to Great: Why Some Companies Make the Leap . . . and Others Don't*. New York: HarperBusiness.

8. Griffith, J. R., and K. R. White. 2005. "The Revolution in Hospital Management." *Journal of Healthcare Management* 50 (3): 170–90.

9. Alexander, J. A., and S.-Y. D. Lee. 2006. "Does Governance Matter? Board Configuration and Performance in Not-for-Profit Hospitals." *Milbank Quarterly* 84 (4): 733–58; Alexander, J. A., Y. Ye, S.-Y. D. Lee, and B. J. Weiner. 2006. "The Effects of Governing Board Configuration on Profound Organizational Change in Hospitals." *Journal of Health and Social Behavior* 47: 291–308.

10. Kane, Clark, and Rivenson (2009).

11. Alexander, J. A., B. J. Weiner, and R. J. Bogue. 2001. "Changes in the Structure, Composition, and Activity of Hospital Governing Boards, 1989–1997: Evidence from Two National Surveys." *Milbank Quarterly* 79 (2): 253–79.

12. Shay, P. D., and K. R. White. 2014. "Executive Compensation in Health Care: A Systematic Review." *Health Care Management Review* 39 (3): 255–67; Joynt, K. E., S. T. Le, J. Orav, and A. K. Jha. 2014. "Compensation of Chief Executive Officers in Nonprofit US Hospitals." *JAMA Internal Medicine* 174 (1): 61–67.

13. Prybil, L., S. Levey, R. Killian, D. Fardo, R. Chait, D. Bardach, and W. Roach. 2012. *Governance in Large Nonprofit Health Systems: Current Profile and Emerging Patterns*, 28. Lexington, KY: Commonwealth Center for Governance Studies.

14. Groves, K. S. 2011. "Talent Management Best Practices: How Exemplary Health Care Organizations Create Value in a Down Economy." *Health Care Management Review* 36 (3): 227–40.

15. Dotson, E., and A. Nuru-Jeter. 2012. "Setting the Stage for a Business Case for Leadership Diversity in Healthcare: History, Research, and Leverage." *Journal of Healthcare Management* 57 (1): 35–44.

16. Ford-Eickhoff, K. D., D. Ashmos, and R. R. McDaniel. 2011. "Hospital Boards and Hospital Strategic Focus: The Impact of Board Involvement in Strategic Decision Making." *Health Care Management Review* 36 (2): 145–54.

17. Chassin, M. R., and J. M. Loeb. 2013. "High-Reliability Health Care: Getting There from Here." *Milbank Quarterly* 91 (3): 459–90.

18. Griffith, J. R. 2015. "How Good Are Baldrige Winners?" *Journal of Healthcare Management* 60 (1): 44–61.

19. Chassin, M. R. 2013. "Improving the Quality of Health Care: What's Taking So Long?" *Health Affairs* 32 (10): 1761–65.

20. Jha, A., and A. Epstein. 2010. "Hospital Governance and the Quality of Care." *Health Affairs* 29 (1): 182–87.

21. Joint Commission. 2015. "Core Measure Sets." [Online information; retrieved 5/24/14.] www.jointcommission.org/core_measure_sets.aspx.

22. Centers for Medicare & Medicaid Services. 2011. "Hospital Quality Initiative." [Online information; retrieved 5/23/14.] www.cms.hhs.gov/HospitalQualityInits/08_HospitalRHQDAPU.asp.

23. *Patrick v. Burget et al.* 1988. 486 U.S. 94, No. 86-1145, Supreme Court of the United States.

24. Greene, J. 2008. "It's a Privilege." *Trustee* 61 (3): 8–11.

25. Hann, D. P. 2001. "Emerging Issues in U.S. Corporate Governance: Are the Recent Reforms Working?" *Defense Counsel Journal* 68 (2): 191–205.

26. Hamilton, R. W. 2000. "Corporate Governance in America 1950–2000: Major Changes but Uncertain Benefits." *Journal of Corporation Law* 25 (2): 349–70.

27. Institute of Medicine, Committee on Quality of Health Care in America. 2001. *Crossing the Quality Chasm: A New Health System for the 21st Century.* Washington, DC: National Academies Press.

28. Centers for Medicare & Medicaid Services. 2013. "CMS-Approved Accreditation Programs." [Online information; retrieved 5/24/14.] www.cms.gov/Medicare/Provider-Enrollment-and-Certification/SurveyCertificationGenInfo/Downloads/CMS-Approved-Accreditation-Organizations.pdf.

29. Public Accounting Reform and Investor Protection Act of 2002, P.L. No. 107-204, 116 Stat. 745 [2002]).

30. Alexander, J. A., G. J. Young, B. J. Weiner, and L. R. Hearld. 2008. "Governance and Community Benefit: Are Nonprofit Hospitals Good Candidates for Sarbanes-Oxley Type Reforms?" *Journal of Health Politics, Policy and Law* 33 (2): 199–224.

31. *Ibid.*; Evashwick, C. J., and K. Gautam. 2008. "Governance and Management of Community Benefit: How Can Hospitals Be Positioned to Address New Challenges?" *Health Progress* (September–October): 10–15.

32. Connelly, M. D. 2004. "The Sea Change in Nonprofit Governance: A New Universe of Opportunities and Responsibilities." *Inquiry* 41 (1): 6–20.

33. American Hospital Association Center for Healthcare Governance. 2014. "GAP Versions," [Online information; retrieved 6/8/14.] www.americangovernance.com/gap/versions.shtml.

34. Millar, R. A., R. A. Mannion, T. B. Freeman, and H. T. O. Davies. 2013. "Hospital Board Oversight of Quality and Patient Safety: A Narrative Review and Synthesis of Recent Empirical Research." *Milbank Quarterly* 91 (4): 738–70.

35. Volunteer Protection Act of 1997. P.L. 105-119.

36. Alexander, J. A., and S.-Y. D. Lee. 2006. "Does Governance Matter? Board Configuration and Performance in Not-for-Profit Hospitals." *Milbank Quarterly* 84 (4): 733–58.

37. Alexander, J. A., S.-Y. D. Lee, V. Wang, and F. S. Margolin. 2009. "Changes in the Monitoring and Oversight Practices of Not-for-Profit Hospital Governing Boards 1989–2005: Evidence from Three National Surveys." *Medical Care Research and Review* 66 (2): 181–96.

38. Bai, G. E., and R. Krishnan. 2015. "Do Hospitals Without Physicians on the Board Deliver Lower Quality of Care?" *American Journal of Medical Quality* 30 (1): 58–65.

39. Goes, J. B., and C. Zhan. 1995. "The Effects of Hospital-Physician Integration Strategies on Hospital Financial Performance." *Health Services Research* 30 (4): 507–30; Molinari, C., M. Hendryx, and J. Goodstein. 1997. "The Effects of CEO-Board Relations on Hospital Performance." *Health Care Management Review* 22 (3): 7–15.

40. Goeschel, C. A., R. M. Wachter., and P. J. Pronovost. 2010. "Responsibility for Quality Improvement and Patient Safety: Hospital Board and Medical Staff Leadership Challenges." *Chest* 138 (1): 171–78.

41. Whitehead, R., Jr., and B. Humphrey. 1997. "IRS Eases Rules for Physician Representation on Governing Boards." *Healthcare Financial Management* 51 (3): 36–39.

42. Jiang, H. J., C. Lockee, K. Bass, and I. Fraser. 2009. "Board Oversight of Quality: Any Differences in Process of Care and Mortality?" *Journal of Healthcare Management* 54 (1): 15–30; Joshi, M. S., and S. C. Hines. 2006. "Getting the Board on Board: Engaging Hospital Boards in Quality and Patient Safety." *Journal on Quality and Patient Safety* 32 (4): 179–87.

43. Burns, L. R., and R. W. Muller. 2008. "Hospital-Physician Collaboration: Landscape of Economic Integration and Impact on Clinical Integration." *Milbank Quarterly* 86 (3): 375–434.

44. Saint Luke's Hospital's application to the Malcolm Baldrige National Quality Award, 2003, vii.

45. Griffith, J. R., and K. R. White. 2003. *Thinking Forward: Six Strategies for Highly Successful Organizations*, 87–118. Chicago: Health Administration Press.

46. Molinari, C., L. Morlock, J. Alexander, and C. A. Lyles. 1993. "Hospital Board Effectiveness: Relationships Between Governing Board Composition and Hospital Financial Viability." *Health Services Research* 28 (3): 358–77.

47. Griffith and White (2003).

48. Millar et al. (2013).

49. Van Dyke, K., J. Combes, and M. Joshi. 2011. *2011 AHA Health Care Governance Survey Report*. Chicago: American Hospital Association.

50. Prybil et al. (2012).

51. *Ibid.*, p. 14.

52. Van Dyke, Combes, and Joshi (2011).

53. U.S. Internal Revenue Service, Ruling 69-383. 1969.

II

CLINICAL

5 FOUNDATIONS OF CLINICAL PERFORMANCE

Critical Issues in Foundations of Clinical Performance

1. *Using patient management protocols to deliver evidence-based patient care:*
   - Assist caregivers in establishing a complete, accurate diagnosis for each patient.
   - Maintain, apply, and update evidence-based patient management protocols.
   - Use interdisciplinary plans of care and case management for individualized, patient-centered care.

2. *Using functional protocols to ensure safe, effective, patient-centered, timely, efficient, and equitable care:*
   - Standardize evidence-based care processes.
   - Train caregivers to achieve uniform care and high-reliability results.
   - Coordinate care processes across professional boundaries.

3. *Continuously improving clinical care:*
   - Develop an individualized plan of care for each patient.
   - Measure and benchmark outcomes and effective care processes.
   - Assist empowered caregivers to identify opportunities and coordinate changes in care.

4. *Supporting an empowered culture of evidence-based medicine and evidence-based management:*
   - Use service lines to organize caregiving teams.
   - Provide a transformational structure for discussion, adaptation, and conflict resolution.
   - Use goal setting and rewards to improve operating performance.

5. *Strengthening population health:*
   - Expand HCO service lines to provide comprehensive care.
   - Understand the costs and benefits of prevention.
   - Develop coalitions to promote population health.

These questions are about applying the chapter content. It's often helpful to discuss them with classmates or mentors, gaining different perspectives on the issues.

1. HCOs use a specific system to achieve excellent care. (The system is the content of Chapter 5.) Leaders must often explain the system to patients, customer stakeholders, and caregivers. Here are four common questions. How can you convey the answers clearly and convincingly?
   - Why should clinical performance be focused on outcomes?
   - Why are six dimensions (safe, effective, patient-centered, timely, efficient, and equitable) of measurement necessary?
   - Does this system generate high reliability and a culture of safety (i.e., an HCO that drives errors and accidents to zero)?
   - Why is it important that medical diagnosis is a heuristic process?

2. All HCO leaders need to understand the structure to achieve excellent care, because they must keep their teams aligned with it. If you were training new first-line managers, how would you help them understand the following:
   - What do patient management protocols contribute to care?
   - How does our HCO establish and update patient management protocols?
   - Do leaders in supplies, accounting, and security really "need to understand the structure to achieve excellent care"?

3. Caregiver leaders need to be able to answer these questions:
   - When and how can a caregiver depart from a patient management protocol?
   - Why are individualized patient care plans and case management important?
   - What are the answers you'd like to hear uniformly across the HCO?

4. How would an HCO develop functional protocols for functions like drug administration, which involve several different accountability units? The chief medical officer would like to develop an HCO-wide procedure for creating, validating, and standardizing functional protocols.
   - How should she proceed?
   - What are some issues that need to be addressed to make sure the procedure is effective?

5. The governing board of every multiple-service-line HCO must answer this question: Is the best mission for our HCO "excellence in patient care" or "healthy community"? What are the important factors the board should consider?

Purpose

The first purpose of any HCO is excellence in healthcare. Specifically, it is expected

to identify and meet each patient's complete healthcare needs. *individuals*

Safe, effective, patient-centered, timely, efficient, and equitable healthcare is the vision that should guide every caregiving team. Excellent HCOs support caregiving teams to make the vision reality, helping each caregiver perform effectively, building teams that collaborate, providing the information and communication, integrating the efforts of the several teams that most patients will need, and maintaining the environment of care. As of 2015, few HCOs come close to the vision.[1] As Mark R. Chassin, MD, president of The Joint Commission, put it, "quality and safety problems in healthcare continue to routinely result in harm to patients. Desired progress will not be achieved unless substantial changes are made to the way in which quality improvement is conducted."[2]

The "substantial changes" to achieve the vision are now well documented. Excellence requires:

1. Skilled physicians and independent practitioners who can diagnose disease from symptoms and complaints
2. Trained interdisciplinary caregiving teams who can respond to patients' needs
3. Complete and timely health records
4. Evidence-based patient care protocols as foundations for integrated care plans
5. Functional protocols that ensure uniform delivery of care
6. Ongoing patient listening and the flexibility to identify and meet each patient's unique needs
7. Effective collaboration within and across teams[3]

Any one of these can fail, and any failure will prevent excellence. Perhaps the biggest challenge is creating an overall culture of high reliability, where each of the seven elements not only happens routinely but is integrated with the other six.[4]

The high-performing HCOs that are models for the *Well-Managed Healthcare Organization* have not achieved perfection, but they have a solid record of better-than-average results.[5] The combination of transformational management (Chapter 2) and continuous improvement (Chapter 3) is the only documented path to a culture of high reliability. Building on them, this chapter explains the evidence-based model of twenty-first-century care. Chapter 6 discusses the arrangements between the HCO and its care leaders—physicians, nurse practitioners, physicians assistants, and other caregivers licensed to manage patient care and lead care teams. Chapter 7 describes the role of nursing; Chapter 8 the contribution of clinical support services, like imaging and pharmacy; and Chapter 9 the extension of excellence in care to population health. The following chapters, on knowledge management, human resources, and environment of care, are also essential to high reliability.

Many excellent HCOs extend their mission to a second, broader purpose: to improve population health, that is,

to identify and meet the community's healthcare needs.   *populations*

Implementing the population health purpose requires the first. It goes beyond excellence in care to minimize unnecessary use of health services through collaborative efforts to promote health, prevent disease, and curtail unnecessary treatment.

Functions

Exhibit 5.1 describes five functions of an HCO's clinical organization that support excellence in care, and move beyond it to population health.

Ensuring Accurate Diagnosis

Diagnosis, the process of determining the nature of disease, drives all of evidence-based medicine. The codification of disease initiated by Sydenham in the seventeenth century and now implemented by the International Classification of Diseases, version 10,[6] provides the foundation for all treatment. Identifying the correct and complete diagnosis is not simple. It integrates information from the patient's complaint, history, physical examination, and diagnostic testing. It is heuristic, that is, it systematically employs a trial-and-error mechanism that recognizes uncertainty and proceeds cyclically as more information is gathered. It continues even after treatment is begun, until the patient is discharged. Exhibit 5.2 shows the major steps in the diagnostic process.

Although Exhibit 5.2 is a useful conceptual model, most real care is substantially more complicated. Several additional considerations are critical to understanding the realities of modern patient care.

1. Diagnosis is subject to improvement until the patient is discharged. Although the diagnosis becomes surer as the patient progresses, revision to the plan of care remains possible. Actual care is much more dynamically heuristic than the figure suggests. The primary caregiver begins constructing the diagnosis when the patient walks in and adds or rules out possibilities almost continuously as examination and care progress. Many patients have multiple complaints and multiple diagnoses. Their diagnosis is an ongoing process. It is more often "current" than "final."

Function	Description	What the HCO Does
Ensuring accurate diagnosis	Diagnosis is the critical contribution of the care leader. It is an ongoing heuristic process driven by observation and interaction with the patient.	Selects effective care leaders Monitors their effectiveness Provides training to maintain and improve clinical skills Supports responsive listening to patients' needs Provides diagnostic clinical support services
Ensure that all treatment is safe, effective, patient centered, timely, efficient, and equitable	Diagnosis establishes the initial treatment plan, using patient management protocols to establish each patient's needs. Individual care activities are performed according to functional protocols so that care needs are uniformly fullfilled.	Updates and maintains protocols Trains caregivers in their use Ensures patient safety and minimizes risks Provides informed consent Maintains logistic support Keeps a record of care Coordinates care
Individualize patient care planning and treatment	Treatment is also heuristic. Patient variability is met by continued monitoring, individualized and interprofessional plans of care, and case management.	Provides specialist consultation Provides nursing care Supports communication between caregivers, patient, family, and subsequent caregivers
Improve community health	Community-wide approaches promote healthy behavior, prevent injury and disease, and promote cost-effective use of services. The HCO builds these collaboratively with other community organizations.	Measures community health with a set of indicators and benchmarks Catalyzes community interest Collaborates with other organizations Promotes effectiveness Discourages unnecessary care
Improve clinical performance and population health	Measurement and benchmarking of clinical outcomes and processes identify OFIs. PITs address them. Training implements improved performance. Success is rewarded.	Supports measurement and benchmarking Supports PITs Uses protocols, training, and incentives to implement improved methods

EXHIBIT 5.1
Functions of the Clinical Organization

excellent care [handwritten annotation]

OFI: opportunities for improvement; PIT: process improvement teams

2. The "differential diagnosis," introduced around the start of the twentieth century, is the key to managing the uncertainty. The care leader lists the several possible diagnoses consistent with the patient's complaint and symptoms, with the most likely first.[7]

3. In all but the simplest cases, nursing provides an additional diagnosis that is often important in reaching full recovery (Chapter 7). The nursing diagnosis follows a different logic and structure from the medical one. It often addresses social, emotional, and attitudinal problems that complicate care, but that must be solved to achieve excellence.

4. Clinical support services provide diagnostic testing to confirm or rule out each of the listed diagnoses. Specialists perform and interpret these tests. They and treatment specialists are available as consultants to the primary caregivers.

5. Definitive treatment for serious disease often involves referral to a treatment specialist. The treatment specialist typically manages a specific diagnosis and returns care to the primary caregiver when that treatment is complete. Ongoing care of chronic illness is typically managed by the primary caregiver, often coordinating several specialists.

For many patients the diagnostic process becomes a team effort, led by the attending physician.

The process meets the IOM goals when:

- No treatable diagnosis is overlooked.
- No diagnosis is treated that should have been ruled out.
- The nursing diagnosis addresses additional needs critical to recovery.
- The patient or patient's advocate is fully informed about the diagnoses and allowed to exercise control over treatment selection.
- All decisions are reached in a timely manner.
- All diagnostic tests are safe, effective, and efficient.

All failures in diagnosis are costly. Some are very costly, and a few shorten life. High-performing HCOs use their clinical, logistic, and strategic support systems to reduce failures.[8] Successful efforts to improve diagnostic accuracy have been reported.[9]

Excellent HCOs reach high performance by relying on the following:

1. Empowerment for all caregivers, establishing a blame-free culture and ensuring that issues impairing each caregiver's best effort are promptly corrected.

2. Credentialing, training, and quality review (Chapter 6) to verify and increase care leaders' qualifications and improve performance.

3. Success as "a great place to give care" to recruit and retain well-qualified caregivers. Steps 1 to 3 create a culture where peer pressure helps every caregiver do his or her best.

EXHIBIT 5.2
Simplified
Diagnostic
Process

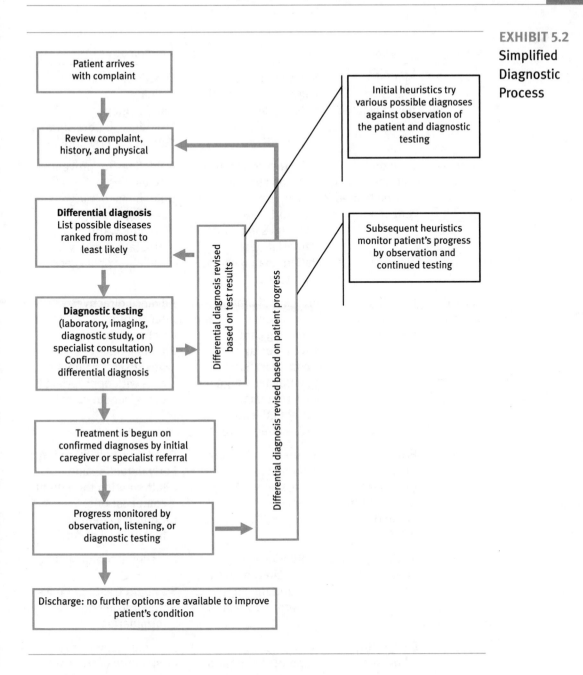

4. Ongoing learning and continuous improvement to improve caregivers' skills. PITs become team efforts to reach benchmark by careful analysis and improvement of processes.

Ensuring Excellent Care

Exhibit 5.3 shows the HCO contribution to "excellent care," care that fulfills each of the IOM aims. The exhibit reflects the broad range of HCO contribution, but two major functions—protocol-driven activities and appropriate and continuous training and education of caregivers—are fundamental.

EXHIBIT 5.3

HCO

Contribution to
Excellent Care

Goal	Purpose	Activity	Examples
Safe	Minimize risk and unanticipated outcomes	Safety practices Engineering controls Safety plans Risk management plans	Functional protocols Training Hand hygiene "Huddles" before surgery Patient fall precautions
Effective	Provide treatment that meets desired outcome	Selecting treatment options based on evidence Monitoring for changes in response to treatment Patient management protocols	Guidelines for preventive screening Guidelines for diagnostic testing Watchful waiting for prostate cancer vs. radiation or surgery
Patient centered	Coordinate care that is individualized	Pre-care planning Nursing diagnosis and nursing care Psychosocial considerations Cultural and language competency Patient education in care alternatives	Advance directives Interpreters Discharge follow-up Planning for postdischarge home care with appropriate caregiver education
Timely	Provide the right treatment at the right time at the right place	Accurate and timely diagnosis Decreasing waiting times	Door-to-intervention time Early detection and intervention for patient complications Prompt transfer to a higher level of care
Efficient	Achieving quality with lowest cost	Evaluating lower-cost alternatives of treatment, supplies, pharmaceuticals	Functional protocols and training Standard treatment packs Standardizing drug formularies
Equitable	Ensure that all persons have equal access to best treatment	Evaluating appropriateness of intervention when resources are scarce, depending on patient's condition, pros, and cons	Uncompensated care Community outreach Cultural competence For certain costly cases (e.g., transplant), refer to ethics committee or similar resource for assistance in making decisions

Clinical activities are specific, often scientific, responses to patient stimuli. For hypothetical identical patients, the diagnoses would be the same, leading to the same **patient management protocols**. For excellence, this uniformity must also be true for every care activity. Every injection requires several specific actions: the patient's name, site, drug, equipment, and skin preparation. Every surgical procedure is checked and double-checked to prevent errors.[10] Uniformity is achieved through functional protocols.

Patient management protocols
Formally established expectations that define the normal steps or processes in the care of a clinically related group of patients at a specific institution.

Protocols present several advantages. First, they make cooperation possible and are essential to sophisticated teamwork. Second, they provide the basis for monitoring processes. Many protocol steps are recorded and can be tallied. Specific completion failures can be identified as opportunities for improvement (OFIs). Third, protocols have become a convenient statement of contracts with patients and insurers.[11] The courts and the marketplace have reinforced the right of consumers to have their care conform to clinical standards developed by professionals.

Patient Management Protocols

Patient management protocols (also called pathways, guidelines, or simply protocols) are now the standard of care for most diseases[12] and are included in continuing medical education programs.[13] Protocols have supported shorter inpatient stays and improved survival rates;[14] the use of less expensive sites for care, such as rehabilitation hospitals, same-day surgery programs, and palliative care options; and the development of alternatives to expensive and dangerous treatments such as spinal fusions for back pain.

Protocols define the normal steps or processes in the care of a clinically related group of patients at a specific institution. Patient management protocols are organized around episodes of patient care, classified by symptom, disease, or condition, such as chest pain, pneumonia, or pregnancy. They specify the components of care, outcomes quality goals, and, by implication, the cost. They are developed by cross-functional teams and are written so that they can be easily communicated among the caregiving professionals, thereby increasing efficiency and reducing the chance of error.

Patient management protocols improve individual caregiver performance in five ways:

1. An evidence-based guideline is supported by training and becomes habitual as a starting point.
2. Several professions can use it to anticipate and coordinate care events.
3. Caregivers can use it as shorthand or an outline to guide their decisions and their communications to others.

4. The protocol defines the measures of performance and incorporates information collection that can be used for its evaluation and improvement. The individualized plans also contribute information for protocol revision.

5. The protocol forms the foundation for the interdisciplinary plan of care (IPOC) developed for each patient; team members modify the protocol to meet individual patients' needs. The individual care plan notes the exceptions to the protocol.

Guidelines as the Source of Protocols   Patient management protocols are adapted from clinical practice guidelines—"systematically developed statements to assist practitioner and patient decisions about appropriate health care for specific clinical circumstances."[15] Several hundred conditions now have nationally promulgated guidelines that serve as a basis for local review and implementation. Many conditions have several published guidelines. The protocol implements the selected guideline at a particular institution. Well-managed inpatient HCOs have protocols in place for several dozens of their most common conditions.

The National Guideline Clearinghouse (NGC) provides a web-based library of guidelines contributed by qualified clinical organizations. Listed guidelines must contain a "systematic review, a rigorous protocol-driven literature review that summarizes evidence by identifying, selecting, assessing, and synthesizing the findings of similar but separate studies." The NGC explains the desired content of the systematic review and expects to expand listing requirements in the future, emphasizing relative benefits and harms of treatment.[16]

Key components of the NGC guidelines include the following:

- Structured abstracts (summaries) about each guideline and its development
- Links to full-text guidelines, where available, and/or ordering information for print copies
- Personal digital assistant downloads of the NGC's "Complete Summary" for all guidelines represented in the database
- A guideline comparison utility for a side-by-side comparison of attributes of two or more guidelines
- Unique guideline comparisons called Guideline Syntheses covering similar topics, highlighting areas of similarity and difference, with international comparisons
- An electronic forum—NGC-L—for exchanging information on clinical practice guidelines and their development, implementation, and use
- An annotated bibliography database on guideline development methodology, structure, evaluation, and implementation
- An expert commentary feature
- Disease-specific outcomes and process measures[17]

As of 2014, the NGC has more than 2,500 guidelines covering most common diseases and conditions and a number of prevention activities. The Center also has several hundred functional guidelines.

No guideline should ever be implemented without careful review of the implications of using it in a specific institution. The review should be undertaken by a PIT representing all potential users. The PIT should explore all the ramifications of the protocol, including trials as necessary. The development process has at least three components: It encourages discussion of the debatable issues and builds consensus. It helps the caregivers learn new approaches. It pilot tests the proposed protocol against current practice and identifies supply, equipment, and training needs.

Translating Guidelines to Patient Management Protocols

Protocols must be reviewed regularly to identify changes in the evidence for specific practices. The NGC's comparison tool makes it easy to identify the changes in guidelines. The local PIT is reassembled periodically to consider these changes.

Exhibit 5.4 outlines the Clinical Highlights portion of the protocol for diagnosis and treatment of chest pain and acute coronary syndrome developed by the Institute for Clinical Systems Improvement (ICSI). Chest pain is the most common symptom of acute myocardial infarction (AMI, or heart attack). The ICSI guideline is one of many AMI guidelines listed by the NGC:

Example of a Patient Management Protocol

> The recommendations for diagnosis and treatment of chest pain and acute coronary syndrome (ACS) are presented in the form of 7 algorithms with 126 components, accompanied by detailed annotations. Algorithms are provided in [https://www.icsi.org/_asset/ydv4b3/ACS-Interactive1112b.pdf] for Chest Pain Screening; Emergency Intervention; ST-Segment Elevation Myocardial Infarction (STEMI); Acute Myocardial Infarction Complications; Special Workup; Non-Cardiac Causes; and Clinic Evaluation. Clinical highlights and selected annotations (numbered to correspond with the algorithm) follow.[18]

Exhibit 5.4 is a summary of the seven algorithms (presented as flowcharts), which are backed in turn by a 91-page documentation and discussion. More than 5 million patients a year will appear at emergency departments (EDs) with this life-threatening symptom, averaging about three patients a day for all the EDs in the nation. Others will appear at other care sites. The guideline begins with "quickly," requires "immediate assessment" to identify chest pains "suggestive of serious illness," and calls for triage "based on a validated risk assessment" (bullets 1 through 3 in Exhibit 5.4). For serious patients, treatment begins "within 30 to 60 minutes of arrival" with definitive treatment (PCI) within 90 minutes (bullet 5). The guideline

EXHIBIT 5.4

Clinical
Highlights of
Guidelines
for Acute
Chest Pain,
Institute for
Clinical Systems
Improvement

- On initial contact with the health care system, high-risk patients need to be identified quickly and referred to an emergency department via the 911 system. (*Annotations #1, 2, 4, 5, 6; Aim #1*)
- Patients whose chest pain symptoms are suggestive of serious illness need immediate assessment in a monitored area and early therapy to include an immediate electrocardiogram (ECG), intravenous access, oxygen, aspirin, and other appropriate medical therapies. (*Annotations #20 and 30; Aims #1 and 3*)
- Triage and management of patients with chest pain and unstable angina should be based on a validated risk assessment system and clinical findings. (*Annotation #39*)
- Patients with low-risk symptoms could be evaluated as outpatients. (*Annotations #39, 49, 50*)
- Thrombolysis for ST-elevation, myocardial infarction (MI) or left bundle branch block (LBBB) should be instituted within 30 to 60 minutes of arrival, or angiogram/primary percutaneous coronary intervention (PCI) should be performed within 90 minutes of arrival, with a target of less than 60 minutes. High-risk patients initially treated at non-PCI-capable facilities who cannot be transferred for PCI within 90 minutes should receive thrombolysis followed by as-soon-as-possible transfer to a PCI-capable facility. (*Annotations #54, 55, 58, 59, 60, 61; Aim #2*)
- Recommend use of the following medications: P2Y12 inhibitor and aspirin (or P2Y12 inhibitor alone if aspirin allergic) at admission. Avoid P2Y12 inhibitor if cardiac surgery is anticipated. Use beta-blockers whenever possible and/or angiotensin-converting enzyme (ACE) inhibitors/angiotensin receptor blockers at 24 hours if stable, nitrates (when indicated), and statins whenever possible. (*Annotations #22, 65, 67; Aim #3*)
- Recommend use of cardiac rehabilitation. (*Annotations #76, 78*)

Source: Davis T, Bluhm J, Burke R, Iqbal Q, Kim K, Kokoszka M, Larson T, Puppala V, Setterlund L, Vuong K, Zwank M. Institute for Clinical Systems Improvement. Diagnosis and Treatment of Chest Pain and Acute Coronary Syndrome (ACS). http://bit.ly.ACS1112. Updated November 2012, https://www.icsi.org/_asset/ydv4b3/ACS-Interactive1112b.pdf, p. 12.

then recommends medications and rehabilitation for follow-up (bullets 6 and 7). Excellence means every patient is correctly diagnosed, and every patient who has a diagnosis of myocardial infarction or left bundle branch block gets every step.

From a management perspective, this guideline is challenging. Here is what must happen to ensure compliance:

- Arrangements must be made to train 911 responders.
- Emergency physicians, other emergency caregivers, cardiologists, and primary care physicians must reach consensus about accepting or modifying the guidelines for local use. This will involve a local review team and a publicized opportunity for those not on the team to comment.

- A triage nurse or physician for each shift must be trained to identify ischemic pain. (Potential AMI patients arrive without notice, on any shift.) The step is critical:

  > Initial errors in ECG interpretation can result in up to 12% of patients being categorized inappropriately (ST elevation versus no elevation), demonstrating a potential benefit of accurate computer-interpreted electrocardiography and facsimile transmission to an expert.[19]

- Twelve-lead ECG equipment must be made readily available in the ED. Supplies and equipment for advanced life support must also be available.
- Several caregivers on each shift must be trained in administering the 12-lead ECG so that one is available when needed. "Code teams" to handle cardiac arrest and manage advanced life support must be trained. For smaller departments, telemedicine coverage for skilled ECG interpretation must be arranged.
- All ED nurses must be trained in the initial care, so that they start it without written orders when the triage person indicates it.
- A mechanism must be in place to deliver the blood draw to the laboratory. The laboratory must respond with blood chemistry analyses within about 20 minutes.
- Arrangements must be made for skilled ECG interpretation, by training emergency physicians, acquiring interpretation software, or forwarding to a cardiologist. The laboratory data must also be interpreted by a skilled physician.
- Consensus must be reached in advance on the criteria for selecting among the treatment options, which vary substantially in cost, effectiveness, and risk of complications depending on the patient's exact condition.
- Provision must be made for thrombolysis reperfusion and PCI within 60 minutes. A team from the cardiology service line usually performs these procedures.
- Informed consent for PCI or open-heart surgery must be obtained from the patient or advocate, if possible.

Taken as a whole, steps on the guideline represented a new level of performance for most EDs when they emerged in the mid-1990s.[20] The guidelines and the evidence are strong enough to suggest a legal standard of care—EDs failing to meet it are at risk for malpractice liability. Several critical elements are about organization and teamwork. Consensus building, training, advance preparation, and practice are the keys to success.

Functional Protocols

Functional protocols are step-wise procedures for specific components of care, ranging from the simplest, like hand washing, to checklists for complex and dangerous treatments, like surgery and cancer therapy. Exhibit 5.5 is an example of a functional protocol.

EXHIBIT 5.5

Functional
Protocol for
Medication
Order and
Fulfillment

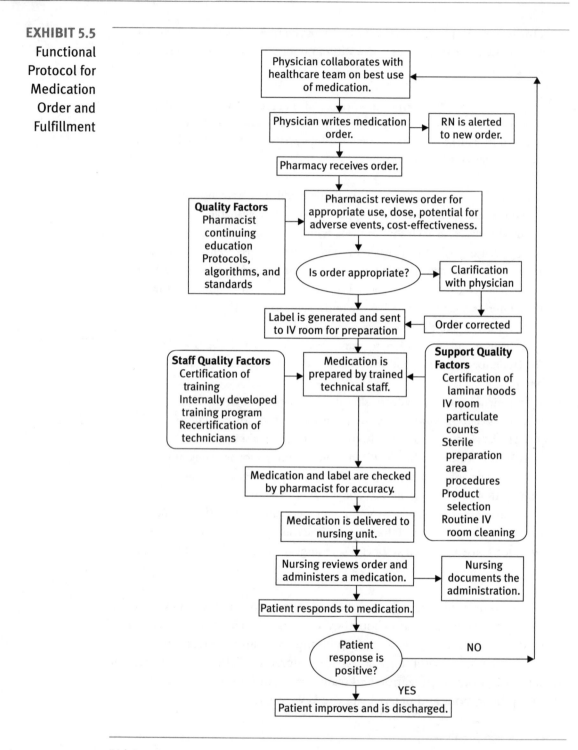

IV: intravenous

Functional protocols exist in large numbers. They are designed to ensure that the activity will have the desired outcome (e.g., the wound dressing will protect the wound, the laboratory value will be correct), but they also provide a basis for teamwork, and they simplify and standardize the medical record. Functional protocols are major contributors to patient safety. Most failures—from falls to infections to wrong-site surgery to drug errors—trace to incomplete, inaccurate, or overlooked functional protocols. These failures cause tens of thousands of undesirable outcomes each year, and the available evidence suggests that little progress has been made toward their correction.[21]

Functional protocols improve processes by several different mechanisms:[22]

- Eliminating unnecessary or redundant tasks—these often appear when different protocols or usual practices are compared.
- Alerting for tasks previously overlooked or omitted—these often improve quality by ensuring the optimal outcome or by preventing a complication.
- Standardizing supplies, with savings through volume discounts, inventory, and training costs.
- Scheduling or sequencing to reduce errors or delays.
- Substituting lower-cost personnel for specific activities.
- Reengineering the care process—the new process may combine several of the preceding opportunities and require substantial investment, but it delivers a better product overall.

Good functional protocols have the following components:

1. *Authorization*—statement of who may order the procedure
2. *Indication*—statement clarifying clinical conditions that are appropriate use of the protocol
3. *Contraindications*—conditions where the procedure must be modified, replaced, or avoided
4. *Required supplies, equipment, and conditions*—all special requirements and how they will be met
5. *Actions*—clear, step-by-step statements of what must be done
6. *Recording*—instructions for recording the procedure and observation of the patient's reaction
7. *Follow-up*—subsequent actions, including checks on the patient's response, measures of effectiveness, indications for repeating the procedure, and disposal or cleanup of supplies

The profession most directly involved usually establishes the functional protocol, often from professional textbooks. Modification may be necessary to accommodate the equipment and facilities or the patient population of a specific HCO. In many cases, the profession involved can apply the protocol without assistance. Some applications will require review by other profession and support personnel to ensure coordination.

Functional protocols tend to be stable over time and between patients and institutions, but they can be modified to improve quality and efficiency.

An important source of improvement is eliminating unnecessary or inappropriate procedures by making the indications or authorizations more restrictive. For example, protocols for expensive drugs and diagnostic tests can require failure of simpler approaches as indications. Some very expensive procedures can require prior approval or a formal second opinion. The activities themselves can be modified to be safer or less expensive; changes in equipment and supplies often require such adjustments. Follow-up specifications can improve patients' reactions by describing specific signs or symptoms and the appropriate response. Computerized order entry and medication reconciliation systems are examples of procedure improvements in drug administration. The new systems have better alerts to guard against prescribing the wrong drug, administering the wrong dose, or recording the dose incorrectly. The result is both lower cost and higher quality.[23]

Sets of interrelated functional protocols have become more commonplace. Surgical care provides several examples. Preoperative care includes obtaining informed consent, instructing the patient, obtaining final diagnostic values from lab and x-ray, completing the pre-anesthesia examination, and administering preoperative medications. To perform surgery without delay, each activity must be orchestrated to occur at the earliest possible time and in the proper order. The preoperative care process requires advance agreement on the tasks and their order among several clinical support and medical professions. Many of these agreements are independent of the patient's specific disease. They become components of patient management protocols for several hundred surgical procedures.

The flow process design of Exhibit 5.5 is popular in guidelines and protocols because it shows the sequencing and conditional relationships of each step. It can be accessible on personal data devices. Reference to the flow process is superior to memory. Other approaches—detailing activity by the calendar or day of stay, for example—are also used. The best form would be the one yielding the best outcomes. The flowchart with detailed documentation is the most prevalent.

Checklists

Checklists are similar to functional protocols, but they are focused on patients rather than procedures. A checklist is used in the surgical time-out to verify several critical elements, such as the right patient, the right surgery, and any relevant additional conditions. A checklist for hospitalized general medical patients, directing the team's attention to pneumococcal immunization, pressure ulcers (bedsores), catheter-associated urinary tract infections, and deep venous thrombosis was associated with "significantly increased documentation and adherence to care processes" for these conditions.[24]

Caregiver Training and Selection

The HCO must have a **credentialing** process, described in Chapter 6, to ensure caregiver competence (knowledge and skill obtained through formal education and experience and regulated by licensure and certification bodies) and proficiency (evidence that the clinician applies the knowledge and skills appropriately). Credentialing applies to specific patient populations defined by treatment, diagnosis, or age. For example, a physician would be credentialed for uncomplicated vaginal deliveries or for care of diabetic patients.

Credentialing
The process of validating a professional's eligibility for medical staff membership and/or privileges to be granted on the basis of academic preparation, licensing, training, certifications, and performance.

Credentialing must be repeated to ensure continued competence and proficiency. Protocols change as new treatment modalities and new technology are developed. For beginning professional caregivers and nonprofessional clinical workers, substantial in-house training programs may be required with a phase-in approach to delivering care independently.

Caregiving professionals must receive refresher courses and updated education on new and established protocols. This is typically accomplished with an in-house education training and development function.

Record Management

Excellence requires that all caregivers have two kinds of knowledge: communication of patients' current needs, and understanding of the clinically indicated responses. The first is now supported by the electronic health record (EHR). The record provides a history for evaluating the patient's current condition and instantaneous communication to all team members. The second is now supported by access to web-based information. Guides to developing the differential diagnosis and evaluating the entries are now easily accessible on handheld devices. The guidelines supporting the protocols can be accessed to understand the underlying science and its limitations. Even moderate-sized HCOs will have several hundred protocols. These are also electronically accessible, increasingly on mobile devices. It is easy to refresh knowledge about less frequently encountered diagnoses and treatments.

Telemedicine is increasingly important in small HCOs. The EHR can be accessed by distant specialists. Audio, video, and processes like the 12-lead ECG in Exhibit 5.3 enhance the interchange with remote specialists. Improved patient outcomes have been documented.[25]

Clinical Support Services and Specialist Consultation

Excellent care requires an array of specialist consultation and referral, including the clinical support services such as laboratory and imaging. The HCO's credentialing process and operational scorecards support excellent services from all clinical support services and specialties. A large team of qualified specialists is obviously an asset, but rural communities cannot support more than a few people. Formal affiliations with larger centers are superior to individual patient referrals. They establish sharing of expensive resources like magnetic resonance imagers, support for measured performance and annual goal setting, and educational services and advice on protocols. Telemedicine and referral linkages are making remote consultation more practical, extending services in rural areas. The anticipated volume of activity can be established using the epidemiologic planning model.

Using Unexpected Events

Chapter 3 noted the importance of a reporting system for "unexpected events," including clinical errors and misadventures, accidents, near accidents, property losses, and any other situations where reality fell short of patients', guests', or associates' expectations. The reports generate a substantial file that is an important resource for continuous improvement. Each incident must be evaluated. Often additional information must be collected. For serious events, a team must establish the HCO's appropriate response to the individuals involved. Many event reports summarize "service recovery" (chapters 11 and 15), where the response is begun at the time of the event.

The reports create a valuable statistical record, revealing when, where, and how unfortunate results occur, and providing OFIs to reduce the incidence. Clinical unexpected events are pursued further:

1. Reporting near misses of serious events is encouraged. These are more frequent than actual events and provide insight into preventive opportunities.
2. Individual events are evaluated to establish the patient harm and HCO's appropriate liability.
3. Individual events causing serious or potentially serious clinical consequences are studied to improve protocols and prevent recurrence.
4. Frequently occurring similar events are pursued as OFIs, using PITs to improve protocols.
5. When appropriate, a financial settlement is offered to the injured party as an alternative to the injured party's right to pursue legal action. In cases where it appears that the harm was unavoidable, no financial settlement is offered.
6. The HCO is prepared to vigorously defend its position in the event the injured party chooses legal action.[26]

These six steps, now common in many leading HCOs, have proven successful. They have essentially eliminated the "malpractice crisis" for HCOs that implement them. Most injured parties accept an immediate settlement that approximates what they would receive in court, after deduction of attorneys' fees. The HCO saves attorneys' fees and court costs.[27]

Individualizing Patient Care Planning and Treatment

Protocols are not mechanistic. Caregivers are obligated to monitor the patient's progress and to modify the protocol to fit the patient's needs, as Exhibit 5.2 shows.

When the evidence behind a protocol step is not conclusive, the IOM aim of patient-centered care and the ethical principle of autonomy on which it is based become critical. For example, for the diagnosis of localized, low-risk prostate cancer, there is an array of treatment options and a lack of evidence that any of the treatment choices is superior. However, the costs are widely variable, as shown in Exhibit 5.6.[28] The patient will choose. Providing him with comprehensive and accurate advice is clearly critical to achieving both patient-centered care and efficiency. Over time, comparative effectiveness research will improve our understanding of prostate cancer care. It is essential for providing better information about alternatives for both patient and physician decision making.[29,30] The underlying uncertainty will be diminished, but it will never disappear. There will always be a frontier of scientific knowledge, where patient counseling will make important differences in total cost of care for a community.

The **interdisciplinary plan of care** is a process that includes the patient, family, and all clinical disciplines relevant to the diagnoses. It should begin

Interdisciplinary plan of care (IPOC)

A documented process that includes the patient, the family, and all clinical disciplines involved in planning and providing care to patients, from system point of entry, throughout the entire acute care episode, and to the next level of care.

Treatment	Explanation	Lifetime Cost
Watchful waiting	Observation without monitoring; palliative treatment when symptomatic	$24,520
Active surveillance	Close follow-up with exams and testing; treatment with curative intent for disease progression	$39,884
Radical prostatectomy	Complete removal of prostate gland	$38,180
Brachytherapy	Implantation of radioactive seeds	$35,374
Intensity-modulation radiation therapy	Advanced radiation beam therapy targeted at tumor	$48,699

EXHIBIT 5.6
Average Lifetime Costs for Treatment of Localized, Low-Risk Prostate Cancer in Men Age 65+

Source: Data from Hayes, J. H., D. A. Ollendorf, S. D. Pearson, M. J. Barry, P. W. Kantoff, P. A. Lee, and P. M. McMahon. 2013. "Observation Versus Initial Treatment for Men with Localized, Low-Risk Prostate Cancer: A Cost-Effectiveness Analysis." *Annals of Internal Medicine* 158: 853–60.

at entry and extend through the entire care episode to the next level of care.[31] The IPOC is not replaced by patient management protocols; every patient's individual needs should be evaluated to make sure the protocol will meet them. The IPOC is a foundation for case management in cases of exceptional complexity.

An IPOC is generally initiated by a nurse beginning with the relevant protocols and developed in collaboration with other members of the caregiving team. It includes input from the patient and family. The caregiving team develops goals for the episode of care and across the trajectory of the illness or condition. The IPOC addresses psychosocial and spiritual support, educational needs, cultural and linguistic needs, home environment, community resources, and postdischarge planning.

The IPOC forms the basis for coordinating multiple therapeutic services, such as surgical or other invasive interventions, intensive care, pharmaceuticals, and rehabilitation therapies (physical, occupational, speech). A good IPOC will address all of the following elements:

1. *Assessment*—comprehensive review of the patient's diagnosis, disabilities, and needs and identification of any unique risks
2. *Treatment goals*—statement of clinical goals, such as "elimination of congestive heart failure," and functional goals, such as "restore ability to dress and feed self"
3. *Component activities*—a list, often selected from relevant care guidelines and functional protocols, of procedures desired for the patient
4. *Recording*—a formal routine for recording what was done and reporting it to others caring for the patient
5. *Measures of progress and a time schedule for improvement*—where possible, measures of improvement should be used and should parallel the goals developed in the assessment
6. *Danger signals and contraindications*—specific events indicating a need to reconsider the plan

The IPOC supports both the patient management protocol and the case management approach to improvement. Two critical aspects are patient listening, being vigilant to subtle changes in the patient's condition, and communicating about the patient's progress with the attending physician and other caregivers.

Case Management

Some patients will have exceptionally complex care needs that will require formalizing a comprehensive clinical strategy. Case management uses expanded IPOCs for complex problems such as multiple concurrent conditions and expensive chronic diseases like end-stage heart failure and multiple sclerosis.

Care for these patients is usually long term and often goes beyond medical assistance. Emotional support is often an issue. Family and community contributions are important, and special equipment and facilities are often necessary. In the most complex cases, the care plan may be a written consensus of professional viewpoints, closely monitored to gain the best possible results while minimizing costs.[32,33] Although case management is routine for very complex long-term conditions, it is not routinely necessary. The evidence does not show that case management reduces overall care costs.[34]

Improving Community Health

An overall population health strategy must address not only excellence in personal care but also disease prevention and health promotion. The issue is central to the control of costs of healthcare.[35] **Prevention** is generally considered to be direct interventions to avoid or reduce disease or disability. Many preventive activities are focused on individuals, such as immunization and healthy lifestyles, but much prevention involves community-wide activities such as pure water, crime, and legislation on firearms and dangerous substances. Population health includes all activities to change patient or customer behavior. It is undertaken by caregivers and by civic agencies such as public health departments, education systems, and voluntary associations. It has become an important topic for employers.

> **Prevention**
> A direct intervention to avoid or reduce disease or disability.

HCOs provide prevention and population health for four reasons:

1. The moral commitment of all caregiving professions is to health, clearly including prevention.
2. Prevention opportunities arise from the same scientific knowledge as treatment opportunities. More than 1,300 of the NGC guidelines reference prevention, and the number is increasing.[36]
3. Healthcare professionals are respected authority figures, and their advice is given at times when the patient is receptive.
4. Prevention helps communities that own HCOs. Each episode of illness prevented translates eventually to reductions in cost of care. A healthier community has more workers and lower health insurance costs, making it a better place to build or expand business. (Ironically, disease prevention reduces hospital and physician revenues. Well-managed institutions do it anyway; it is probably essential to avoid bankrupting the major healthcare financing programs.)

Prevention

Prevention can be categorized as primary, secondary, or tertiary, and health promotion tools can be used to change behavior on all three levels. **Primary prevention** activities are those that take place before the

> **Primary prevention**
> Activities that take place before the disease occurs to eliminate or reduce its occurrence.

Secondary prevention
Activities that reduce the consequences of existing disease, often by early detection and treatment.

Tertiary prevention
Activities that reduce or avoid complications or sequellae in existing disease or disability.

disease occurs to eliminate or reduce its occurrence. Immunizations, use of seat belts and condoms, sewage treatment, and restrictions on alcohol sales are examples. **Secondary prevention** reduces the consequences of disease, often by early detection and treatment. Self-examinations for cancer; routine dental inspections; mammographies; colonoscopies; and management of chronic diseases like diabetes, hypertension, and asthma are examples. **Tertiary prevention** is the avoidance of complications or sequelae. Early physical therapy for strokes, retraining in activities of daily living, and respite services to help family caregivers are examples. Secondary and tertiary prevention are done mainly by caregivers and the patients themselves.

Functional and patient management protocols should incorporate prevention and health promotion. For example, functional protocols for injections, surgical interventions, and other treatments prevent both hospital-acquired infections and injury to caregivers. Home care visit protocols include inspection for hazards and discussion of patient needs and symptoms with family members. Diabetic and cardiovascular care protocols include selection of the optimal pharmacological treatment and guidance to the patient in lifestyle and nutrition. Prenatal, postnatal, and child care protocols include immunizations; checks for potential developmental disabilities; and education for the mother on child development, nutrition, home safety, and domestic violence.

Population Health

HCOs differ in the extent to which they pursue population health. Those with an excellence-in-care mission focus on those services that occur between the caregiver and the individual patient. Those with a community health mission extend their efforts to broader initiatives to minimize disease and its impact. The Affordable Care Act stimulated transition to community health missions. Chapter 9 addresses the distinction and its implications as well as strategies for improving population health.

Improving Clinical Performance

Each service line has specific performance measures, benchmarks, negotiated goals, and OFIs for team performance, with detail distributed to each of its operating units. It uses PITs to pursue the OFIs and keep the protocols updated. Success requires a cultural (Chapter 2) foundation as well so that the following become true and are believed by most associates:

- The values of the organization are advertised. Recruitment emphasizes the philosophy of the organization so that it attracts caregivers and employees who believe in its mission and who are committed to excellence.

- The culture encourages individual judgment to identify unique patient needs and unusual circumstances. It encourages informal consultation and collaboration to provide individualized care.
- All workers and managers understand the importance of respect for each individual's contribution, open exchange of information, cooperation, and prompt response to questions.
- Participation in the development of goals is widespread.
- The climate is blame free. It encourages change while also reassuring associates of their personal security. The major components of reassurance include consistent procedures and processes; well-understood avenues for comment with prompt, sensitive response; and recognition of the importance of dissent.
- Compliance with cultural expectations (e.g., scheduling, documentation, timeliness, courtesy) is accepted as essential. Violations are discouraged, with measured sanctions promptly applied. For example, the penalty for incomplete medical records (usually a temporary loss of privileges) is automated and routine. As a result, well-run organizations have few incomplete records.
- Sanctions are used reluctantly but predictably in the case of repeated unjustifiable practice.

Lengthy as this list is, it is clearly doable, and excellent HCOs do it. Fulfilling this list creates a culture of high reliability[37] or of "continuously learning healthcare."[38]

As discussed in Chapter 2, senior leaders establish an organizational culture of quality and safety and focus priorities on clinical performance and quality outcomes. Clinical managers integrate quality and safety principles into the workplace. They should also serve as examples by modeling quality principles in their interactions with staff, patients, and guests.[39]

People

Building an Engaged Workforce

The service excellence model (Chapter 2) is critical in patient care.[40] It commits the HCO to meeting caregivers' needs, maintaining "a great place to give care." Doing that systematically builds a cadre of like-minded, engaged caregivers who help one another to achieve excellence. The result is a culture where team expectations help individuals and vice versa. The pursuit of excellence becomes a routine and rewarding part of life. The HCO management uses the servant leadership model to maintain the culture.

In the daily care of patients, caregiving teams tend to be small and transient. They change composition as the attending physician, hospitalist, nurses, and pharmacy and therapy professionals change. Many teams have physician or advanced practice providers as leaders. Nonprofessional caregivers are important contributors. These teams "huddle" frequently to resolve questions and coordinate care. They are drawn from larger and more permanent accountability units that participate in the formal goal-setting, performance measurement, and reward system activities and that have resources to support them.

Clinical unit managers play a critical role in supporting the culture of clinical excellence.[41] They must be trained in servant leadership, in understanding the performance measures, and in the continuous improvement process. Much of this training is ongoing, but several hours of classes and a formal system of just-in-time assistance, mentoring, and review are important.[42]

Organization of Clinical Units

Clinical units are organized by grouping patients with similar needs. Service lines, the largest clinical units, generally parallel major clinical specialties. Smaller units are also built around clinical similarity, creating work teams that become skilled in specialized care.

The complexities of excellent care are such that many HCOs use specialized internal consulting activities to support their work teams and clinically oriented PITs. Internal specialists in quality management have additional education in quality monitoring and statistical issues, and often continuous improvement systems such as Lean. Healthcare quality management professionals may complete special training and pass an examination sponsored by the National Association for Healthcare Quality to be designated a Certified Professional in Healthcare Quality.[43] Infection preventionists are generally nurses or other clinicians with advanced education in epidemiology and microbiology. They may be certified by the Association for Professionals in Infection Control and Epidemiology and earn the Certification in Infection Prevention and Control credential.[44] Physicians are certified by the Infectious Disease Society of America, through the American Board of Internal Medicine. Similarly, risk management professionals may earn certification sponsored by the American Society for Healthcare Risk Management.[45] The specialists and their staffs are truly consultants. They do not have authority over accountability units. Such authority is known to erode the empowerment of the clinical teams.[46]

Exhibit 5.7 shows a possible organization of service lines supported by several centralized functional services and an internal consulting unit. Reality is far more dynamic than the exhibit depicts. In effective HCOs, associates collaborate constantly both in clinical teams around individual patients and in improvement teams to design protocols and work processes. The exhibit's framework provides a mechanism for setting improvement goals, achieving the collaboration those goals require, and resolving issues arising in the implementation.

Interprofessional Conflicts

Clinical professionals are recognized in a formal process of certification, licensure, or registration. Several hundred such processes exist in healthcare, more

EXHIBIT 5.7
Organization of
Clinical Services

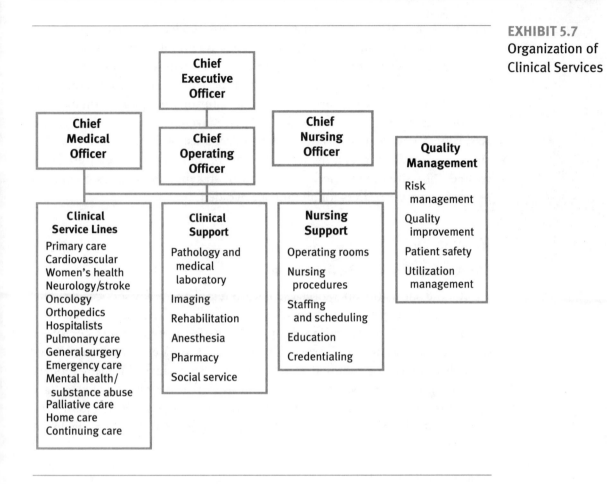

than 100 in medicine alone. They typically require both classroom and experiential education, as well as continuing education to maintain competencies. Many caregiving teams have several professionals. Disputes over professional rights are common, especially when fees are involved.

Professionalism is justified as protecting the consumer by establishing knowledge and skill requirements. It is important to understand that it also creates economic monopolies that increase the profession's income and the customer's cost of care.[47] Thus the questions of professional domain—what requirements are necessary for a given task—is one in which customer stakeholders have a profound interest. One role of the HCO management is to exercise that interest wisely. Protocols create many opportunities to substitute less expensive nonprofessionals for professionals. Most applicable law makes this acceptable so long as professional supervision is available. Part of the negotiation to translate guidelines to protocols should include establishing the clinically necessary level of training for each task, as opposed to the political position of the professions involved. The evidence-based rules of medicine and management are the correct drivers; tasks should be completed by the lowest level of skill required to do them safely. When a higher skill is necessary, the HCO should supply it. That need can arise collectively from published concern or individually from a caregiver's assessment of a patient's need.

These substitutions often create potential income losses for the practitioners. Well-managed organizations must be sensitive to income concerns, but they must press forward with sound solutions in spite of them. The criterion must be evidence of safety and effectiveness. The rules under the Resolving Disagreements section in Chapter 2 must be applied in clinical discussions. The disputants must leave the debate thinking that they were fairly treated. The situations where one group of stakeholders uses its economic power to stymie progress for all must be avoided.

Measures

Measuring Clinical Performance

Exhibit 5.8 shows the operational scorecard template for any service line. The operational scorecard can be applied to units within service lines, such as specific primary care offices or inpatient care units for acute care services, often with specific outcome and process measures. Automated processing allows immediate reporting of any deterioration in performance. Monthly reports can track goal achievement, while other measures remain available in the data warehouse. When the service line is separately incorporated, as in a joint venture, a strategic scorecard (Exhibit 1.10) is required as well, adding financial performance.

Demand and Output

Output—the use of services—is captured in accounting systems, which generate detailed data on the kind of service (or occasionally product, such as a drug). Demand for care is often inferred from output, but it can be measured in patient scheduling and intake systems. Direct measurement permits identification of scheduling delays and lost cases, valuable quality and marketing indicators.

The epidemiologic planning model constructs demand forecasts from available community information. Forecast demand provides a denominator for market share. It can support detailed analysis of community sectors selecting the HCO for specific services. It is also useful in evaluating effectiveness. The model can construct expectations for major clinical events. These can be compared to actual demand to identify overuse or underuse.

Quality Assessment

Both outcomes and process quality measures have expanded substantially in recent years. The new measures often contain sophisticated adjustments to remove factors beyond the service's control. They have become practical as electronic record keeping has expanded.

EXHIBIT 5.8
Profile of
Service Line
Operational
Scorecard

Dimensions	Examples
	Input Measures

Demand

Requests for care	Patient arrivals, appointment requests, consultation and referral requests; often specified by patient age, service, and location
Market share	Percent of total demand from community
Appropriateness of service	Percent of expected or benchmark demand from epidemiologic planning model
Logistics of service	Hours of availability

Cost/Resources

Total costs	Labor, supplies, plant, indirect costs for service line
Resource condition	Occupancy and percent of capacity rates, age of equipment, failure rates of equipment

Human Resources

Supply	Staffing levels, staffing shortfalls, vacancy rates
Training	Average hours of training per associate
Associate satisfaction	Associate loyalty, retention or termination, absenteeism, work loss days from accident or injury

Output Measures

Output/Productivity

Patients treated	Discharge counts by specified group
Cost per case	Total costs/discharges by specified group
Cost per treatment	Costs for specific activity such as surgical operations or examinations/patients receiving

Quality

Clinical outcomes	Mortality, patient safety events, readmissions, patient condition at discharge
Procedural quality	Procedural measures assessing completion of specific tasks or events
Structural quality	Structural measures assessing availability and adequacy of service, particularly staffing and facility safety

Customer Satisfaction

Patient satisfaction	Postdischarge surveys, counts of "Caught in the Act," complaints, service recovery, and unexpected incidents
Referring physician satisfaction	Survey, rounding, complaints
Other customer satisfaction	Community surveys, boundary-spanning activities
Access	Delays for service, unfilled demand

The National Quality Measures Clearinghouse, a service of the federal Agency for Healthcare Research and Quality, provides detailed information on definitions, adjustments, scientific foundation, and rationale. Many measures are used by several sites and can be benchmarked. As of August 2014, the clearinghouse had 2,179 disease-specific measures. A hierarchical array associates related measures. Most of the measures are outcomes. Some measure appropriateness of care or procedural compliance. The clearinghouse is the starting point for any discussion of clinical performance measurement.[48]

Outcomes quality measures are aggregated from groups of patients with similar diseases. Disease specificity is often a key to improving patient management protocols. In general, specific measures should be available for the smallest groups that are statistically meaningful.

Good guidelines and protocols contain their own measurements of quality. For the chest pain guideline in Exhibit 5.4, the principal outcome measure is percentage of patients with AMI surviving at discharge or at a specific time after discharge. A second outcome measure is an error rate: a count of patients turned over to other care at the first-bullet phase whose diagnosis was later revised to AMI.

The Joint Commission National Patient Safety Goals promote specific improvements in patient safety. Updated each year since 2003, the goals include both outcomes and process measures:

- Accuracy of patient identification
- Communication among caregivers
- Medications safety
- Infections
- Medication management
- Patient falls
- Response to changes in a patient's condition
- The Universal Protocol for invasive diagnosis or treatment (conducting a preprocedure verification process, marking the procedure site, and performing a time-out)[49]

In addition, The Joint Commission looks for evidence that the HCO encourages patients' active involvement in their own care as a safety strategy and explicitly identifies and addresses safety risks.[50]

Quality is increasingly publicly reported. The Leapfrog Group publishes a hospital safety score.[51] The National Quality Forum publishes its *Field Guide*, cataloguing several hundred outcomes and process measures, with information on users and sources of benchmarks.[52] WhyNotTheBest.org publishes a wide range of hospital-specific values, drawn mainly from the Centers for Medicare & Medicaid Services (CMS) Medicare data.[53] CMS plans to publish hospital quality rankings.[54] These measures usually incorporate several service lines, more like the governing board's strategic scorecard than a unit's or a service line's. They are useful in benchmarking and goal setting.

Quality measures must be carefully handled statistically. Extensive specification and adjustment are necessary to make "apples to apples" comparison, more accurately described as adjusting for factors in the patient population that are beyond the unit's control. Size and sensitivity can be a problem.[55] A small ED with 250 AMI admissions per year might have only three deaths per month. Adjustment of the survival rates for risk factors such as comorbid conditions, obesity, or smoking would be appropriate, but the high success rates will make any detection of change difficult. Process measures are useful supplements. They would cover completion of various steps such as administration of aspirin and oxygen, percentages of patients meeting timelines, delays for patients failing to meet timelines, and other process failures. The expectations would be that compliance approached 100 percent and that individual failures could be investigated for correctable causes. The process measures will be sensitive where the outcomes are not, but it is important to select processes that are important and scientifically justified.

Structural measures of quality, basically counts of availability of appropriate resources, are now rarely useful for quality assessment.

Quality Measures and Pay for Performance

A growing number of private and public healthcare payers, including Medicare, have embraced pay for performance (P4P) as a means to improve the health of patients and foster new behaviors from physicians.[56] As stated in Chapter 1, P4P initiatives are collaborations with providers and other stakeholders to ensure that valid quality measures are used, outcomes measures are true indicators of quality of care, providers are not being pulled in conflicting directions, and providers have reward for achieving actual improvement. P4P is intended to foster new behavior from physicians by providing incentives that improve care for people with chronic illnesses. P4P also enables health plans to treat sicker populations without spending more, although more research is needed to gauge long-term results.[57,58] It is expected that P4P, as a national health policy initiative, will change physician and hospital behaviors, improve healthcare quality, and decrease costs,[59,60] without unintended consequences such as overtreatment or a focus on the incentive to the exclusion of other mitigating factors.[61] This expectation may be more hope than reality.[62] Measures that can be used to identify OFIs often lack the reliability and sensitivity necessary for incentive compensation. Small sample sizes, unusual populations, and simple random variation plague many proposed applications.[63]

Patient Satisfaction and Associate Engagement

Satisfaction data are now collected by contract with companies specializing in patient discharge surveys. Reliable information requires careful monitoring of the sample, rigorous and standardized question design, deliberate efforts to improve response rates, statistical analysis, and benchmarking. Patient satisfaction data now includes Hospital Consumer Assessment of Healthcare Providers and Systems (HCAHPS) measures of patient perception of quality of care as a condition of Medicare participation, with specific questions to address the larger functional services such as nursing and rehabilitation therapies. The HCAHPS questions (available at www.hcahpsonline.org) identify several specific elements of the patient experience that are controlled by the organization, such as pain management and explanation of pharmaceuticals. The questions must be incorporated in commercial patient satisfaction surveys, and public reporting is required and posted on government (U.S Department of Health and Human Services) and other websites.[64] Respondents are identified by disease group, allowing easy tallying for accountable teams.

Clinical associates are also formally surveyed. Their engagement is closely linked to high outcomes performance, retention, and the return on training investments. Physicians are generally associated with service lines; their response is an important source of marketing and quality insight. It is common to supplement surveys with focus groups and rounding to identify OFIs.

Managerial Issues

The issues that trap hospitals in mediocrity are failures of the transformational and evidence-based management process. Over recent decades, evidence-based management has made substantial gains. Arguments about protocols and measurement have been resolved; a governing board that fails to implement these approaches and set improvement goals is increasingly at risk for financial or legal difficulties. As the measures reveal OFIs, management must successfully focus on two issues: sustaining a culture of teamwork and respect, and supporting the system of continuous improvement.

Sustaining a Culture of Teamwork and Respect

Serious illness requires not just teams, but teams of teams. Many of the caregivers contributing to the same patient never meet one another; they are in different locations or on different shifts. Coordination within and between teams becomes an important issue. Breakdowns are most common not within the activities of a single caregiver but in the "handoff" from one caregiver to another and one team to another. Critical information is lost, causing something to be done wrong, delayed, or left undone. Effective team communication is a function of both system and culture. The systems are built around the electronic record and continuous improvement. The electronic record can clearly and succinctly summarize needs, accomplishments, and next steps. It provides the data for many performance measures structured around patient management and functional protocols. Continuous improvement, with its celebrations and financial rewards, reinforces a culture based on commitment to a common mission and values. These systems build confidence that encourages communication among teammates. Leadership that is highly visible and that models appropriate behavior supports the systems and the culture, focusing the teams on patient need.

Maintaining Continuous Clinical Improvement

The record of clinical failure in U.S. HCOs shows quite clearly that the path to excellence is not easy. It requires a solid foundation: protocols, measures, goal setting, continuous improvement, and a culture of empowerment. Behind these lie substantial hidden investments: excellence in knowledge management, statistical expertise, solid processes for negotiating goals, training, a reward system. Behind those lie solid financial management, providing the reserves that support the investments.[65] The record of Baldrige recipients and others committed to excellence shows that progress can be made incrementally; early steps build resources for later, larger ones.

A key factor is leadership commitment. Senior leadership cannot falter. Goals must be achieved; it is far better to achieve a modest goal than to fail at an overly ambitious one. Obvious problems must be addressed. Dishonesty and intractable incompetence must be eliminated. Debate must be encouraged, obstructionism removed. In short, governance and senior leadership must be unequivocally committed.

With that commitment in place, clinical excellence is profitable. The service excellence business model works.[66] High-performing HCOs work strategically with markets and money. Delays are eliminated, quality is improved, and cost is minimized by sizing each service according to its epidemiologic needs. Market share is enhanced because patients are delighted with their service. New equipment is available because funds were on hand to buy it. Credentialing standards can be upheld because the organization is "a great place to give care," but also because it pursues recruitment and individual associate development aggressively.

High-performing HCOs understand both *why* financial success is important and *how* it can be obtained. The underlying reason is that care that meets IOM goals is inherently less costly than care that falls short.

Additional Resources

Carroll, R. (ed.). 2010. *Risk Management Handbook for Health Care Organizations, Student Edition*, 6th ed. San Francisco: Jossey-Bass.

Fallon, Jr., L. F., J. W. Begun, and W. Riley. 2013. *Managing Health Organizations for Quality and Performance*. Burlington, MA: Jones and Bartlett Learning.

Gawande, A. 2009. *The Checklist Manifesto: How to Get Things Right*. New York: Metropolitan Books; American Hospital Association. 2014. "Hospitals in Pursuit of Excellence." [Online information; retrieved 2/6/15.] www.hpoe.org/.

Iezzoni, L. 2012. *Risk Adjustment for Measuring Health Care Outcomes*, 4th ed. Chicago: Health Administration Press.

Institute for Healthcare Improvement. 2015. Home page. [Online information; retrieved 2/6/15.] www.ihi.org/Pages/default.aspx.

Joint Commission. Various years. *Accreditation Standards*. Oakbrook Terrace, IL: Joint Commission.

Joshi, M. S., E. R. Ransom, D. B. Nash, and S. B. Ransom. 2014. *The Healthcare Quality Book: Vision, Strategy, and Tools*, 3rd ed. Chicago: Health Administration Press.

Smith, M. (chair). 2012. *Best Care at Lower Cost: The Path to Continuously Learning Health Care in America*. [Online report; retrieved 8/27/14.] www.iom.edu/Reports/2012/Best-Care-at-Lower-Cost-The-Path-to-Continuously-Learning-Health-Care-in-America.aspx.

Notes

1. WhyNotTheBest.org. 2015. Home page. [Online information; retrieved 8/12/14.] www.whynotthebest.org/.
2. Chassin, M. R. 2013. "VIEWPOINT: Improving the Quality of Health Care: What's Taking So Long." *Health Affairs* 32 (10): 1761–65.
3. Institute of Medicine. 2014. "Establishing Transdisciplinary Professionalism for Improving Health Outcomes: Workshop Summary." Washington, DC: National Academies Press.
4. Begun, J. W., K. R. White, and G. Mosser. 2011. "Interprofessional Care Teams: The Role of the Healthcare Administrator." *Journal of Interprofessional Care* 25: 119–23.
5. Griffith, J. R. 2015. "How Good Are Baldrige Winners?" *Journal of Healthcare Management* 60 (1): 44–61.
6. World Health Organization. 2014. *International Statistical Classification of Diseases and Related Health Problems*, 10th revision, version for 2014. [Online information; retrieved 8/14/14.] www.who.int/classifications/icd/en/.
7. Cabot, R. C. 1911. *Differential Diagnosis*. Philadelphia, PA: W. B. Saunders.
8. Swenson, S. J., J. A. Dilling, D. S. Milliner, R. S. Zimmerman, W. J. Maples, M. E. Lindsay, and G. B. Bartley. 2009. "Quality, the Mayo Clinic Approach." *American Journal of Medical Quality* 24 (5): 428–40.
9. Graber, M. L., R. Trowbridge, J. S. Myers, C. A. Umscheid, W. Strull, and M. H. Kanter. 2014. "The Next Organizational Challenge: Finding and Addressing Diagnostic Error." *Joint Commission Journal on Quality & Patient Safety* 40 (3): 102–10.
10. American Academy of Orthopaedic Surgeons. 2015. "Guidelines for Implementation of the Universal Protocol for the Prevention of Wrong Site, Wrong Procedure and Wrong Person Surgery." [Online information; retrieved 2/6/15.] www3.aaos.org/member/safety/guidelines.cfm.
11. Peterson, E. D., N. M. Albert, A. Amin, J. H. Patterson, and G. C. Fonarow. 2008. "Implementing Critical Pathways and a Multidisciplinary Team Approach to Cardiovascular Disease Management." *American Journal of Cardiology* 102 (5A): 47G–55G.
12. Montori, V. M., and G. H. Guyatt. 2008. "Progress in Evidence-Based Medicine." *Journal of the American Medical Association* 300: 1814–16.
13. Mazmanian, P. E., D. A. Davis, and R. Galbraith. 2009. "Continuing Medical Education Effect on Clinical Outcomes: Effectiveness of Continuing Medical

Education: American College of Chest Physicians Evidence-Based Education Guidelines." *Chest* 135 (3, Suppl.): 49S–55S.

14. Peterson et al. (2008).

15. Field, M. J., and K. N. Lohr (eds.). 1990. *Clinical Practice Guidelines: Directions for a New Program*, 38. Washington, DC: National Academies Press.

16. National Guideline Clearinghouse. 2013. "Introducing the National Guideline Clearinghouse Revised Inclusion Criteria." [Online information; retrieved 8/15/14.] www.guideline.gov/expert/expert-commentary.aspx?id=46924.

17. National Guideline Clearinghouse. 2014. "Guidelines by Topic." [Online information; retrieved 8/15/14.] www.guideline.gov/browse/by-topic.aspx.

18. National Guideline Clearinghouse. 2008. "Diagnosis and Treatment of Chest Pain and Acute Coronary Syndrome." Institute for Clinical Systems Improvement guideline. [Online information; retrieved 5/27/09.] www.guideline.gov/summary/summary.aspx?doc_id=13480&nbr=6889#s23.

19. Ryan, T. J., J. L. Anderson, E. M. Antman, B. A. Braniff, N. H. Brooks, R. M. Califf, L. D. Hillis, L. F. Hiratzka, E. Rapaport, B. J. Riegel, R. O. Russell, E. E. Smith III, and W. D. Weaver. 1996. "ACC/AHA Guidelines for the Management of Patients with Acute Myocardial Infarction: A Report of the American College of Cardiology/American Heart Association Task Force on Practice Guidelines (Committee on Management of Acute Myocardial Infarction)." *Journal of the American College of Cardiology* 28 (5): 1340.

20. Katz, D. A. 1999. "Barriers Between Guidelines and Improved Patient Care: An Analysis of AHCPR's Unstable Angina Clinical Practice Guideline, Agency for Health Care Policy and Research." *Health Services Research* 34 (1, Pt. II): 377–89.

21. Longo, D. R., J. E. Hewett, B. Ge, and S. Schubert. 2005. "The Long Road to Patient Safety: A Status Report on Patient Safety Systems." *Journal of the American Medical Association* 294 (22): 2858–65.

22. Spath, P. L. (ed.). 1997. *Beyond Clinical Paths: Advanced Tools for Outcomes Management*. Chicago: American Hospital Publishing.

23. Agrawal, A., and W. Y. Wu. 2009. "Reducing Medication Errors and Improving Systems Reliability Using an Electronic Medication Reconciliation System." *Joint Commission Journal on Quality and Patient Safety* 35 (2): 106–14.

24. Aspesi, A. V., G. E. Kauffmann, A. M. Davis, E. M. Schulwolf, V. G. Press, K. L. Stupay, J. J. Lee, and V. M. Arora. 2013. IBCD: Development and Testing of a Checklist to Improve Quality of Care for Hospitalized General Medical Patients." *Joint Commission Journal on Quality & Patient Safety* 39 (4): 147–56.

25. Hilty, D. M., D. C. Ferrer, M. B. Parish, B. Johnston, E. J. Callahan, and P. M. Yellowlees. 2013."The Effectiveness of Telemental Health: A 2013 Review." *Telemedicine Journal & E-Health* 19 (6): 444–54.

26. Boothman R., M. M. Hoyler, A. Kachalia, and S. R. Kaufman. 2013. "The University of Michigan's Early Disclosure and Offer Program." *Bulletin of the American College of Surgeons* 98 (3): 21–25.

27. Boothman, R., S. Anderson, K. Welch, S. Saint, and M. A. Rogers. 2010. "Liability Claims and Costs Before and After Implementation of a Medical Error Disclosure Program." *Annals of Internal Medicine* 153 (4): 213–21.

28. Hayes, J. H., D. A. Ollendorf, S. D. Pearson, M. J. Barry, P. W. Kantoff, P. A. Lee, and P. M. McMahon. 2013. "Observation Versus Initial Treatment for Men with Localized, Low-Risk Prostate Cancer: A Cost-Effectiveness Analysis." *Annals of Internal Medicine* 158: 853–60.

29. Conway, P. H., and C. Clancy. 2009. "Comparative-Effectiveness Research: Implications of the Coordinating Council's Report." *New England Journal of Medicine* 361 (4): 328–30.

30. Conway, P. H., and C. Clancy. 2009. "Transformation of Health Care at the Front Line." *Journal of the American Medical Association* 301: 763–65.

31. Lewis, C. K., M. L. Hoffmann, A. Gard, J. Coons, P. Bichinich, and J. Euclide. 2005. "Development and Implementation of an Interdisciplinary Plan of Care." *Journal for Healthcare Quality* 27 (1): 15–23.

32. Christianson, J. B., L. H. Warrick, F. E. Netting, F. G. Williams, W. Read, and J. Murphy. 1991. "Hospital Case Management: Bridging Acute and Long-Term Care." *Health Affairs* 10 (2): 173–84.

33. Williams, F. G., L. H. Warrick, J. B. Christianson, and F. E. Netting. 1993. "Critical Factors for Successful Hospital-Based Case Management." *Health Care Management Review* 18 (1): 63–70.

34. Huntley, A. L., R. Thomas, M. Mann, D. Huws, G. Elwyn, S. Paranjothy, and S. Purdy. 2013. "Is Case Management Effective in Reducing the Risk of Unplanned Hospital Admissions for Older People? A Systematic Review and Meta-analysis." *Family Practice* 30 (3): 266–75; You, E. C., D. R. Dunt, and C. Doyle. 2013. "Case Managed Community Aged Care: What Is the Evidence for Effects on Service Use and Costs?" *Journal of Aging & Health* 25 (7): 1204–42.

35. Commission on a High Performance Health System. 2009. "The Path to a High Performance U.S. Health System: A 2020 Vision and the Policies to Pave the Way." New York: Commonwealth Fund.

36. National Guideline Clearinghouse. 2009. Search results: "prevention." [Online information; retrieved 5/27/09.] www.guideline.gov/search/search. aspx?term=prevention.

37. Chassin, M., and J. M. Loeb. 2013. "High-Reliability Health Care: Getting There from Here." *Milbank Quarterly* 91 (3): 459–90.

38. Institute of Medicine. 2013. *Best Care at Lower Cost: The Path to Continuously Learning Health Care in America*. Washington, DC: National Academies Press.

39. Proenca, E. J. 2007. "Team Dynamics and Team Empowerment in Health Care Organizations." *Health Care Management Review* 32 (4): 370–78.

40. Vaughn, T., M. Koepke, S. Levey, E. Kroch, C. Hatcher, C. Tompkins, and J. Baloh. 2014. "Governing Board, C-suite, and Clinical Management Perceptions of Quality and Safety Structures, Processes, and Priorities in U.S. Hospitals." *Journal of Healthcare Management* 59 (2): 111–28.

41. Pronovost, P. J., M. R. Miller, R. M. Wachter, and G. S. Meyer. 2009. "Perspective: Physician Leadership in Quality." *Academic Medicine* 84 (12): 1651–56.

42. Bohmer, R. M. 2010. "Fixing Health Care on the Front Lines." *Harvard Business Review* 88 (4): 62–69.

43. National Association for Healthcare Quality. 2014. "Commit to Quality. Commit to the CPHQ." [Online information; retrieved 8/25/14.] www.nahq.org/certify/content/index.html.

44. Association for Professionals in Infection Control and Epidemiology. 2014. Home page. [Online information; retrieved 8/25/14.] www.apic.org.

45. American Society for Healthcare Risk Management. 2014. Home page. [Online information; retrieved 8/25/14.] www.ashrm.org/.

46. Wardhani, V., A. Utarini, J. P. van Dijk, D. Post, and J. W. Groothoff. 2009. "Determinants of Quality Management Systems Implementation in Hospitals." *Health Policy* 89 (3): 239–51.

47. Starr, P. 1982. *The Social Transformation of American Medicine*, 21–24. New York: Basic Books.

48. National Quality Measures Clearinghouse, Agency for Healthcare Research and Quality. 2009. Home page. [Online information; retrieved 8/14/14.] www.qualitymeasures.ahrq.gov/.

49. Joint Commission. 2014. "National Patient Safety Goals." [Online information; retrieved 8/22/14.] http://www.jointcommission.org/standards_information/npsgs.aspx.

50. Joint Commission. 2009. "National Patient Safety Goals." [Online information; retrieved 8/25/14.] www.jointcommission.org/PatientSafety/NationalPatient SafetyGoals/09_hap_npsgs.htm.

51. Leapfrog Group. 2014. "Hospital Safety Score." [Online information; retrieved 8/25/14.] www.hospitalsafetyscore.org/.

52. National Quality Forum. 2014. *Field Guide to NQF Resources.* [Online information; retrieved 8/25/14.] www.qualityforum.org/field_guide/.

53. WhyNotTheBest.org (2014).

54. Centers for Medicare & Medicaid Services. 2014. "Quality Initiatives—General Information." [Online information; retrieved 8/25/14.] www.cms.gov/Medicare/Quality-Initiatives-Patient-Assessment-Instruments/QualityInitiativesGenInfo/index.html?redirect=/qualityinitiativesgeninfo/.

55. Smith, K. A., J. B. Sussman, S. Bernstein, and R. Hayward. 2013. "Improving the Reliability of Physician 'Report Cards.'" *Medical Care* 51 (3): 266–74.

56. Thomas, F. G., and T. Caldis. 2007. "Emerging Issues of Pay-for-Performance in Health Care." *Health Care Financing Review* 29 (1): 1–4.

57. Jones, R. S., C. Brown, and F. Opelka. 2005. "Surgeon Compensation: 'Pay for Performance,' the American College of Surgeons National Surgical Quality Improvement Program, the Surgical Care Improvement Program, and Other Considerations." *Surgery* 138 (5): 829–36.

58. Rosenthal, M. B., R. G. Frank, Z. Li, and A. M. Epstein. 2005. "Early Experience with Pay-for-Performance: From Concept to Practice." *Journal of the American Medical Association* 294 (14): 1821–23.

59. Commonwealth Fund. 2005. "Early Experience with Pay-for-Performance: From Concept to Practice. In the Literature." [Online article; retrieved 12/12/05.] www.cmwf.org/publications/publications_show.htm?doc_id=307183.

60. Hasselman, D. 2009. "Provider Incentive Programs: An Opportunity for Medicaid to Improve Quality at the Point of Care." Center for Health Care Strategies. [Online information; retrieved 5/28/09.] www.chcs.org/usr_doc/P4P_Resource_Paper.pdf.

61. Damberg, C. L., K. Raube, K. K. Teleki, and E. Dela Cruz. 2009. "Taking Stock of Pay for Performance: A Candid Assessment from the Front Lines." *Health Affairs* 28 (2): 517–25.

62. Hayward, R. A. 2007. "Performance Measurement in Search of a Path." *New England Journal of Medicine* 356: 951–53.

63. Hayward, R. A. 2008. "Access to Clinically-Detailed Patient Information: A Fundamental Element for Improving the Efficiency and Quality of Healthcare." *Medical Care* 46 (3): 229–31.

64. Centers for Medicare & Medicaid Services. 2011. "Hospital Quality Initiative." [Online information; retrieved 8/24/14.] www.cms.gov/Medicare/Quality-Initiatives-Patient-Assessment-Instruments/HospitalQualityInits/index.html.

65. White, K. R., S. Thompson, and J. R. Griffith. 2011. "Transforming the Dominant Logic of Hospitals." *Advances in Health Care Management* 11: 133–45.

66. Griffith, J. R. 2009. "Finding the Frontier of Hospital Management." *Journal of Healthcare Management* 54 (1): 57–72; discussion 72–73; Griffith (2015).

6 THE CLINICAL STAFF ORGANIZATION

Critical Issues in the Clinical Staff Organization

1. *Achieving excellent care:*
   - Build a network of communication so that every clinical staff member is confident of her or his empowerment.
   - Establish clinical staff accountability.
   - Meet clinical needs effectively and promptly.
   - Develop effective clinical staff leadership.

2. *Credentialing:*
   - Verify the preparation and skills of each clinical staff member for appointment.
   - Monitor and improve individual performance.
   - Maintain periodic review for reappointment.

3. *Planning and recruiting:*
   - Plan clinical staff capacity to ensure excellent care.
   - Recruit and retain qualified clinical staff.
   - Provide continuing education to clinical staff.

4. *Compensating clinical staff:*
   - Assure clinical staff of a competitive income.
   - Reward excellent practice.

Questions for Discussion

These questions are about applying the chapter content. It's often helpful to discuss them with classmates or mentors, gaining different perspectives on the issues.

1. The clinical staff member provides the diagnoses that drive each patient's plan of care and also has a professional commitment to represent the patient and fulfill the patient's needs. A trustee who runs a successful manufacturing company says, "That's a lot of authority in one person. How do we know these people are really fulfilling our excellence-in-care mission?" Identify the key phrases he needs to take away, and explain them to him.

2. "Yale-New Haven Hospital pursued organization-wide method changes . . . standardizing the discharge process, using status boards for visual control, and accuracy and timeliness of data entry" (see Pursuing High Reliability section). Your CMO says, "We should do that here." What should she do to get started?

3. The process for credentialing and clinical staff appointment (Exhibit 6.2) looks overwhelming to many starting clinical staff members. What should you say to reassure one of them who expresses concern?

4. You will be lunching with the newly appointed clinical staff members. How will you explain to them why and how the HCO plans its clinical staff supply and what the advantages are to them?

5. Some flash points in clinical staff relations are recurring and predictable. In an interview for a new position, you are asked, "How should our HCO deal with these issues?"
   - Interspecialty disputes: orthopedics and imaging, surgery and cardiology, or nonphysicians and physicians?
   - Emergency referrals: providing specialist care to emergency patients, who often arrive at inconvenient times and without insurance or financing?
   - Impaired or obstructive clinical staff members?

Purpose

The purpose of the clinical staff organization is

to recruit and retain physicians and other qualified providers and support them to deliver excellent care.

Clinical staffs are groups of professionals licensed and specialty-certified to lead patient care. They provide the diagnoses that drive the care processes, undertake interventions like surgery and obstetrical delivery, monitor the patients' progress, and transition patients to different levels of care when acute care is no longer needed. Physicians were the original clinical staff members. Historically, physicians were ascribed magical powers, granted extraordinary privileges and confidences, and expected to assume extra moral obligations since the dawn of human existence. As evidence-based medicine has progressed, they have pursued specialties and sub-specialties, and they have been joined by several other licensed independent practitioners (LIPs). Specific practitioner lists differ by state. Nurse practitioners, physician assistants, psychologists, dentists, and podiatrists are commonly included. The privileges, confidences, and moral obligations continue.

The clinical staff organization addresses how hospital HCOs support these professionals, including processes to promote excellence, to ensure qualifications and skill, to provide an adequate supply, and to arrange compensation. Smaller HCOs must complete the same tasks. They tend to rely on less formal arrangements than the chapter describes, although the basic principles are still applicable.

The purpose implies a contract between the community stakeholders who own the HCO and individual clinical staff members that deliberately specifies excellent care as the HCO's expectation. The community brings substantial dowry to the contract. It provides facilities, equipment, and trained personnel essential to successful practice. It provides marketing to build patient volume and facilitates the clinical staff's compensation through contracts with health insurers. In return, it asks for the clinical staff's commitment to its mission, compliance with its rules and procedures, and maintenance of professional competence. Although physicians traditionally worked as independent professionals paid by patients or their insurers, the basic contract is increasingly an employment relationship through the HCO or one of its subsidiaries. Even if the clinical staff is not employed, the contract is enforced by law. HCOs are liable for errors committed by their clinical staff members as they are for their employees, even if the clinical staff members are not employed.[1]

Like all relationships, the contract must be robust enough to withstand the stresses that arise and respond to them in a constructive manner. In fact, examples of excellence are rare. Several studies show that only about half of all patient–physician encounters result in optimal treatment.[2,3] Large HCOs do not automatically improve clinical staff performance.[4] At the same time, Baldrige recipients and others have reported success implementing the functions outlined in this chapter. Their model is a combination of empowerment, measured performance, continued improvement—and, increasingly—direct financial incentives. It creates an environment where both individual and collective clinical excellence are prized and where collegial commitments reinforce personal ones, so that clinical staff members can rely on colleagues and form effective teams to achieve patient care goals.

Functions

In excellent HCOs, the purpose is fulfilled in six major functions, summarized in Exhibit 6.1.

Achieving Excellent Care

Although different service lines provide very different kinds of care, the management actions that promote excellence are the same. Excellent care is built on evidence-based foundations—the right protocols—and healthcare teams that are well trained and empowered. Clinical staff members are critical in both. They lead the protocol design, make the diagnoses, initiate the interdisciplinary plan of care (IPOC), and implement it through their own efforts and the team's. Each clinical staff member accepts responsibility for the care of his or her patients, including supervision of the care teams involved. Leading HCOs are also using clinical staffs to address high reliability, the concept that clinical errors should be driven to zero by improvement of care processes and their application.

Expectations of Clinical Staff as Clinical Team Leaders

The clinical staff is expected to believe and exemplify the ancient commitments of the physicians' Hippocratic Oath, to support their patients and "do no harm." In the twenty-first century, those commitments are to safe, effective, patient-centered, timely, efficient, and equitable care. The Accreditation Council for Graduate Medical Education (ACGME) accredits residency programs based on physician mastery of six competencies:

1. *Patient care* that is compassionate, appropriate, and effective for the treatment of health problems and the promotion of health
2. *Medical knowledge* about established and evolving biomedical, clinical, and cognate (e.g., epidemiological and social-behavioral) sciences and the application of this knowledge to patient care
3. *Practice-based learning and improvement* that involves investigation and evaluation of their own patient care, appraisal and assimilation of scientific evidence, and improvements in patient care

Function	Contribution	Examples
Achieving excellent care	Supporting each clinical staff member to provide excellent healthcare	Empowerment, effective protocols, use of the IPOC, team leadership, "high reliability" PITs
Reviewing credentials and delineating privileges	Ensuring continued effectiveness and clinical competence of clinical staff members	Verification of individual clinical staff credentials Ongoing review of clinical staff performance
Planning and implementing clinical staff recruitment	Ensuring an adequate, but not excessive, supply	Identify and respond to shifts in demand and supply of clinical staff
Providing clinical education for physicians and other professionals	Ensuring a well-trained body of care providers	Use case reviews, protocol development, PITs, and continuing education to help clinical staff and other care team members remain current
Negotiating compensation arrangements	Allowing each caregiver a competitive financial reward	Employ or contract with individual clinical staff members Negotiate risk-sharing contracts with payers and intermediaries
Improving the clinical staff organization continuously	Identifying, communicating, and resolving opportunities for improvement in clinical staff relationships	Ongoing, responsive communication with individual clinical staff Governing board, strategic planning, budgeting participation

EXHIBIT 6.1
Functions of the Clinical Staff Organization

IPOC: interdisciplinary plan of care; PIT: process improvement team

4. *Interpersonal and communication skills* that result in effective information exchange and teaming with patients, their families, and other health professionals
5. *Professionalism*, as manifested through a commitment to carrying out professional responsibilities, adherence to ethical principles, and sensitivity to a diverse patient population
6. *Systems-based practice*, as manifested by actions that demonstrate an awareness of and responsiveness to the larger context and system of healthcare and the ability to effectively call on system resources to provide care that is of optimal value[5]

Only patient care, medical knowledge, and professionalism were emphasized in the twentieth century. Learning and improvement, interpersonal skills, and systems-based practice were added to adapt to the changing needs. Thus an

HCO can expect both basic understanding and commitment from its younger clinical staff. More experienced physicians—with the most robust clinical practices, which are important to HCOs—often have learned all these skills, but some may need assistance mastering the recent additions. HCOs provide assistance and reinforce these basic professional commitments principally by example and selection.

1. All the HCO's nonphysician clinical staff members share the commitment, are trained in the skills, and are expected to model them at all times.
2. Clinical staff members are frequently assisted by nonphysician leaders who can informally coach empowerment concepts and effective leadership.
3. Senior leadership makes extensive contacts with clinical staff members in a deliberate effort to empower them and meet their professional needs.
4. Clinical staff members accepting leadership in service lines are selected for these skills in addition to their clinical acumen. These leaders provide role models and mentors for colleagues.

Creating and Managing Protocols

Clinical protocols are designed by performance improvement teams (PITs) or protocol planning committees built around the relevant service lines that assemble and review guidelines, examine the practicality of each step, modify the guideline or operating practices as necessary, test the protocol, and recommend the final protocol.

1. Leadership of the committee is usually assigned to the clinical staff who treats the largest percentage of patients with the disease or condition.
2. Committee leaders are supported by managerial staff trained in committee management; in Lean or similar problem analysis; and in using financial analysis, knowledge management, and training resources.
3. Each committee has a charge, membership, and a timetable.
   a. The charge is to establish the initial set of care procedures for typical patients with a specific disease or condition.
   b. Membership must represent all potential users.
   c. The timetable is flexible but requires evidence of progress.
4. The committee's recommendations must meet criteria:
   a. Clinical indications and contraindications for assigning the protocol to patients must be clear.
   b. Each step of the protocol must be achievable by the designated team members, meaning that they must have the training, information, supplies, and equipment they need every time the step arises.
   c. Several versions of the protocol may result, reflecting the needs of patient subsets.
5. In most cases, the protocol must be tested in realistic settings.

6. Managerial staff must plan to acquire necessary equipment, provide new training, and review scheduling to see that caregivers are available when patients need the care.

7. The committee's recommendation must be reviewed and approved at a medical staff meeting of the appropriate service lines.

Active clinical staff participation throughout these steps empowers individual members, improves the resulting protocols, and speeds smooth implementation.

Pursuing High Reliability

Leading HCOs report substantial success using clinically oriented PITs focused on high reliability, improving outcomes measures such as mortality or readmissions. The concept is strongly endorsed by The Joint Commission.[6] PITs that focus on high reliability cross service lines and often involve several HCOs. They require a strong supporting organization that can identify specific opportunities, address them through protocol revisions, and implement the changes using training, incentives, and team leadership.[7] For example:

- "With support from leadership and a conceptual model to communicate goals, use robust improvement methods, and ensure accountability, The Johns Hopkins Hospital achieved high reliability for The Joint Commission accountability measures."[8]
- "Implementation of Complete Care at [Kaiser Permanente Southern California] was followed by six-year quality gains that outpaced changes in the . . . national percentiles for many measures."[9]
- Yale-New Haven Hospital (YNHH) pursued "Organization-wide method changes . . . standardizing the discharge process, using status boards for visual control, and improving accuracy and timeliness of data entry. . . . Between FY 2008 and FY 2011, YNHH experienced an 84% improvement in discharges by 11:00 A.M. . . . The average length of stay decreased from 5.23 to 5.05 days."[10]
- The University of Pennsylvania Health System established the Mortality Review Committee, a hospital wide, systematic process to review and address inpatient deaths. "During the committee's first six years of activity, the . . . observed mortality decreas[ed] from 2.45% to 1.62%."[11]
- "Sutter Medical Center, Sacramento [California] chartered a multidisciplinary Perinatal Data Committee to improve and simplify data capture for six obstetric quality measures. . . . All six quality measures showed significantly improved trends from 2010 through 2012."[12]
- Memorial Hermann Health System (MHHS) "partnered with the Joint Commission Center for Transforming Healthcare . . . to establish reliable hand hygiene behaviors, which improved MHHS's average hand hygiene compliance rate from 44% to 92% currently. Soon after compliance exceeded 85% at all 12

hospitals, the average rate of central line-associated bloodstream and ventilator-associated pneumonias decreased to essentially zero."[13]

These document substantial shifts in important outcomes, demonstrating practical implementation of The Joint Commission's campaign for high reliability.

Reviewing Credentials and Delineating Privileges

The governing board of each hospital HCO is responsible for granting qualified individuals clinical staff privileges to participate in the medical staff organization and to provide specific treatment within her or his training and experience and within the capabilities of the HCO. (Nonhospital HCOs must still review clinical staff credentials and performance. They follow a simplified version of the hospital model, usually omitting the formal bylaws and the appeals procedure.) Each clinical staff member's credentials and recent performance are evaluated by several clinical staff peer review bodies with a recommendation to the governing board, permitting privileges for up to two years.

Privileging fulfills the HCO's obligation to patients to ensure that each clinical staff member meets minimum levels of competence and proficiency. It is important to the clinical staff as well. Each clinical staff member can rely on all colleagues to have the necessary skills and diligence. Privileging is a small but critical component of a larger strategy to improve clinical care.[14] It is a safeguard against serious clinical staff failure, a foundation for a general program of quality improvement.

Elements of Privilege

The hospital privilege agreement is nationally standardized by the accrediting organizations—the National Committee for Quality Assurance and The Joint Commission—and by various court decisions. It is a contract with four critical elements:

1. *Bylaws.* The clinical staff collectively establishes mutually acceptable rules and regulations, subject to governing board approval. These define the rights to participate in the clinical staff organization and to provide care with HCO teams, and the obligations to meet ethical standards, to ensure quality and economy of care to their own patients, and to participate in educational and quality improvement activities. The bylaws define how the clinical staff organization makes decisions, its accountability hierarchy, and how the rules may be amended. They may also define rules for compensation. Given the complexity of most of these issues, the bylaws themselves are supplemented by various procedural statements included by reference. Clinical staff accept the bylaws as part of the privilege agreement.

The bylaws are the principal source of due-process protection for the clinical staff. They establish all procedural elements of privileging, including application requirements, timing, review processes, confidentiality, committees and participants, methods of establishing expectations, sources of data, and appeals procedures. Regular review and updating of bylaws are important.

2. *Privileges.* The organization extends the privilege of treating patients within the HCO to clinical staff willing to accept the bylaws and judged competent to participate. The initial appointment and granting of privileges is for specific kinds of patient care matching the individual's training, specialty certification, and demonstrated capability. Reappointment is based on peer review of actual clinical performance as well as completion of appropriate continuing education. The review process leading to privileges is frequently called *credentialing.* Those privileged to practice were traditionally called attending physicians.

3. *Independent patient relationship.* Each clinical staff member establishes her or his own relationship to each patient and is expected to pursue diligently the obligations of that relationship. The contract recognizes clinical staff agency, that the clinical staff has explicit obligations to his or her patients as individuals, including an obligation to represent the patient and see that the patient's needs are fulfilled. Agency is independent of clinical staff compensation; that is, salaried clinical staff have the same obligations to patients as those who work under fee-for-service.

4. *Continuous improvement and peer review.* Clinical staff receiving privileges are expected to participate in the ongoing activities of the organization, including continuous improvement assignments such as PITs. They are also expected to participate in review of the quality of care of their peers and be the subject of such review. The concept of peer review is a central element of professional autonomy. It is highly prized by most clinical staff, and they invest much time and energy in carrying out their obligations.

For hospitals and all HCOs, the contractual consideration is access to HCO resources; on the part of the clinical staff, it is willingness to practice good medicine and accept the obligations.

Criteria for Privileges

An HCO may deny or discontinue the right of clinical staff privileges on grounds that the expected demand or the HCO's available resources are inadequate to provide acceptable quality of care. Thus, an HCO is not obligated to privilege a cardiac surgeon if it has no cardiologist or no cardiopulmonary laboratory. It may reject a qualified applicant if evidence suggests that it has insufficient demand to support a high-quality practice. If it has forecasted demand and determined that demand does not support an additional specialist (see below), it is not obligated to accept an application.

Denial Based on Forecast of Insufficient Demand

Specialty Certification

It is increasingly common to insist on full certification by the appropriate national specialty board as a condition of privileges. In the case of clinical staff still completing their training, a program and timetable for earning certification is specified. The clinical activities normally included in the certification become a prototype for privileges. Well-run HCOs have additional constraints for privileges:

- Maintenance of specialty certification. Most specialty boards have continuing education requirements to ensure that clinical staff keep up with scientific advances.
- Maintenance of a minimum number of cases treated annually to ensure that the skills of both the clinical staff and the hospital support team remain up-to-date.

The judgments of national specialty boards cannot be the sole criterion for assigning a specific privilege to a given specialty or specialties. First, the issue of quality is not as simple as it first looks. Primary care clinicians argue that they can handle a great many uncomplicated cases without referral, while obstetricians, pediatricians, and medical subspecialists argue that their specialized skills are more likely to promote quality. There are two issues involved. The first is correctly identifying the patient's total needs, placing the excellence of a specific treatment in a context of overall recovery. The higher the value placed on comprehensive care, the stronger the generalists' argument. Many thoughtful analysts believe that comprehensiveness is undervalued in U.S. healthcare and that the balance has shifted too far toward specialization.

The second issue is its effect on clinical staff income. Decisions to limit obstetrics to obstetricians and newborn care to pediatricians transfer income. By reducing the income of primary care clinicians, the decisions may reduce primary care availability in the community. It will also increase the fees charged per delivery.

Developing a Sound Privileging Strategy

Well-managed HCOs address the complexity of issues using the following process to establish eligibility for specific privileges.

1. Scientific evidence takes precedence. Privileges are normally extended to any specialty whose performance is documented as safe and effective.
2. Criteria for specific procedures are developed by PITs with broad membership.
3. Deliberate effort is made to hear and discuss a broad range of options and opinions.
4. Review and approval by the governing board ensures that all viewpoints have been considered and the final decision is in the customer stakeholders' best interests.

Privilege Review Process

Privileges are granted only through a precisely defined process intended to protect the rights of all parties. The major steps are specified in detail in the bylaws and are shown in Exhibit 6.2. The first substantive decision is by the service line or specialty department, thus ensuring review by peers, clinical staff whose clinical practice is similar to the applicant's. For new applicants, the reviewers rely on references, certifications, and the applicant's portfolio of previous work. For recertification, they rely on evidence of continuing education, measures of quality of care, reports of unexpected events, and in some cases, direct observation.

The credentials committee review is the first of several steps beyond specialty review to ensure objectivity and equity in the process. The committee represents the HCO as a whole, covering all service lines. The ideal member of the credentials committee possesses the attributes of a good judge: he or

Role of the Credentials Committee

EXHIBIT 6.2
Flowchart of Clinical Staff Credentialing

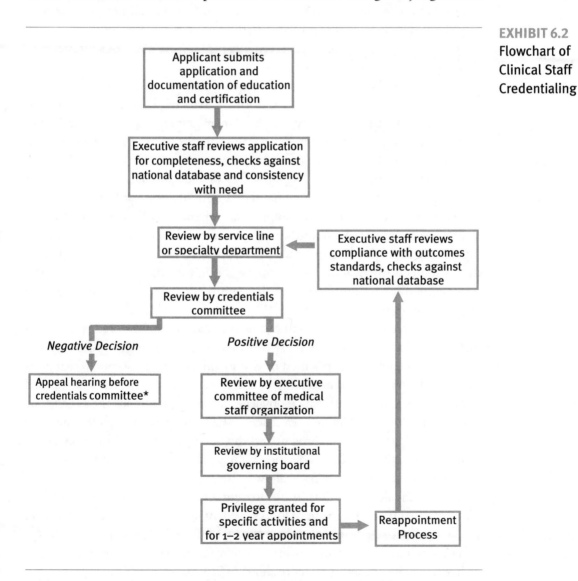

*Both positive and negative decisions by the appeals body are subject to further review by the governing board.

she is patient, consistent, thorough, factual, and considerate. Clearly, clinical knowledge and skill are useful, but detailed clinical evaluation should occur in specialty review. Committee members should be widely respected. Clinical staff with other important leadership tasks should not serve simultaneously on the credentials committee, and membership should rotate fairly frequently. The committee may seek additional opinions from specialists outside the HCO.

The committee must follow the bylaws rigorously. HCOs are liable for failure to provide due process, failure to remove incompetent clinical staff, and failure to establish appropriate standards of practice.[15] The individuals participating in the credentialing process must practice the duty of fundamental fairness, which includes constitutional provisions, when applicable; state non-discrimination statues; the public policy of fundamental fairness as expressed in judicial decisions; state and federal antitrust statutes prohibiting unlawful restraints of trade; and tort law precedents prohibiting malicious interference with a physician's right to practice.[16]

A management representative, usually the vice president for medical affairs, should staff the committee, both to assist with the workload and to ensure compliance with the bylaws. The management representative implements all procedures under the bylaws and the direction of the chair. Formal procedures for advance notice, agenda, attendance, minutes, and appeal mechanisms are mandatory. The summary of the candidate's activities must be compiled in writing and documented.[17] Candidates must have the opportunity to see the information compiled about them and to comment on it. Because the committee should function at a secondary level, evaluating the report of the service line or specialty department rather than actual patient care, the need for new direct testimony is minimized. When necessary, the statements must be carefully identified and recorded. Participation by legal counsel is desirable.

Should either management or the candidate appeal the credentials committee decision, the grounds must be documented. Both the HCO and the clinical staff should be represented by counsel in the appeals session. Final decision must be made by the governing board, again subject to the rules established in the bylaws. Clinical staff denied privileges not infrequently sue the HCO. The documentation is the defense. Excellent HCOs prevent lawsuits through the careful maintenance of due process and the documentation of sound evidence in support of the committee's decisions. They also protect committee members and others in the credentialing chain with insurance and legal counsel.

The Health Care Quality Improvement Act of 1986, Title IV of P.L. 100-177, mandates reporting of loss of credentials or other disciplinary action to a federal information bank. The purpose of the act is to reduce the chance of incompetent clinical staff moving to a new location and misrepresenting his or her skills. Specifically, the act requires HCOs to

1. notify the National Practitioner Data Bank of
    *   any clinical staff reduction or loss of privileges for any period greater than 30 days,
    *   any voluntary surrender of privileges to avoid investigation,
    *   any requirement for medical proctoring or supervision imposed as a result of peer review, or
    *   any malpractice settlement against any member of the medical staff or "other health practitioner" as defined in the act and
2. check the information bank prior to initial privileging.

The act also protects any person reporting to or working for a professional review body, such as an accredited organization's credentialing committee, by raising the standard of proof for any legal action by the individual disciplined.[18] Although the act was well intended, there is little or no evidence that it changed behavior. It appears that many credentialing committees seek alternatives that evade the reporting requirement.[19]

Standards for Granting and Renewing Privileges

The use of scientifically based protocols and measured clinical performance, as discussed in Chapter 5, effectively simplifies the credentialing review to five questions:

1. Does the clinical staff member comply with general requirements for continuing education, professional certification, and meeting minimum levels of activity?
2. Does the clinical staff member correctly perform the procedures that are his or her direct responsibility, including appropriate selection of, compliance with, and departure from protocols?
3. Does the clinical staff member achieve outcomes consistent with the expectations of the community, with due consideration of differences in the population being treated?
4. Has the clinical staff member avoided all activity that directly threatens the rights or safety of patients or colleagues?
5. Does the clinical staff member have appropriate interpersonal communication skills and abstain from disruptive behavior?[20,21]

The committee seeks evidence that the candidate substantially affirms the five questions, and that any circumstances prompting negative answers are unlikely to be repeated. In reviews of new applicants, the first question is verified directly, and references are sought as evidence on the others. In subsequent reviews, emphasis is placed on the clinical staff's recent actual performance. The best credentials process limits its review to only these questions. Other issues of quality, patient satisfaction, team participation, and cost-effectiveness are handled by ongoing training and counseling. The credentialing activity is deliberately separated from those activities.

Information and Data Support

The record required by the credentials committee has two major components. Initial reviews require the credentials themselves—documents and references testifying to the education, licensure, certification, experience, and character of applicants. The applicant is often charged with collecting the documents. Reappointments require information on the clinical performance of current staff members. Clinical staffs' clinical performance assessment systems may be used to quantify their performance based on the rates at which their patients experience certain outcomes of care and/or the rates at which clinical staffs adhere to evidence-based protocols during their actual practice of medicine.[22] Two groups of processes—the service line organization and HCO processes for quality review, and utilization and the risk management processes—monitor clinical activity and prepare reports during the year on clinical outcomes. Dual reporting safeguards the process; it requires the service line to act on problems.

Failure to Renew Privileges

Properly run, the credentials process will not be a prominent element in HCO operations. A sound monitoring process at the service line level will identify clinical staff who need help quickly. Service line leadership, working in a supportive culture, will assist any clinical staff encountering difficulty well before credentialing review. In fact, failure to renew privileges will be rare. In extreme cases, resignation or leave of absence is an option to avoid loss of privileges.

Clinical Staff Impairment

The credentials committee faces certain predictable problems, among them the impaired clinical staff member. Clinicians, like other human beings, can be disabled by age, physical or mental disease or condition, declining cognitive ability, personal trauma, or substance abuse. The prevalence of these difficulties among practicing physicians is hard to estimate, but it is generally conceded to be between 5 percent and 15 percent.[23] Thus, a medium-sized HCO could have a dozen clinical staff either impaired or in danger of impairment at any given time. The response of the service line and the credentials committee should be tailored to the kind of problem. Aging and uncorrectable physical or mental disability must force reduction of privileges. Depression and substance abuse should be treated, and programs designed especially for clinical staff can be reached through state medical societies. Arrangements can be made to assist impaired clinical staff with their practices during the period of recovery, thus ensuring that patients receive acceptable care without unduly disrupting the clinical staff–patient relationship or the clinical staffs' income. Larger organizations often have a committee or group set up specifically to deal with this problem. Although it usually keeps affected clinical staffs' identities secret, its activities must be coordinated with those of the credentials committee. While every reasonable effort at rehabilitation should be made, the credentials committee is ultimately accountable for recommending the suspension or removal of privileges.

Clinical staff must uphold the HCO values, including respect for members of their team and other associates. Privileges can be withdrawn for repeated failure. The best programs to support this requirement train service line leaders to recognize disruptive behavior and act promptly to assist the associate to more appropriate actions. Training programs and professional counseling are available when the individual does not immediately respond. These programs are appropriate for clinical staff, and successful application has been reported.[24]

Disruptive Behavior

Trends in Credentialing and Privileging

The privilege system has robust flexibility. It can cover care in various settings, be tailored to unique geographic needs or special markets, be simplified but not abandoned by small HCOs, and adapt to any insurance or clinical staff payment system. It differs from the usual employment relation between an organization and its associates principally in providing more adequate protection to the clinical staff. It formally implements empowerment. The CEO and the management staff, for example, serve at the pleasure of the governing board and can be discharged at any legally constituted meeting for any grounds not discriminatory or libelous. Only civil service, some union contracts, and the tenure system of professors provide individuals rights similar to credentialing.

Determining and Recruiting for Clinical Staff Need

A successful clinical staff organization must be properly sized to the community it serves. If it is too large, individual clinical staff income and professional satisfaction goals will not be met, skills may be lost through lack of practice, and clinical staffs may face strong temptations to pursue unnecessary treatment.[25] If it is too small, patients will be unable to get timely service and an adequate choice of practitioners. The clinical staff may be overworked, endangering quality and the satisfaction of both practitioners and patients. One solution is to leave the clinical staff supply to the market, essentially allowing the clinical staff to come and go as they individually evaluate the community's willingness to support their service. A better alternative is to plan the staff size as part of the strategic and long-range planning of the institution. The HCO cannot deny a clinical staff the right to open or close a practice. But it can deny access to the hospital, and it can recruit for needed specialists. Well-managed HCOs do this, using the best available planning information to assist their clinical staff in the most critical business decisions. Because they do it effectively, they help their communities overcome shortages, maintain quality of care, and avoid excess cost.

The HCO's medical staff planning activity is an indirect control over fee-for-service income. It is based on assumptions that the clinical staff involved will fulfill demand for effective care and will avoid unnecessary procedures. By putting planned goals and recruitment strategies in place, the

HCO makes a clear statement about the kind of medical practice it wants for the community. It also begins to implement the underlying philosophy of compensation that any associate's income should be the same as she or he could earn for equivalent effort elsewhere.

Forecasting Future Need for Clinical Staff

The conceptual model for forecasting is an extension of the general epidemiologic planning model discussed in Chapter 3. It is applied to each specialty. In Model 1, the epidemiologic model forecasts equation (1). The services provided per clinical staff year can be estimated from history. The clinical staff involved are surveyed about their work intentions, such as retirements, leaves, and plans to change their HCO affiliation. They can also comment on trends in treatment and market share.

Model 1

$$(1) \quad \left\{ \begin{array}{c} \text{Number} \\ \text{of services} \\ \text{needed} \end{array} \right\} = \left\{ \begin{array}{c} \text{Population} \\ \text{at risk} \end{array} \right\} \times \left\{ \begin{array}{c} \text{Average services} \\ \text{per patient year} \end{array} \right\} \times \left\{ \begin{array}{c} \text{Market} \\ \text{share} \end{array} \right\}$$

$$(2) \quad \left\{ \begin{array}{c} \text{Number of} \\ \text{care leaders} \\ \text{needed} \end{array} \right\} = \left\{ \begin{array}{c} \text{Number} \\ \text{of services} \\ \text{needed} \end{array} \right\} \div \left\{ \begin{array}{c} \text{Services provided} \\ \text{per care leader} \end{array} \right\}$$

$$(3) \quad \left\{ \begin{array}{c} \text{Care leader} \\ \text{recruitments} \\ \text{needed} \end{array} \right\} = \left\{ \begin{array}{c} \text{Number of} \\ \text{care leaders} \\ \text{needed} \end{array} \right\} - \left\{ \begin{array}{c} \text{Number of} \\ \text{care leaders} \\ \text{available} \end{array} \right\}$$

While Model 1 works well with major clinical events, like neurosurgery and advanced cancer treatment, it is impractical for primary care and the more general specialties. An alternate model, Model 2, uses standard ratios of clinical staff per population based on the aggregate service experience of existing health systems and communities.[26]

Model 2

$$(1) \quad \left\{ \begin{array}{c} \text{Number of} \\ \text{care leaders} \\ \text{needed} \end{array} \right\} = \left\{ \begin{array}{c} \text{Population} \\ \text{at risk} \end{array} \right\} \times \left\{ \begin{array}{c} \text{Standard} \\ \text{care leaders} \\ \text{per population} \end{array} \right\}$$

$$(2) \quad \left\{ \begin{array}{c} \text{Care leader} \\ \text{recruitments} \\ \text{needed} \end{array} \right\} = \left\{ \begin{array}{c} \text{Number of} \\ \text{care leaders} \\ \text{needed} \end{array} \right\} - \left\{ \begin{array}{c} \text{Number of} \\ \text{care leaders} \\ \text{available} \end{array} \right\}$$

Model 2 still requires the survey of clinical staff intentions.

The models have a number of limitations. They assume that the current care protocols will continue to be used. New technology, prevention, and improved protocols can change the incidence, the treatment, and the specialty required. For example, changes in the U.S. Preventive Services Task Force recommendations for breast cancer screening reduced the potential need for screening by more than half.[27] Market share is also difficult to forecast. The prior breast screening criteria were only implemented by about half of eligible women. Changes in the payment system can have an important impact. Prepaid group practices have witnessed an increased use in specialist physicians while maintaining an overall physician-to-population ratio that is 22 percent to 37 percent below the national rate.[28] Even with these limitations, the HCO is better positioned to make constructive decisions about clinical staff recruitment.

Developing a Clinical Staff Supply Plan

The clinical staff supply plan allows the hospital to move to meet community needs in a timely manner. It also allows the hospital to protect the income of its clinical staff.

Good practice calls for a careful analysis of the present situation and anticipated changes using the models with varying assumptions to explore a range of possible outcomes and their consequences. A forecast of treatments based on local history is usually obtained through the cross-functional teams and the specialties involved. One based on national data should also be used, with due regard to benchmarks and published scientific opinion. Several referents, such as values used by staff-model health maintenance organizations, conditions in similar-sized cities, and means adjusted for anticipated insurance trends, should be considered to evaluate current levels and show the implications for clinical staff supply.

The analysis and the alternative forecasts should be used to stimulate discussion among clinical staff and the governing board. Widespread understanding of the opportunities will improve individual decision making. Discussion may prompt early retirements or deliberate recruitment. The governing board is obligated to address indications of undersupply and severe oversupply.

Few communities have a surplus of primary care providers. A recruitment strategy is essential to remain competitive. It must specify the need by type of provider and location and then consider incentives necessary to attract qualified applicants. A sound approach will promote discussion of the issue among all affected groups, leading to recommendations from the medical staff organization and final acceptance by the institutional board.

High-volume specialties (e.g., cardiology, endocrinology, obstetrics) should be individually forecast. High-cost, low-volume specialties (e.g., neurosurgery, neonatology) should be carefully justified before the institution commits capital and personnel. A plan to provide a specific referral specialty service affirms that sufficient local demand will exist to maintain the quality and to justify the cost. In general, highly specialized treatment of disease incurs high fixed costs that must be spread over large populations to be cost-effective. The income expectations of the specialists themselves are high, and substantial clinical support is necessary. Unit cost falls rapidly as volume increases. It is also true that treatment teams caring for higher volumes of patients will have better-quality results.[29] As Exhibit 6.3 shows, for any given treatment there is an increasing quality structure, a declining cost structure, and increasing specialist incomes as volume increases. There are also competitive standards for all three. If competitive standards are not met, patients and payers will select other sources, after allowing for any inconvenience such as travel to a remote site. The standards dictate a critical volume, V_q, V_i, V_c. An HCO that operates a specialty below its critical volumes faces poor quality, inefficiency, and often financial losses.

Coronary artery bypass surgery provides a useful example. The need is dependent on the population of the community, its age, and health habits. The United States averaged 1.8 operations per thousand in 2000 to 2002, but the rate is declining and was only 1.4 per thousand in 2008, the most recent year reported.[30] A population of about 80,000 is necessary to maintain a volume of at least two procedures per week. The HCO that does not have a service population of 80,000 per privileged surgeon faces high unit costs. The surgeons who work in that HCO face lower-than-average income. Both face the problem that outcomes may be below achievable levels because the team does not get enough practice.

The medical staff plan protects clinical staffs against new competitors, because the HCO will decline privileges to applicants exceeding the planned numbers. If clinical staffs were to do this themselves, it would be collusion in restraint of trade, a violation of anti-trust law. Because of this, although medical staff comment should be solicited on the plan, final approval must rest with the governing board.

EXHIBIT 6.3
Critical Volumes for Specialty Services

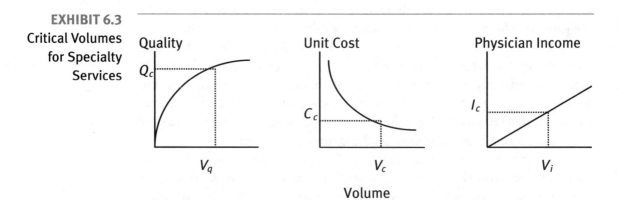

Establishing a critical, or target, level of quality, unit cost, or clinical staff income also establishes a critical volume of patients.

Integrating the Clinical Staff Recruitment Plan with Other HCO Plans

The healthcare institution must make capital investments to support the clinical staff supply. The investment decisions are part of the strategic or long-range plan of the institution discussed in Chapter 14. Decisions are made first on the question of scope of service—"Should we have a cardiovascular surgery program?"—and second on the actual facilities and number of clinical staff required.

The advantages of formal planning are summarized in Exhibit 6.4. These help sell the HCO to clinical staff and, when backed by an effective plan of service, make the HCO "a great place to give care."

Recruiting Clinical Staff

In most communities, population growth, aging, and retirements create vacancies that must be filled. Good clinical staff members have their choice of practice location, and they are actively recruited even in times of relative surplus. A recruitment offer frequently includes arrangements for office facilities and services, income guarantees, health insurance participation contracts, malpractice coverage, membership in a medical partnership or group, and introductions to referring clinical staff or available specialists. A substantial capital resource is necessary to assemble these elements. At the same time, the

Advantage	Clinical Staff Benefit	Institution Benefit
Restriction on entry of competing clinical staff	Protection against excessive competition; assurances of "fair" income	Medical staff commitment to effective care
Shared information and cooperative analysis allow more accurate forecasts	See future sooner and more clearly, have more time to react	Improve safety, return, and market attractiveness of investments
Facility and employee needs integrated with physician needs	Support available when needed	Volumes adequate to keep costs and quality competitive
Better management of clinical supply	Facilitate potentially painful transitions	Meet community demand for access Reduce pressure for inappropriate treatment
Better management of insurance contracts	More options for insurance contracts More income stability More market share	Broader array of options for customers More market share

EXHIBIT 6.4
Advantages of Clinical Staff Supply Planning

clinical staff wants to work where their colleagues are capable and friendly; complex offers require early assurance that medical credentials are acceptable; and selecting the right candidate involves assessment of clinical skills.

Recruitment has become a relatively well-codified activity, carried out by a search committee of the clinical staff organization. It includes the following components:

1. Establishment of criteria for the position and the person sought
2. Establishment of compensation and incentives
3. Advertising and solicitation of candidates
4. Initial selection
5. Interviews and visits
6. Final selection and negotiation

Recruitment is commonly a collaborative activity with existing clinical staff members. The HCO's support contributes to success.

Providing Clinical Education

All HCOs have two educational functions; larger HCOs usually have three. All staffs are responsible for promoting the continuing education of their own members and for assisting in the clinical education of other associates. Many larger HCOs and academic medical centers have responsibilities for postdegree and occasionally degree medical education as well.

The interrelation of education, continuous improvement, and protocol development should not be overlooked. Analysis of past performance, benchmarking, the design of new processes, and the preparation of protocols are educational activities in themselves, affecting the quality improvement, credentialing, planning, and educational functions simultaneously. Increasingly, the educational function is driven by the continuous improvement process.

Continuing Medical Education (CME)

Continuing education for the clinical staff is routinely required for licensure and specialty certifications. Many educational programs are offered outside the HCO; these do not substitute for the continued study of the HCO's own patients. Much education now occurs through the protocol development teams. Education helps ensure that every caregiver fully understands the protocols; develops group pressure to encourage compliance; and, by changing behavior beforehand, eliminates blame for failures.

Continuing education need not be limited to clinical subjects. Programs to help the clinical staff understand the corporate approach to decision making; to gain skills in organized activities such as team building; and to learn fundamentals of technologies, such as quality control and cost accounting, are also important.

How much to invest in staff education is a difficult judgment. It is worth noting that large successful organizations, like Kaiser Permanente, Sentara Healthcare, Henry Ford Health System, and Intermountain Healthcare, invest heavily in education. They use their size to assemble programs that might not be cost-effective for smaller institutions. Programs for clinical staff are often expensive to mount, but they are more expensive to attend. The opportunity cost of clinical staff time is very high, and educational time must be judged in the context of other demands from practice, family, and other organizational demands on the clinical staff time. The Joint Commission and all clinical staff professional associations agree that all clinical staffs should have access to sufficient educational opportunity to stay current. This requires, and The Joint Commission specifies, at least monthly educational meetings with required attendance.

Education of HCO Associates

By tradition, preparation, and law, the clinical staff member is the leader of the healthcare team. With this leadership comes an obligation to educate others, not only other clinical professionals but also trustees, executives, and other management personnel. A particularly important part of this education deals with new clinical developments. New approaches to care frequently require retraining for personnel at several levels, and clinical staff should participate in that education. In addition, trustees and planners rely on the medical staff to identify new opportunities for care and to make clinical implications clear in terms that promote effective decisions. Many of these educational requirements are met through participation on various committees and day-to-day associations.

Postgraduate Medical Education

Medicine has acknowledged its obligation to train new generations since Hippocrates. Clinical training of medical students occurs in a limited number of institutions that incorporate such training in their mission. In 2014, there were nearly 400 teaching hospitals and health systems offering postgraduate medical education programs for 110,000 **residents** and **fellows**—licensed physicians completing specialty education.[31] (Residents and fellows are also called house officers.) Many of these sites were in academic medical centers, but most were in larger HCOs.[32]

Residents
Licensed physicians who pursue postgraduate education in a medical specialty.

Fellows
Residents who pursue advanced study, usually in a subspecialty.

The content of this education is controlled through certification by individual specialty boards and is coordinated through the ACGME. House officers are paid stipends during their residencies because they provide important direct service, because hospitals feel they are a valuable source of recruits, and because their presence has long been thought to improve overall quality of care. An important benefit to both the community and the attending staff is that house officers are expected to cover patient needs at times when attending clinical staff are not present. In addition, many of the programs suitable for house officers are appropriate continuing education for attending clinical staff, and educating house officers is educational in itself.

Negotiating and Maintaining Compensation Arrangements

All HCOs rely on their clinical staff to accept patients for care, but the financial relationship with clinical staff was and is complex. The underlying goal is to provide each clinical staff member with compensation equal to that she or he could earn in another, equivalent setting. This is a market criterion; departing from it is unwise. Paying more than market wastes customers' money and can jeopardize tax-exempt status. Paying less than market will make recruiting of qualified applicants difficult and could cause valued associates to leave. That said, "market" is difficult to determine, and it does not address the structure of the compensation contract.

The early twentieth-century tradition of financial independence between the physician and HCO has eroded steadily and seems almost certain to erode further. Although the tradition is imbedded in Medicare, it too often fails to provide either patients or buyers with safe, effective, patient-centered, efficient care. Various corporate structures have arisen over the past 50 years. It is now estimated that more than 50 percent of practicing physicians, and probably a larger percentage of all clinical staff, are employees of corporations. Smaller HCOs moved to limited liability corporations. For hospitals and larger HCOs, multispecialty physician corporations or direct payment from the HCO are emerging as the dominant employment models. Joint venture corporations, linking a not-for-profit hospital and a small physician group, remain common.

In these corporate forms, the trend has been to provide a base salary with incentives for desirable performance. The financial relationship should be designed to reinforce the organizational functions shown in Exhibit 6.1, providing incentives for clinical staff to act consistently and aggressively in pursuit of the HCO's mission. A growing body of evidence supports the use of incentives; they help clinical staff meet quality,[33] patient satisfaction,[34] and length-of-stay goals. One study found incentives effective among low-performing physicians.[35] Best practice on clinical staff compensation is unclear, but a solid contract will be built around

1. a base salary;
2. incentives for meeting quality-of-care goals;
3. incentives for meeting patient volume needs, such as a payment for each patient;
4. incentives for meeting patient satisfaction goals; and
5. incentives for team leadership and participation in continuous improvement activities.

Individual contracts will vary. Service line and unit chiefs will have a different distribution of incentives from clinical staff within the units.

Lee and Cosgrove suggest that clinical staff compensation must be imbedded in a broader strategy. It should have four "levers":

1. Begin with clear goals that can be shared by individuals and the HCO, such as the mission and values.
2. Appeal to the clinical staff's self-interests, recognizing that offers must be competitive with other alternatives.
3. Earn the respect of colleagues, by which they mean routine sharing of quality scores of individual clinical staff among their peers.
4. Embrace the HCO's traditions. Their examples, from Mayo and Cleveland Clinics, are from long-standing tradition of the highest clinical and ethical standards. They note:

> [O]rganizations must be willing to part company with physicians who refuse to work with their colleagues toward a shared purpose.[36]

Lee and Cosgrove also offer four guidelines for compensation design:

1. Avoid attaching large sums to any single target. They have found small incentives surprisingly effective.
2. Watch for conflicts of interest. The incentive must remain in the patient's best interest. Programs that rewarded physicians for cost saving have not been successful; they create a conflict between patient needs and HCO costs.
3. Reward collaboration. Although physicians prefer incentives that they alone control, it is better to use incentives that encourage teamwork.
4. Communicate. They suggest that good incentives are "continually modified."[37]

Financial contracts between HCOs and physicians are subject to important legal constraints. Explicit payment for increasing the profit of the HCO is illegal under a ruling of the Office of Inspector General of the U.S. Department of Health and Human Services.[38] Specific arrangements that might have the impact of increasing profits to the HCO or earnings to the physician fall under Stark law and fraud and abuse provisions of the Medicare contract.[39] Many states have laws that regulate physician incentive compensation.[40] Excellent HCOs always obtain legal counsel for financial contracts with physicians.

Improving the Clinical Staff Organization

Continuous improvement focuses on empowerment of the clinical staff. The emphasis that transformational management places on two-way communication applies to the clinical staff. Excellent HCOs make several systematic efforts to build a communicating culture:

1. Clinical staff voices are included in all major decision discussions, as shown in Exhibit 6.5.
2. Senior managers devote significant time to individual and group contact with the clinical staff.
3. Formal surveys are used to measure clinical staff satisfaction, as with other associates.
4. Clinical staff members in management roles are trained to empower their colleagues and pursue servant leadership.
5. Clinical staff members are invited to serve on the governing board.
6. A complex accountability structure (see Exhibit 6.6 later in the chapter) provides two avenues for discussion of most issues.
7. Formal mechanisms for conflict resolution are built into the medical staff bylaws but are used as a last resort.

Building a Communicating Culture

The goal is a structure where all clinical staff members are empowered and are confident that their voice will be heard in decisions affecting their practice. This means not only listening but also taking effective action to identify issues, discuss implications, and resolve conflicts.[41] Trust between the parties is a critical factor.[42] Success requires a robust network of communications that identifies issues promptly, solicits and organizes opinion about them, and resolves them fairly.[43] All clinical staff members should be close to someone whom they respect and who can hear their concern and either resolve it for them or explain how they can participate in the resolution. Encouraging comment and discussion and resolving it openly creates an environment where issues can be aired, discussed, and decided. Ideally, all clinical staff members should be convinced that they have heard the issue, that they have had a fair opportunity to be heard about the issue, and that the final decision optimizes market realities.

The major constraint is clinical staff time. Efforts outside their practice reduce the time they have for patient care. Many prefer the latter, and all generate income from it. Some specialties are more constrained than others. Primary care clinicians may have offices some distance away and full calendars in their clinics. Specialists are more likely to be nearby and, because they earn more per minute of clinical effort, are more able to devote time to management issues. This creates an imbalance that must be explicitly addressed. Clinical staff time is saved by training leadership and by preparation and flexibility in committee activities. Meetings and meeting agendas should be designed with respect for clinical staff time. Advance preparation and distribution of relevant background material make a noticeable difference, so does proper preparation by the chair. Teleconferencing and attendance as needed should be encouraged. Special efforts should be made to hear the primary care viewpoint.

EXHIBIT 6.5
Clinical Staff
Representation
on Decision
Processes

Decision Type	Example	Physician Participation
Mission/vision	Visioning exercise	Extensive individual participation Review committees Governing board membership
Resource allocation	Environment assessment Strategic plans	Governing board membership Leaders participate in annual review
	Services plan Financial plan	Membership on board planning and finance committees
	Facilities and human resources plans	Representation on committees and consultation for services directly involved
	Clinical staff recruitment plan	Advice from each specialty unit Opportunity for individual comment
	Budgeting	Participation between line units and services particularly involved
	Capital budgeting	Major voice in ranking all clinical equipment purchases Participate in general ranking of capital equipment
Clinical care issues	Process design	Participation by service line in all patient management protocol development Review of relevant functional protocols Participation or consultation in clinical PITs
Organizational	Personnel selection	Credentialing of all clinical staff Participation on executive search committees
	Implementation plans	Participation by service line
	Information plan	Participation in plan and relevant pilot programs
	Conflict resolution	Membership in mediation efforts and appeals panels

PIT: process improvement team

Most clinical staffs learn the communications culture by experience. Just-in-time training and reviews of processes at the start of major discussions are helpful. Where communication and trust are supported by a strong formal system, informal devices can be used to great advantage. If all staff members are confident of their empowerment, much can be accomplished through informal discussions. In well-run HCOs, nonmedical managers make a deliberate effort to maintain informal communications with the medical staff, including going to their offices to meet them. Many successful CEOs and chief operating officers undertake the monitoring function personally. By visiting clinical staff in their offices, hospital managers and executives demonstrate their understanding of the value of a clinical staffs' time and show a willingness to become acquainted with clinical staff on a more personal level.[44]

People

There is an average of almost three clinical staff (700,000 physicians, 150,000 advanced practice nurses,[45] and 80,000 physician assistants[46]) for every 1,000 persons in the United States. They tend to concentrate in urban areas, although most disadvantaged areas have shortages.[47] Larger HCOs have several hundred clinical staff representing a wide variety of specialties and growing numbers of non-physician practitioners.[48] Technology and economics have increased the differences among clinical staff. Less than half are in primary care, which is believed to be a shortage area. Most are specialists who work mostly in institutional settings and, by definition, see a limited range of conditions in which they are expert.

Clinical Staff Organization

Clinical staffs in larger HCOs are organized by service line. The service lines form the foundation for performance measurement and goal setting, privileging, continuous improvement, and compensation negotiations. HCOs also maintain a medical staff organization that serves to address issues that cross service lines, such as the credentials committee (Exhibit 6.2), participation in strategic planning, and ranking capital budget proposals. Exhibit 6.6 shows the basic concept. The medical staff executive committee serves as a coordinating body, with powers delegated in the bylaws. Senior management interacts frequently with the service lines, their subordinate units, and the clinical staff themselves. Senior management attends meetings of the medical staff and advises the governing board on all matters reaching the board, including privileging. The vice president of medical affairs and other leaders in the clinical organization are almost always credentialed and privileged in their specialty, and sometimes retain a small active practice. In larger organizations, their time is largely committed to leadership duties.

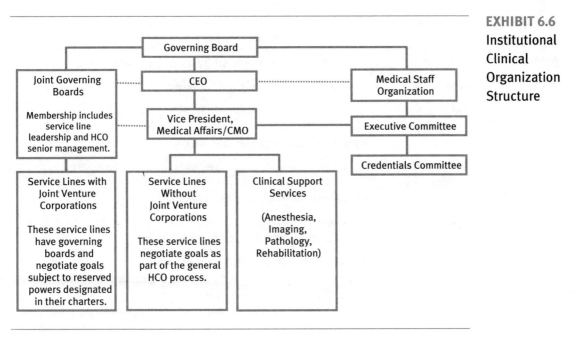

EXHIBIT 6.6
Institutional
Clinical
Organization
Structure

CMO: chief medical officer

Clinical Staff Leadership

Medical leaders form the backbone of the service line organization, filling the key positions and forming the communications network. Leaders are not difficult to identify. They emerge naturally in informal discussions and on PITs. Most clinical staff will declare their leadership candidates. There is surprising consensus. A sound program identifies leaders early in their careers and begins assigning activities appropriate to their skills. As the clinical staff matures, his or her experience deepens and assignments become more complex. Clinical staff members are appointed by the governing board. They progress through the ranks, toward the critical committee assignments, executive positions, and board membership. They join the HCO's nonclinical leadership team. They are deliberately nurtured and trained, often relying on mentors and coaches with just-in-time training as their duties expand and they gain experience.

Measures

Like any other accountable unit of the HCO, the clinical staff organization should have measures of performance and formal expectations for the coming year. The service lines and clinical support services shown in Exhibit 6.6 will have strategic scorecards if they are separately incorporated and unit scorecards if they are part of the HCO corporation. The medical staff organization should also have a unit scorecard. Exhibit 6.7 suggests some approaches that will identify opportunities for improvement (OFIs).

EXHIBIT 6.7
Operational
Measures of
Clinical Staff
Organization
Performance

Dimension	Applicable Measures
Demand	Difficult to measure except by associate satisfaction
Cost	Cost budgets for assigned functions
Associate satisfaction	Surveys of clinical staff satisfaction Meeting attendance Incidents causing excessive disruption
Outcomes and efficiency	Cost/clinician served can be calculated and compared to similar organizations Review by internal or external consultants
Operations	Review by internal or external consultants Items arising from associate satisfaction
Customer satisfaction	The service lines monitor patient quality and satisfaction. The customers of the medical staff organization components are the associates they serve. The customers of clinical support units are both patients and associates.

Managerial Issues

Clinical staff–HCO relations are a traditional "hot spot" in HCO management. Much about the clinical staff organization is in flux as of 2015. Major reforms in the insurance structure are likely to lead to increased collaboration between clinical staff members and between the clinical staff and the HCO. Small HCOs are likely to diminish in number and importance. Large hospital-oriented systems will continue to grow. The foundations outlined in this chapter seem likely to endure. Evidence-based medicine provides a solid foundation for identifying and resolving issues. Clinical measures, benchmarks, and protocols show what is possible and make collaboration more attractive than adversarial relations. Actions by the medical profession, such as the efforts by the American College of Physicians and American College of Surgeons, to stimulate higher quality and the changes in residency competencies will help younger clinical staff. Above all, transformational cultures will help HCOs identify and correct causes of stress in the relationship.

Three areas are likely to need ongoing management attention. They are the potential conflict in values, governing board relations with clinical staff, and clinical staff recruitment.

Managing Conflicting Values

Evidence-based medicine and the IPOC described in Chapter 5 and the processes for credentialing and planning eliminate a number of areas of potential conflict. Clinical staff are ethically committed to act as agents for their patients. HCO managers are ethically committed to act as agents for the community or the owners. These commitments are usually synergistic, a commitment to a common mission of excellent care. There are situations where they can conflict. Resolution must recognize clinical staff empowerment but enforce commitment to basic rules and values.

In a national report on physician perspectives on U.S. hospitals, three of the top five listed physician priorities on what affects the physician–hospital relationship the most dealt with how well the HCO's senior leaders communicate, respond, and collaborate with physicians to meet their practice needs.[49] Engaged clinical staff members demonstrate the following psychological traits:

- *Investment*—The clinical staff have an emotional relationship with the hospital, share in its mission and values, and feel a sense of pride in their association with the organization.
- *Involvement*—The clinical staff take an active role in improving hospital performance and join with the HCO in providing excellent care.
- *Advocacy*—The clinical staff demonstrate behaviors that build the brand of the HCO by recommending the HCO to patients, clinical staff colleagues, and the community at large.[50]

In order to engage the clinical staff, HCO leaders must listen attentively to their needs and concerns; involve them in decision making; make an effort to understand the language of medicine, advanced practice nursing, and other professions and what their clinical staff contributes to excellent patient care; and show that they are valued by the HCO's senior leaders. Organizations with high levels of clinical staff engagement

- receive higher revenue and earnings per admission and per patient day,
- increase referrals from engaged clinical staff,
- reduce clinical staff recruiting costs, and
- sustain significant growth and profitability.[51]

Most important, an engaged clinical staff with higher levels of satisfaction contributes to the overall mission of providing excellent patient care. That is a restatement of the service excellence concept discussed in Chapter 2.

One example of conflict avoided is the caregiver's obligation to act in the individual patient's best interest, possibly departing radically from the patient management protocol or the IPOC. The issue is a common cause for clinical staff concern.[52] The system eliminates the conflict by encouraging the clinical staff to revise the IPOC whenever he or she believes it is in the patient's best interest. At the same time, the unit outcomes measures and goals demand progress toward high reliability. The system reinforces both the clinical staff's and the governing board's ethical commitment, because the clinical staff's judgment is assessed by outcomes measures and subject to peer review.

A second example is concern over staffing or equipment adequacy. The question "Do we have enough (nurses, beds, EKG machines, surgical robots, etc.)?" is virtually inevitable. The system accepts the question as an OFI. It should quickly be transformed to "If we added more, what would be the impact on our unit scorecard outcomes, quality, patient satisfaction, and associate satisfaction?" The question "Can we afford it?" is secondary and is addressed through the service excellence chain. Continued serious outcomes failure may be more expensive than the proposed expenditure. A PIT investigating the OFI will allow all concerned to be heard and is likely to reach a realistic, possibly innovative, answer. The goal is not to get every caregiver to agree with the PIT's recommendation but rather to get every caregiver to agree that the question was fully and fairly explored. ~~licensed independent practitioner~~

A third is representation of nonphysician LIPs. The structure for credentialing and communicating with clinical staff is traditionally called the *medical staff organization*, a term remaining from when physicians were the only clinical staff who were LIPs. A new term is needed; it must emerge from practice. More important, a new perspective is needed, assuring the LIPs of a continued voice in critical decisions. We propose the term *care leaders* to replace *clinical staff* to focus on the leadership of the patient-centered care delivery team.

Representing Clinical Staff on the Governing Board

The practice of providing designated positions on the board for physicians has become almost universal among large, community-based HCOs. Exceptions are mainly limited to those institutions whose corporate charters or enabling legislation precludes such participation. The clinical staff nominates their colleagues in many organizations. To satisfy tax-exemption rules, the board majority must remain nonphysicians; rarely do physicians constitute more than a substantial minority. These few individuals, with only a fraction of the specialties, ages, and financial arrangements of the staff as a whole, cannot represent the complex needs of all clinical staff members. Like other board members, they are expected to vote for the best interests of the community rather than for any short-term advantage to themselves or to the clinical staff. They serve the medical staff more by making sure the clinical staff opinions are fully and fairly heard than by any specific representation.

The potential conflicts are avoided by following the procedures outlined in Chapter 4, with particular attention to all board members' obligation to represent the community as a whole, and strict observation of conflict-of-interest rules. A stronger solution builds an overall relationship with clinical staff, empowers them, and resolves their concerns through continuous improvement. When that strategy is effective, there is less need to resolve conflicts at the board level. The clinical staff can join the community members in seeking to advance the mission. Issues will be disputed in the goal-setting and capital budget processes, where the board will select among competing proposals. Again, the test for the minority is not whether the decision was correct but whether the decision was fair and fully explored.

Ensuring Adequate Clinical Staff Supply

It is likely that most HCOs will work in an environment of shortages for care. Research by the Association of American Medical Colleges predicts increasing physician supply shortages to keep pace with baseline demand, with an estimated shortfall of close to 20 percent by 2025.[53] The aging population, who consume more healthcare services, is the major contributor to this demand.

HCOs that delight their clinical staff will recruit successfully. Delighted clinical staff stay with the organization. They are more open to the experimentation that will be necessary to meet the future. They also become effective recruiters. The key to clinical staff satisfaction is clear enough: It is a network of communication and effective response to issues of concern. Excellent HCOs achieve this by maintaining the culture and system described in this text. Clinical staff are delighted when they are sure that they are empowered, that their patients get what they need, that they can rely on their colleagues, and that income and patient satisfaction goals will be met. In other words, the solution to delighting clinical staff is to implement all 15 chapters of *The Well-Managed Healthcare Organization*.

Additional Resources

Burroughs, J. 2015. *Redesign the Medical Staff Model: A Guide to Collaborative Change.* Chicago: Health Administration Press.

Cullen, S. J., M. J. Lambert, and J. J. Pizzo. 2012. *A Guide to Physician Integration Models for Sustainable Success.* Health Research & Educational Trust and Kaufman Hall. [Online report; retrieved 9/5/14.] www.hpoe.org/physician-integration-models.

Joint Commission. Various. *Comprehensive Accreditation Manual for Hospitals.* Oakbrook Terrace, IL: Joint Commission Resources.

Showalter, J. S. 2015. *The Law of Healthcare Administration,* 7th ed. Chicago: Health Administration Press.

Starr, P. 1982. *The Social Transformation of American Medicine,* 198–232, 420–49. New York: Basic Books.

Todd, M. K. *Physician Integration and Alignment—IPA, PHO, ACO's and Beyond.* Medical Group Management Association. [Online report; retrieved 9/5/14.] www.mgma.com/store/books/printed/physician-integration-and-alignment.

Vukmir, R.V. *Physician Contract Guidebook—Electronic Version.* Medical Group Management Association. [Online publication; retrieved 9/5/14.] www.mgma.com/store/books/electronic/physician-contract-guidebook.

Notes

1. *Darling v. Charleston Community Memorial Hospital,* 33 Ill.2d 326, 211 N.E.2d 253, 14 A.L.R.3d 860 (Ill. Sep 29, 1965).

2. McGlynn, E. A., S. M. Asch, J. Adams, J. Keesey, J. Hicks, A. DeCristofaro, and E. A. Kerr. 2003. "The Quality of Health Care Delivered to Adults in the United States." *New England Journal of Medicine* 348 (26): 2635–45.

3. Casalino, L., R. R. Gillies, S. M. Shortell, J. A. Schmittdiel, T. Bodenheimer, J. C. Robinson, T. Rundall, N. Oswald, H. Schauffler, and M. C. Wang. 2003. "External Incentives, Information Technology, and Organized Processes to Improve Health Care Quality for Patients with Chronic Diseases." *Journal of the American Medical Association* 289 (4): 434–41.

4. McWilliams, M. J., M. E. Chernew, A. M. Zaslavsky, P. Hamed, and B. Landon. 2013. "Delivery System Integration and Health Care Spending and Quality for Medicare Beneficiaries [Review]. *JAMA Internal Medicine* 173 (15): 1447–56.

5. Accreditation Council for Graduate Medical Education. 2014. "ACGME Common Program Requirements." [Online information; retrieved 9/14/14.] www.acgme.org/acgmeweb/Portals/0/PFAssets/ProgramRequirements/CPRs2013.pdf.

6. Chassin, M. R., and J. M. Loeb. 2013. "High-Reliability Health Care: Getting There from Here." *Milbank Quarterly* 91 (3): 459–90.

7. Perla, R. J., E. Bradbury, and C. Gunther-Murphy. 2013. "Large-Scale Improvement Initiatives in Healthcare: A Scan of the Literature." *Journal for Healthcare Quality* 35 (1): 30–40.

8. Pronovost, P. J., R. Demski, T. Callender, L. Winner, M. R. Miller, J. M. Austin, S. M. Berenholtz, and National Leadership Core Measures Work Groups. 2013. "Demonstrating High Reliability on Accountability Measures at the Johns Hopkins Hospital." *Joint Commission Journal on Quality & Patient Safety* 39 (12): 531–44.

9. Kanter, M. H., G. Lindsay, J. Bellows, and A. Chase. 2013. "Complete Care at Kaiser Permanente: Transforming Chronic and Preventive Care." *Joint Commission Journal on Quality & Patient Safety* 39 (11): 484–94.

10. Jweinat, J., P. Damore, V. Morris, R. D'Aquila, S. Bacon, and T. J. Balcezak. 2013. "The Safe Patient Flow Initiative: A Collaborative Quality Improvement Journey at Yale-New Haven Hospital." *Joint Commission Journal on Quality & Patient Safety* 39 (10): 447–59.

11. Barbieri, J. S., B. D. Fuchs, N. Fishman, C. C. Cutilli, C. A. Umscheid, C. Kean, S. Koshy, P. G. Sullivan, P. J. Brennan, and R. R. Kelz. 2013. "The Mortality Review Committee: A Novel and Scalable Approach to Reducing Inpatient Mortality." *Joint Commission Journal on Quality & Patient Safety* 39 (9): 387–95.

12. Gilbert, W. M., M. C. Bliss, A. Johnson, W. Farrell, L. Gregg, and C. Swanson. 2013. "Improving Recording Accuracy, Transparency, and Performance for Obstetric Quality Measures in a Community Hospital-Based Obstetrics Department." *Joint Commission Journal on Quality & Patient Safety* 39 (6): 258–66.

13. Shabot, M. M., D. Monroe, J. Inurria, D. Garbade, and A. C. France. 2013. "Memorial Hermann: High Reliability from Board to Bedside." *Joint Commission Journal on Quality & Patient Safety* 39 (6): 253–57.

14. Gardner, L. A., V. Snow, K. B. Weiss, G. Amundson, E. Schneider, D. Casey, E. R. Hornbake, S. Manaker, L. G. Pawlson, P. Reynolds, M. Sha, and D. Baker. 2010. "Leveraging Improvement in Quality and Value in Health Care Through a Clinical Performance Measure Framework: A Recommendation of the American College of Physicians." *American Journal of Medical Quality* 25 (5): 336–42.

15. Showalter, J. S. 2014. *The Law of Healthcare Administration*, 7th ed., 245–64. Chicago: Health Administration Press.

16. *Ibid.*, pp. 247–48.

17. Ramsey, P. G., M. D. Wenrich, J. D. Carline, T. S. Inui, E. B. Larson, and J. P. LoGerfo. 1993. "Use of Peer Ratings to Evaluate Physician Performance." *Journal*

of the American Medical Association 269 (13): 1655–60; Norman, G. R., D. A. Davis, S. Lamb, E. Hanna, P. Caulford, and T. Kaigas. 1993. "Competency Assessment of Primary Care Physicians as Part of a Peer Review Program." *Journal of the American Medical Association* 270 (9): 1046–51.

18. Health Care Quality Improvement Act of 1986, P. L. 99-177.

19. *Credentialing and Peer Review Legal Insider*. 2009. "Lack of NPDB Reporting Brings Peer Review Practices into Question." *Credentialing and Peer Review Legal Insider* 6 (8): 1542–1600.

20. Rosentein, A. H., and M. O'Daniel. 2008. "A Survey of the Impact of Disruptive Behaviors and Communication Defects on Patient Safety." *Joint Commission Journal on Quality & Patient Safety* 34 (8): 464–71.

21. McLaren, K., J. Lord, and S. Murray. 2011. "Perspective: Delivering Effective and Engaging Continuing Medical Education on Physicians' Disruptive Behavior." *Academic Medicine* 86 (5): 612–17.

22. Landon, B. E., S. L. Normand, D. Blumenthal, and J. Daley. 2003. "Physician Clinical Performance Assessment: Prospects and Barriers." *Journal of the American Medical Association* 290 (9): 1183–89.

23. Williams, B. W. 2006. "The Prevalence and Special Educational Requirements of Dyscompetent Physicians." *Journal of Continuing Education in the Health Professions* 26 (3): 173–91.

24. Hickson, G. B., J. W. Pichert, L. E. Webb, and S. G. Gabbe. 2007. "A Complementary Approach to Promoting Professionalism: Identifying, Measuring, and Addressing Unprofessional Behaviors." *Academic Medicine* 82 (11): 1040–48.

25. Rice, T. H., and R. J. Labelle. 1989. "Do Physicians Induce Demand for Medical Services?" *Journal of Health Politics, Policy and Law* 14 (3): 587–600.

26. Holm, C. E. 2004. "A Guide to Medical Staff Development Planning." In *Allies or Adversaries: Revitalizing the Medical Staff Organization*, 27–52. Chicago: Health Administration Press.

27. U.S. Preventive Services Task Force. 2009. "Breast Cancer: Screening." [Online information; retrieved 9/1/14.] www.uspreventiveservicestaskforce.org/uspstf/uspsbrca.htm.

28. Weiner, J. P. 2004. "Prepaid Group Practice Staffing and U.S. Physician Supply: Lessons for Workforce Policy." *Health Affairs* (Web Exclusive): W4-43–W4-59.

29. Post, P. N., M. Kuijpers, T. Ebels, and F. Zijlstra. 2010. "The Relation Between Volume and Outcome of Coronary Interventions: A Systematic Review and Meta-analysis." *European Heart Journal* 31 (16): 1985–92.

30. U.S. Census Bureau. 2014. *Statistical Abstract of the U.S., 2012*, Table. 171. [Online information; retrieved 9/1/14.] www.census.gov/compendia/statab/2012/tables/12s0171.pdf.

31. Association of American Medical Colleges. 2014. "Council of Teaching Hospitals and Health Systems." [Online information; retrieved 9/1/14.] https://www.aamc.org/about/.

32. Association of American Medical Colleges. 2005. *AAMC Databook: Statistical Information Related to Medical Education*, Table G7. Washington, DC: AAMC.

33. Gilmore, A. S., Y. Zhao, N. Kang, K. L. Ryskina, A. P. Legorreta, D. A. Taira, and R. S. Chung. 2007. "Patient Outcomes and Evidence-Based Medicine in a Preferred Provider Organization Setting: A Six-Year Evaluation of a Physician Pay-for-Performance Program." *Health Services Research* 42 (6, Pt .I): 2140–59.

34. Kirschner, K., J. Braspenning, R. P. Akkermans, J. E. A. Jacobs, and R. Grol. 2013. "Assessment of a Pay-for-Performance Program in Primary Care Designed by Target Users." *Family Practice* 30 (2): 161–71.

35. Chen, J. Y., N. Kang, D. T. Juarez, K. A. Hodges, and R. S. Chung. 2010. "Impact of a Pay-for-Performance Program on Low Performing Physicians." *Journal for Healthcare Quality* 32 (1): 13–22.

36. Lee, T. H., and T. Cosgrove. 2014. "Engaging Doctors in the Health Care Revolution." *Harvard Business Review* 92 (6): 104–16.

37. *Ibid.*, p. 112.

38. Wiehl, J. G., and S. L. Murphy. 1999. "Gainsharing: A Call for Guidance." *Journal of Health Law* 32 (4): 515–63.

39. Centers for Medicare & Medicaid Services. "Report Fraud &Abuse." [Online information; retrieved 11/6/14.] www.medicare.gov/forms-help-and-resources/report-fraud-and-abuse/fraud-and-abuse.html.

40. Stauffer, M. 2000. "Finance Issue Brief: Bans on Financial Incentives." *Issue Brief: Health Policy Tracking Service* (June 1): 1–10.

41. Gillies, R. R., H. S. Zuckerman, L. R. Burns, S. M. Shortell, J. A. Alexander, P. P. Budetti, and T. M. Waters. 2001. "Physician-System Relationships: Stumbling Blocks and Promising Practices." *Medical Care* 39 (7, Suppl.): I-92–I-106.

42. Zazzali, J. L. 2003. "Trust: An Implicit Force in Health Care Organization Theory." In *Advances in Health Care Organization Theory*, edited by S. S. Mick and M. E. Wyttenbach, 233–52. San Francisco: Jossey-Bass.

43. Holm, C. E. 2004. "Techniques to Foster Effective Working Relationships." In *Allies or Adversaries: Revitalizing the Medical Staff Organization*, 85–103. Chicago: Health Administration Press.

44. *Ibid.*

45. U.S. Bureau of Labor Statistics. "Physicians and Surgeons." [Online information; retrieved 9/2/14.] www.bls.gov/ooh/healthcare/physicians-and-surgeons.htm.

46. American Academy of Physician Assistants. 2014. "Milestones in PA History." [Online information; retrieved 9/2/14.] www.aapa.org/WorkArea/DownloadAsset.aspx?id=789.

47. U.S. Department of Health and Human Services, Health Resources and Services Administration. "Shortage Designation: Health Professional Shortage Areas & Medically Underserved Areas/Populations." [Online information; retrieved 2/6/15.] www.hrsa.gov/shortage/.

48. White, K. R., and D. G. Clement. 2014. "Healthcare Professionals." In *Human Resources in Healthcare: Managing for Success*, 4th ed., edited by B. Fried and M. Fottler. Chicago: Health Administration Press.

49. Press Ganey. 2008. *Hospital Check-Up Report—Physician Perspectives on American Hospitals*. South Bend, IN: Press Ganey Associates.

50. Paller, D. 2009. "Physician Partnership: Creating Powerful Relationships." [Online information; retrieved 7/14/09.] www.pressganey.com/galleries/default-file/Physician_Partnership_Creating_Powerful_Relationships.pdf.

51. Gallup. 2009. "Physician Engagement." [Online information; retrieved 7/14/09.] www.gallup.com/consulting/healthcare/15385/Physician-Engagement.aspx.

52. Wachter, R. M., and P. J. Pronovost. 2009. "Balancing 'No Blame' with Accountability in Patient Safety." *New England Journal of Medicine* 361 (14): 1401–6.

53. Association of American Medical Colleges. 2014. "GME Funding: How to Fix the Doctor Shortage." [Online information; retrieved 9/3/14.] www.aamc.org/advocacy/campaigns_and_coalitions/fixdocshortage/.

CHAPTER

7 NURSING

Critical Issues in Nursing

1. *Delivering excellent care:*
   - Build effective nursing and interdisciplinary teams to deliver individualized, patient-centered care.
   - Plan, deliver, and evaluate care that is safe, effective, and evidence based.
   - Provide training and logistic needs.
   - Measure and improve nursing team performance.

2. *Communicating for comprehensive patient care:*
   - Ensure full transfer of knowledge between nurses, physicians, and other team members.
   - Use team huddles for patient safety and quality.
   - Use the electronic health record to integrate care from direct and indirect care providers.

3. *Educating patients, families, and communities:*
   - Use the patient–HCO encounter to address preventive and continuing needs.
   - Consider cultural and linguistic competence.
   - Support community health initiatives.

4. *Sustaining the supply of nurses:*
   - Ensure healthy work environments.
   - Promote nursing as a career choice in elementary, middle, and high school.
   - Provide learning and advancement opportunities for nursing personnel.
   - Reach out to groups previously underrepresented in nursing.

Questions for Discussion

These questions are about applying the chapter content. It's often helpful to discuss them with classmates or mentors, gaining different perspectives on the issues.

1. You are thinking about taking a senior management position at an HCO you've not known at all. You're meeting tomorrow morning with the chief nursing officer (CNO). What are some "trigger" comments or questions you want to make, so that he discusses achievements and opportunities for improvement in patient care?

2. In your conversation with the CNO (Question 1), he remarks that "a couple service lines seem to have trouble coordinating with their physicians" and asks what you think could be done about that. What do you need to know to make a constructive response? What questions do you ask?

3. As this conversation develops, it turns out that these units are the lowest scoring in patient satisfaction, nursing satisfaction, and readmissions. Suggest to the CNO what you would do if you were in senior management.

4. How would you select and prepare nurses for managerial roles? What does a nurse manager need to know? How does he or she get that knowledge?

5. In view of the national threat of a nursing shortage, outline a strategy to ensure an adequate supply of nurses in your HCO. What short-term and long-term actions would you propose to senior management?

Purpose

The purposes of nursing are

to deliver safe and excellent evidence-based care to each patient

and

to maintain a work environment that ensures nursing associates' competence and engagement.

Nursing is by far the largest clinical profession. Its contribution is clearly recognized by patients. In its annual survey on the honesty and ethical standards of various professions, Gallup reports that Americans rate nurses at the top of the list.[1] Most people, when asked to evaluate their inpatient care, speak first not of the doctor but of the nurse. Furthermore, if they think well of the nursing care, they tend to rate the whole experience, even the bill, more favorably.

Florence Nightingale saw the nursing role as stretching from emotional support to control of hazards in the environment. She articulated the objective of assisting the patient to **homeostasis**—a state of equilibrium with one's environment—when she said in 1859 that nursing consists of those activities

> *Homeostasis*
> A state of equilibrium with one's environment.

that "put the patient in the best condition for nature to act upon him."[2] This concept prevails in most of the more modern definitions, with the added goal of restoring the patient's independence[3] and nursing advocacy for individuals, families, communities, and populations through participation in shaping health policy and creating patient and health systems management.[4]

Obviously, preventing the loss of equilibrium is better than trying to regain it. Prevention of illness and promotion of health have always been important in nursing. Nurses' work with well individuals and families includes immunization, education, environmental safety, and disease screening. For persons who are ill or injured, the route to homeostasis includes a nursing assessment or diagnosis, the development of an individualized care plan, the implementation of the plan, and the evaluation of the plan by specific nursing care or activities requested of other services. Even for the person who is ill, preventing the spread of disability is as important as correcting losses. Nurses instruct patients and their families in adapting to disease and disability, speeding their recovery, and minimizing the risk of further impairment.

The role of the nursing organization is to see that the purposes are uniformly implemented for all patients across the HCO's spectrum of outpatient, inpatient, and continuing care.

Functions

As shown in Exhibit 7.1, nurses must perform five functions, beginning with the provision of excellent patient care. Nurses must also coordinate inter-disciplinary team–based care. Nurses provide the bulk of patient and family education and much of community health education. As the day-to-day leaders of most patient care teams, nurses must have managerial skills, including the ability to sustain and improve the transformational environment, plan staffing and resource management, and provide staff development. The nursing voice is critical on most planning committees, protocol selection committees and process improvement teams (PITs). Nurses are expected to improve their own performance as well as to engage in clinical research to improve patient care.

Delivering Excellent Care

The extensive contribution of nursing and the breadth of nurses' roles make nursing a critical focal point for high-performing HCOs. In meeting the Institute of Medicine's goals of safe, effective, patient-centered, timely, efficient, and equitable care, nursing contributes to higher levels of per-formance.[5] The leading institutions are achieving this with a sophisticated program of knowledge management; enhanced education and development; improved protocols; better logistic support; and, above all, attention to an organizational culture that promotes nurses' value, autonomy, personal and professional needs, and job satisfaction. Exhibit 7.2 summarizes the contribu-tions of nursing in delivering excellent care.

Implementation of the Nursing Process

Nurses deliver excellent care by implementing the **nursing process**, a system of assessing patients, diagnosing individual nursing care needs, planning care, implementing plans, and evaluating care. Exhibit 7.3 shows the elements of the nursing process with knowledge management resources and examples.

Nursing process
A system of assessing patients, diagnosing individual nursing care needs, planning care, implementing plans, and evaluating care.

Assessment

Upon the patient's admission, the nurse assesses the patient, using the nursing process (see Exhibit 7.3), and takes into consideration the patient's total set of diseases and disabilities, general physical and emotional condition, family and social history, and the medical history. Family views are important, and a description of the patient's home environment is frequently required. At this time, the nurse also notes medication allergies and advance directives (e.g., living will, durable power of attorney for healthcare).

The nursing assessment includes objective and subjective information. Objective criteria are based on facts, such as visual inspection, palpation, and

EXHIBIT 7.1 Nursing Functions

Function	Activities	Results
Delivering excellent care	Implement the nursing process: Identify patients' needs, nursing diagnosis, and care plan. Integrate nursing process with IPOCs. Coordinate IPOC implementation. Evaluate patient progress. Use case management for complicated cases.	Optimal outcomes are achieved for safe, effective, patient-centered, timely, efficient, and equitable care. Each patient has a nursing diagnosis and care plan. The plan is coordinated with patient management protocols and IPOCs. Progress toward maximal function is monitored. Nursing care is evidence based.
Coordinating and monitoring interdisciplinary care	Ensure effective communication and integration with physicians, other CSS, and other service lines. Pursue and correct gaps or problems in care management.	Interdisciplinary patient rounds and IPOC are used to coordinate care. Schedule coordinates diagnostic testing and therapeutic interventions. Patient and family needs for spiritual care, social services, palliative care, ethics consultation are identified and met.
Educating patients, families, and communities	Meet or exceed expectations of patients, other stakeholders. Consider cultural, literacy level, and linguistic competencies. Participate in discussions about palliative care and advance care planning.	Patient education materials are available for appropriate cultural and literacy level and language. Knowledge gaps are identified and teaching plans are carried out. Prevention and continuing care needs are identified and applied to care plans and documented in the EHR. Patients and families will have knowledge of advance care planning options. Inpatient readmissions are minimized.
Maintaining the nursing organization	Use shared governance to plan, organize, and evaluate the work and outcomes of nursing. Maintain professional nursing model and advancement in knowledge and skill-based competencies. Project future personnel and facility needs; budget; ensure appropriate number and skill of staff complement. Recruit, select, retain, and motivate an effective workforce based on participation, HCO decision involvement, and empowerment.	Nursing practice councils are in place for improvement, education, research, standards. Effective skill mix (RN, unlicensed assistive personnel, contract) and expertise (specialty certified, experienced) and numbers of personnel to match patient needs are achieved. All nurses participate in practice decisions. Facility, equipment, and supply needs are met.
Improving nursing performance	Commit to continuous improvement of nursing practice. Offer in-house nursing education programs. Participate in clinical nursing research. Translate nursing research into practice improvements. Integrate organizational structures and management processes with plan and deliver nursing care. Inspire shared vision, commitment, creative responses to challenges. Participate in professional nursing organizations.	Pursuit of professional certifications and advancement is supported. Management and leadership development programs are offered. Mentoring and residency programs are in place. Performance reviews are conducted regularly. Competitive salaries and benefits are offered. Positive relationships are established within HCO and community. Budgets, facilities, equipment plans, emergency preparedness plans and drills, and marketing strategies are in place. Professional development plans are offered to all nursing staff. Patient and nursing advocacy is practiced through professional organizations.

CSS: clinical services support; EHR: electronic health record; IPOC: interdisciplinary plan of care; RN: registered nurse

	Goal	Nursing Role	Examples
EXHIBIT 7.2 Nursing and the Goals of Excellent Care	Safe	Eliminate biological, physical, human, and psychological risks in both the inpatient and home environments Maintain safety of diagnosis and treatment	Any safety hazard that nursing identifies in a patient care setting is corrected by nursing or by the appropriate support unit. Nurses work with patients and families in home settings to promote safety. Nursing administers drugs and monitors all treatments, promotes hand washing, and assesses patient mobility and psychological status.
	Effective	Monitor the care process and provide the early warning for any deviation from the plan Evaluate patient progress toward comprehensive recovery; identify and remove barriers	In intensive settings, nurses are in virtually constant contact with patients. As recovery progresses, nurses set recovery goals and milestones, teach, motivate, and celebrate progress.
	Patient-centered	Identify each patient's unique characteristics and adapt protocols to accommodate them	Nurses evaluate tastes and preferences as well as allergies and sensitivities. Nursing identifies cultural variations and adapts to provide culturally competent care.
	Timely	Minimize the duration of the patient's disability	Nursing schedules and coordinates many treatments and activities. Effective nursing speeds recovery and eliminates complications. It shortens length of stay and prevents relapse.
	Efficient	Minimize the total cost of care and disability	Nursing cost is measured by correctable disability as well as its direct cost. Drug errors, falls, adverse events, delays in care, and failures to respond are all partially within nursing's control. These occurrences make inadequate nursing care expensive.
	Equitable	Ensure that care is equally available without regard to ethnicity, culture, gender, or sexual orientation Ensure patients' rights, including the right to refuse treatment	Nurses monitor their own and other caregivers' behavior to eliminate prejudice and unjust responses. Nurses explain care options to patients and families, help them reach decisions, and implement those decisions.

Elements of the Nursing Process	Resources and Guidelines	Example
Assessment	Objective and subjective data	Vital signs, breath sounds, observation of difficulty breathing; laboratory results; physical examination
Nursing diagnosis	NANDA	Ineffective airway clearance and excess thick secretions as evidenced by abnormal breath sounds; crackles, wheezes; change in rate and depth of respiration; and effective cough with sputum
Plan of care	IPOC	Effective airway clearance as evidenced by normal breath sounds, no crackles or wheezes, respiration rate 14–18 per minute, and no cough by within 1 week
Implementation of care	NIC	Instruct and assist patient to TCDB for assistance in loosening and expectorating mucus every 2 hours.
Evaluation of care	NOC	Monitor improvements in breathing, expectorating mucus, and objective measures of oxygen profusion by physical examination and results of diagnostic tests; adjust goals, communicate with physician and CSS for modifications to patient management; and provide education on stopping smoking, if applicable.

EXHIBIT 7.3
Nursing Process Example for Airway Management

CSS: clinical services support; IPOC: interdisciplinary plan of care; NIC: Nursing Interventions Classification; NOC: Nursing Outcomes Classification; TCDB: turn, cough, deep breathe

vital signs (temperature, pulse, respirations, blood pressure). Subjective information is also obtained based on the experienced and intuitive observations of the nurse and the patient's verbal and nonverbal responses to questions, such as "On a scale of 1 to 10, what is your level of pain now?"

Nursing Diagnosis

After an assessment is completed, the nurse identifies one or more nursing diagnoses. A **nursing diagnosis** is a standardized statement about the health of a client (who can be an individual, a family, or a community) for the purpose of providing nursing care. Nursing diagnoses are identified from a master list of nursing diagnosis terminology maintained by NANDA International.[6] Nursing diagnoses provide the basis for a common language in identifying interventions and measuring outcomes, thus a more evidence-based approach to nursing care.

Nursing diagnosis
A standardized statement about the health of a client for the purpose of providing nursing care; identified from a master list of nursing diagnosis terminology.

Plan of Care

The nursing care plan establishes nursing procedures and expectations for outcomes. It is established for each encounter, such as a hospitalization or an emergency department visit, or over the course of a disease or condition, such as ongoing ambulatory or chronic care. It expands and individualizes the patient management protocol to reflect nursing's more comprehensive assessment. The care plan is more formal in inpatient and extensive outpatient care and is often left unwritten in brief, uncomplicated outpatient encounters. A good care plan does the following:

- adapts the care protocol to the specific needs of the patient;
- anticipates individual variations to prevent complications;
- establishes a plan for nursing interventions from the Nursing Interventions Classification (NIC) (patient-specific nursing treatments are defined and standardized by a NIC list and may be classified according to 554 interventions);[7]
- organizes the major events in the hospitalization or disease episode to minimize overall duration;
- establishes realistic clinical outcomes based on the Nursing Outcomes Classification (NOC) and a timetable for their achievement (the NOC is a comprehensive, standardized classification of 490 patient/client outcomes developed to evaluate the effects of nursing interventions);[8]
- incorporates a discharge plan;
- identifies potential barriers to prompt discharge, and plans to investigate and remove them; and
- is integrated into the IPOC with the care leader's modifications to the patient management protocol.

Throughout the encounter (episodic care) or over the course of a disease or condition (ambulatory or chronic care), the nurse evaluates the effectiveness of the nursing interventions and adapts or modifies the plan as needed. With input from the patient, family members, and physicians and other clinical professionals, the nursing care plan is integrated into the IPOC. Advance planning on potential barriers to goal attainment are effective ways to improve quality while potentially reducing length of stay and cost per case.

Care plans are also written for "at risk" problems as well as for "wellness." These follow a similar format, only designed to prevent problems from occurring and to continue or promote healthy behavior.

A major role for nurses in planning care is to recognize early signs of a patient's changing or worsening condition and to communicate those changes to the physician or another provider for early intervention and modification of patient care management protocols. If a patient's condition worsens quickly, nurses may contact a **rapid response team** to intervene with preapproved emergency treatment protocols. Rapid response teams have additional training in critical care patient management and teamwork and have been shown to improve patient outcomes when nurses feel safe and supported in deploying the teams.[9]

Information technology significantly aids patient care plan development. Models for specific diseases, analogous to the clinical protocols discussed in Chapter 5, may be incorporated. Components of the care plan can be assembled from standard nursing practice protocols. Nurses can develop a plan more quickly and with less risk of omission by modifying a disease model to individual needs. They can control the specific content of several thousand activities by relying on approved nursing practice protocols.

> **Rapid response team**
> Care providers with advanced training in critical care management and emergency treatment protocols; deployed when a patient's condition suddenly worsens.

Implementation and Evaluation

The nursing care plan, like medical care, is heuristic. The evidence of the patient's progress is reviewed regularly, and the care plan is modified as necessary. With many diseases and conditions, the patient is returned to health, and the plan is fulfilled. With chronic conditions, the plan is modified regularly as the patient progresses, or in some cases fails. The nursing care plan is fully compatible with palliative care, hospice care, and acceptance of death. Standardized language developments that classify and measure nursing diagnoses, interventions, and associated outcomes (e.g., NANDA, NIC, NOC) have strengthened an evidence-based foundation for nursing.[10] The American Nurses Credentialing Center's (ANCC) Magnet Recognition Program recognizes organizations that provide quality patient care and evidence-based nursing excellence.

Case Management

For patients with multiple diseases or complex conditions that exceed the scope of patient management protocols, case management is used for managing care across the span of illness and various sites of care. Case management has emerged as an effective device for managing complicated disease processes, for patients who require long courses of convalescence, and for those at risk for costly care. Case management begins with a sophisticated IPOC, often developed by a multidisciplinary team of caregivers and often integrating several protocols. The plan identifies specific goals, clinical support services (CSS) and medical services to meet them, measures of improvement, and timetables. Nurses often manage the cases once the plan has been agreed on, working to see that the various services are effectively coordinated.

Coordinating and Monitoring Interdisciplinary Care

Major medical care is a multiple-team event. Nurses generally coordinate and monitor the teams throughout the episode of care, whether it is in an inpatient, outpatient, or home setting. The goal is to organize all elements of care in the least costly and most patient-satisfactory elapsed time. Nursing's oversight responsibility includes recording progress against the IPOC, sequencing and scheduling CSS diagnostic and treatment interventions (including transportation), and monitoring for irregularities in logistics and patients' responses to interventions.

Maintaining Progress of the IPOC

During the patient's episode of inpatient or outpatient care, it is necessary to maintain a comprehensive, current record of the activities contributing to diagnosis and treatment. The patient record, also called the medical record, is increasingly computerized as the electronic health record (EHR). The patient's EHR is accessible to all caregivers and is constantly being updated. In critical care environments, much data are entered directly from monitoring equipment. The IPOC includes symptoms and problems, concurrent disease or complication, working diagnosis, medical orders, and the nursing care plan. The IPOC must also include safety alerts, such as hearing deficits, patient allergies, and language or literacy barriers. The medical record also summarizes diagnostic orders and results, treatment to date, and the patient's response. The professional members of the patient care team are responsible for their own entries into the record, as well as considering what has been entered by other care team members.

Nurses are responsible for monitoring patients' progress toward the IPOC goals of care through the following activities:

- Ensure that the patient's physician has completed diagnosis, treatment, and appropriate follow-up activities in an appropriate and timely manner.
- Report clinical observations to the physician and other members of the caregiving team.
- Identify progress of patient goals as identified in the IPOC.
- Assess and report relevant psychosocial and family-related factors.
- Assess effectiveness of nursing interventions.
- Know where patients are, and receive them from the CSS.
- Receive and transmit results of reports from the CSS.
- Prepare and forward unexpected-events reports.

Nurses use the information to identify omitted, inconsistent, and incorrect actions and actions that had unintended outcomes.[11] Nurses are often the first to detect unexpected results and unsatisfactory responses to treatment, and they intervene to manage the unexpected—a quality of high-reliability organizations.[12] Swift intervention with clear communication techniques is often necessary to improve the situation or to prevent it from further escalation.[13]

The nurse as a patient advocate is expected to take appropriate action diplomatically and effectively. Nurses catch omitted, wrong, lost, conflicting, and delayed reports and orders on a daily basis. Organizational cultures that are group oriented, with a greater extent of quality improvement program implementation, tend to promote higher reporting of quality assessment and risk management data, such as medication administration errors.[14]

Patient Scheduling

Inpatient and outpatient support service scheduling is generally performed via computer scheduling systems that are integrated with other support service functions, such as the laboratory, radiology, and surgery. Nurses or scheduling personnel obtain information directly from patients and coordinate care with support service departments. Scheduling must accommodate limitations in the patient's physical condition and competing demands of various support services. Most of the services require direct physical contact with the patient, and many of the services have sequencing requirements (e.g., perform before meals or before certain other services).

Nursing's responsibility is shifting to active monitoring of the automated process and to more effective preparation of each patient. For improved quality, advance scheduling permits prospective review of compliance with the patient management protocol, even though it may be only a few hours before the events are to take place. Monitoring can reduce duplicated and unusable tests and orders. Prompt fulfillment of scheduled orders also reduces stat (or immediate) requests. All these activities reduce the cost of care.

Patient Transportation

Nursing may also be responsible for the safe transport of inpatients. Although many outpatients can follow wayfinding services to reach the various CSSs, inpatients are frequently impaired by their illness and must be moved by hospital associates. The task is time consuming but important to patient safety and satisfaction. Transportation associates may be supplied by nursing or a unit of guest services (see Chapter 12). They should be trained to follow protocols in patient transfer, in guest relations, and in handling the medical emergencies that may arise while the patient is in transit.

Educating Patients, Families, and Communities

Nursing's constant contact with patients and their visitors contributes to a prime role in educating and communicating. Nursing's prominent role in satisfaction surveys stems from the fact that patients and families see more of nursing than any other caregivers and from the supportive nursing role. People expect nurses to be sympathetic and sensitive to human needs. They are vocally grateful when nurses are sympathetic, and sensitive and disappointed when they are not. Patient satisfaction is a powerful marketing tool, as satisfied customers are less likely to switch provider services and more likely to recommend services to others.[15]

Nurses' success in communicating with the patient and family or other significant persons in the patient's life is a critical element of patient-centered care and overall patient satisfaction. Nurses must evaluate and be sensitive to the patient's cultural, literacy, and language needs in order for interventions to be patient centered and family focused. The patient and family are involved in the broad outline of the care plan, including the anticipated dates of key events such as surgery and discharge. Whenever possible, the patient and family participate with the interdisciplinary team in discussions about treatment choices and goals of care.

For patients with life-limiting illnesses, goals of care are particularly important. Nurses can improve the effectiveness of advance care planning and the discussion about advance directives and patient advocacy, both by encouraging patients and families to address the issues involved and by supporting the patient's advocate in stressful decisions. When curative treatments are no longer effective, palliative care focuses on pain and symptom management (such as shortness of breath, anorexia, nausea, fatigue, depression, and insomnia) to allow a natural death to be as peaceful as possible, whether it occurs at home or in an institution.[16] Nursing support for the patient and family during the dying process and afterward is useful to promote and manage healthy grief and bereavement.

Nursing has extensive educational responsibilities relating to the management of disease. HCO nurses teach individual patients and their families about the role of prevention and risk-factor management. Community health nurses teach prevention and health promotion to groups of citizens for primary prevention and advocate appropriate secondary prevention. If these activities are performed well, future disease is reduced. Patient, professional, and community satisfaction levels improve. Thus, expectations for prevention are an essential part of care plans. As a consequence of much shorter hospital stays, the site for health education is shifting to ambulatory care settings, particularly the patient-centered medical home and the accountable care organization. When education and communication are appropriately carried out with patients, inpatient readmissions are minimized.

General education, offered to the public at large and usually provided to group settings, is another vehicle. Nurses provide educational programs and counseling and organize and assist disease- or disability-oriented support groups (e.g., ostomy care, alcohol abuse, hemophilia) and stressful events other than disease (e.g., divorce, childbirth, caregiving) have become popular following the disease-oriented model.

Maintaining the Nursing Organization

Sustaining the Transformational Culture

The nurse manager plays a central role in the unit culture and is accountable for goals in patient care quality and safety and nurse satisfaction, engagement, and retention. To achieve and sustain a high-performing nursing organization, the nurse manager must be specifically trained in transformational management: how to encourage associates, respond to recurring questions, implement process and protocol changes, and celebrate gains. These skills are taught through programs in human resources, nursing education, or organizational development.

Leading HCOs have implemented systems of care that promote nurse empowerment. **Shared governance** is a nonhierarchical organizational structure that balances power between managers and staff nurses and brings them together in both purpose and discipline.[17] A matrix of councils with authority and accountability for professional practice and decision making work interdependently with organizational leadership and authority to achieved desired outcomes.[18] Shared governance gives nurses more control over their practice and accountability at the point of care. This increased engagement of nurses in practice decisions at the bedside is a key component of autonomous practice, a requirement of Magnet designation.[19]

Shared governance

A nursing model in which staff nurses share the authority and accountability for practice decisions and other activities that influence their work environment.

Nurse managers back up formal education with responsive listening by superiors and senior leadership. They routinely assign coaches and mentors to new nurse managers, and they use a mentoring system or nurse residency program to develop new staff nurses. They use personal development programs for their nurses and other nurse managers and carefully monitor their own satisfaction. The result is that these HCOs have low turnover, attractive work sites, and a stable nursing associate group that gains skills from experience and training. These systems have substantially increased nurse retention while elevating quality and cost outcomes.[20]

Nurse managers must be skilled in the importance of effective listening and celebration. They are supported and coached by both senior and HCO nursing leaders. They are expected to carry out the practices of servant leadership, as described in Chapter 2. Because the interface often involves interdisciplinary collaboration, nurse managers maintain proficiency in teamwork, mediation, and consensus building.

Staffing

Staffing decisions establish the number of professional, technical, and clerical nursing associates required for each nursing unit. The results of staffing decisions establish scheduling and daily assignment requirements and set the nursing expense budget. Combined with forecasts of patient demand, they generate long-range human resource plans. The American Nurses Association recommends that nurse staffing be tailored to the specific needs of each unit, based on factors including patient acuity, the experience of the nursing staff, the skill mix of the staff, available technology, and the support services available to nurses.[21] Although California has had mandated minimum nurse staffing levels since 2004 and other states have attempted to follow suit,[22] there is little evidence that regulatory approaches are effective in improving quality.[23,24] Involving nurses in the decision-making role in the care they provide is the most important consideration in developing staffing approaches.

Given that up to 90 percent of nursing costs are labor costs, getting the right number of nurses for the patients' immediate needs is a critical management function. The nursing care functions are time-consuming activities that cannot be properly performed when nurses are in short supply.

The staffing process establishes expectations for hours of care per patient day, by skill level. It is based on forecasts of demand and patient need (acuity) and generates a forecast of fixed staffing and, in some units, variable staffing. Inpatient nurse staffing decisions are made for each nursing unit and shift. They establish the number and mix of personnel (e.g., registered nurses [RNs], unlicensed assistive personnel, coordinators) required for the expected range of acuity and census. The decision about the level of staff is negotiated; increases in staffing must be justified by the marginal improvement in quality, cost per case, or patient and worker satisfaction. The labor expense budget is determined almost automatically once the staffing pattern and the forecasts of demand are selected.

Fixed staffing is used in settings where demand does not vary (such as outpatient clinics and long-term care) and where demand cannot be predicted (such as in the obstetrics and inpatient care units). Flexible labor budgets use variable staffing models to adjust the actual staff according to patient need, usually on a shift-by-shift schedule. Staffing models use a nursing hours per patient day productivity ratio, which will vary depending on the occupancy rates and acuity of patients. Because not all patients require the same amount of care, adjustments are often made for "weighting" of some staffing plans. For example, the intensity of nursing care for a critically ill infant in the neonatal intensive care unit may be weighted as three times the required nursing hours compared to a nursing unit with uncomplicated care.

Patient requirements are radically different in long-term care, critical care, emergency departments, and surgical services such as the operating room and the post-anesthesia care unit. In many of these areas, requirements differ by day of week and by random variation in patient arrivals and acuity. Team approaches are aimed at reducing costs by substituting less skilled personnel under the supervision of professional nurses.[25]

Scheduling

The budgeted staffing plan must be translated to work schedules for specific employees. Predictable absenteeism, educational leaves, holidays, and non-patient-care assignments must be accommodated in the schedule. A well-designed scheduling system has the following characteristics, listed in approximate order of importance:

- Desired staffing mix is ensured for safe patient care; overstaffing and understaffing are minimized.
- Time and effort required to create complex staff schedules are minimized.
- Overtime, float, and agency usage is reduced, and personnel are scheduled according to their designated specialization, professional competence, and agreed-on work commitment (i.e., full time or part time).
- Schedules for individuals are maintained four or more weeks in advance, but with the ability to manage staffing on a daily basis.
- Weekends, late shifts, and other less desirable assignments are equitably distributed. ("Equitably" is usually not "equally"; one nurse's preferences are not the same as another's.)
- Personal requests for specific days off are accommodated equally, so long as they are submitted in advance, can be met within cost and quality constraints, and do not exploit other workers.

Assignment

Assignment makes the final adjustment of staff on each unit and shift, based on the best available estimate of immediate need, by changing the number of personnel on a given unit or, in some cases, by changing the number of patients on a unit. Some variation can be handled by the ability of the nursing staff to adapt to higher workload demands. Although nurses may be expected to increase productivity in dealing with workload peaks, it is not sustainable and contributes to fatigue and burnout, and eventually turnover. Higher nurse-to-patient ratios enhance job satisfaction, thereby contributing to recruitment and retention strategies.[26]

Census management can also be used to reduce variation in nurse staffing requirements. Many leading HCOs employ sophisticated bed-management systems and specially trained personnel to assign patients to units with adequate nurse staffing levels, appropriate professional competencies of nurses, and proximity of the patient to important CSSs. When possible, patients are scheduled to reduce variation in weighted census. In organizations with several similar treatment units, incoming patients can be placed in units with surplus staff.

Remaining staffing variation is usually met by calling in part-time or backup nurses, requesting overtime from available workers, and transferring cross-trained workers between units. The use of backup staff and transfers may be necessary, but it should be minimized. Agency personnel brought in on contract are expensive, and training is outside the HCO's control. Transfer of nurses from one location to another within the hospital presents similar difficulties. Most nurses do not like to be transferred, and the problems of cross-training and unfamiliar work reduce job satisfaction. Quality may deteriorate as a result.

Improving Nursing Performance

Improvement goals can be negotiated with the specific unit or for groups such as service lines or several service lines. All nursing unit leaders are responsible for maintaining the transformational culture and for improving individual and unit performance. They monitor the operating scorecard of their unit as described below. In addition, the nursing organization must monitor and improve overall clinical performance. It does this by aggregating the individual unit data on common measures. Care must be taken to ensure similarity, but many quality measures, patient satisfaction measures, and staff satisfaction measures can be reviewed across multiple nursing units. Improvements often involve new functional protocols or enhanced training to raise compliance across the HCO.

Improving Individual and Unit Performance

Nurse unit leaders are expected to monitor individual performance as well as performance of their units, identify areas that lag behind similar units or goals that might be in danger, and help team members improve performance. When opportunities for improvement (OFIs) are identified, training programs are developed to improve knowledge and skill development. For individual development and advancement, additional skills attainment and professional certifications are encouraged.

Nursing managers are actively supported by both the nursing organization and senior management, who are frequent visitors and responsive listeners. Support is provided by knowledge management (Chapter 10) and internal consultants (Chapter 14) skilled in identifying root causes, devising new processes, and testing them.

The nursing organization includes clinical specialists who can assist with nursing process issues. Many excellent HCOs also provide nurse managers with resource specialists—more experienced nurses who are not in the direct accountability hierarchy. Under this system, each team has support for any kind of problem, as shown in Exhibit 7.4.

Improving Protocols and Multiple-Unit Performance

Nurses implement evidence-based practices that lead to improved patient outcomes. This involves participation in clinical nursing research and translation of research into practice improvements. The nursing organization manages a large number of functional protocols that define the nursing activities. Nursing is responsible for the continuous improvement of its functional protocols. It is so central to most complex care that it is a major contributor to patient management protocols. Its central position gets it involved with many CSS functional protocols. Campaigns focused on new functional protocols would

EXHIBIT 7.4
Assistance
Available to
Nursing Teams

Problem	Support Available
Equipment, supply, or facilities failure	Plant services associates are trained to respond promptly. Their operating scorecards assess both delays and nurse satisfaction as customers.
Personal difficulty of team member	Human resources has counseling and retraining services.
Harassment or inappropriate behavior toward a team member	Harassment is defined by the associates. Human resources, the nursing organization, and senior management are trained in effective responses.
Staffing shortage	The nursing organization runs the staffing model and is committed to an effective solution. The solution may involve a PIT addressing ways to improve staff productivity or reduce variability in patient demand.
Unexpected clinical event	Reporting is mandatory. The unit team is trained to make emergency response. It may participate in service recovery, further analysis, or a PIT addressing risk management.
Unexpected customer or associate event	The unit team is expected to pursue appropriate service recovery, emergency response, and reporting for review of trends. Reporting is mandatory.

Note: In all of these examples, an unanswered call can be reported either to the nursing organization or senior management, who are expected to correct the problem and eliminate recurrence.

include all nursing units where the protocols are used, often crossing several service lines. Changes in nursing protocols are carried forward in a sophisticated program of training and development of associates, demonstrated proficiency of revised protocols, and inclusion of the required competencies in evaluations of performance. These activities usually take place across multiple nursing units.

The service lines manage patient management protocols. Adopting a patient management protocol without active participation by nurses is probably impossible. Nurse specialists have a particular role here because their specialization makes them experts on particular diseases and conditions. Managers must ensure that appropriate consultation occurs and is constructive.

People

Team Members

Nursing as a profession and as a unit of HCOs is almost as diverse as medicine. Nurses have careers that reach from high-tech in the operating room and intensive care unit (ICU) to high-touch in the home and hospice and to general and public health services that do not involve individual patient care. In addition, there are significant numbers of managerial jobs. The patterns of education, specialization, and practice sites reflect this diversity.

Educational Levels

Nursing has a broad scope of educational programs, practice boundaries, and licensure restrictions. Within nursing are certified nursing assistants, licensed practical nurses (LPNs), RNs, and advanced practice nurses (APRNs). RNs have a variety of educational backgrounds—a two-year associate's degree, a three-year hospital diploma, a four-year baccalaureate degree—or for advanced practice, a master's degree in nursing, as can be seen in Exhibit 7.5.

An Institute of Medicine (IOM) report entitled *Future of Nursing: Leading Change, Advancing Health*, recommends higher levels of education in the nursing profession.[27] The purpose of this recommendation was to prepare nurses for more complex care needs of sicker patients and the sophisticated technologies available for providing care. This report was followed by a federal goal to increase the proportion of baccalaureate-prepared nurses to 80 percent by 2020. In 2013, 55 percent of the RN workforce held a baccalaureate degree or higher.[28] Nurse executives have indicated they have a preference for hiring baccalaureate-prepared nurses, and many organizations have tuition assistance programs to facilitate baccalaureate degree attainment.[29] Job satisfaction and career retention have been shown to be more positive in bachelor's-level nurses than in associate's-level nurses.[30] In Magnet-designated hospitals, bachelor-of-nursing preparation and specialty certification are strongly promoted and required in certain specialty areas.

Types of Specialization

Advanced Practice Nurses   An APRN is a nurse

1. who has completed an accredited graduate-level education program preparing him or her for one of the four recognized APRN roles;
2. who has passed a national certification examination that measures APRN-role and population-focused competencies and who maintains continued competence as evidenced by recertification in the role and population through the national certification program;
3. who has acquired advanced clinical knowledge and skills preparing him or her to provide direct care to patients;
4. whose practice builds on the competencies of RNs by demonstrating a greater depth and breadth of knowledge, a greater ability to synthesize data, increased complexity of skills and interventions, and greater role autonomy;
5. who is educationally prepared to assume responsibility and accountability for health promotion and/or maintenance as well as the assessment, diagnosis, and

management of patient problems, which include the use and prescription of pharmacologic and nonpharmacologic interventions; and

6. who has obtained a license to practice as an APRN in one of the four APRN roles: certified registered nurse anesthetist, certified nurse midwife, clinical nurse specialist (CNS), or certified nurse practitioner.[31]

EXHIBIT 7.5
Educational Levels of Nurses

Title	Education Required	Certification/Examination Required
Registered nurse	Diploma	NCLEX
	Associate degree in nursing (ADN)	NCLEX
	Baccalaureate degree in nursing (BSN)	NCLEX
Advanced Practice Nurses—Master's Degree Required		
Nurse anesthetist	MSN, DNP, DNA	Certified registered nurse anesthetist (CRNA)
Nurse practitioner	MSN, DNP	Primary care or acute care that is population specific (adult/gerontology, pediatric, neonatal) Family nurse practitioner (FNP) Adult nurse practitioner (ANP) Adult/gerontology acute care nurse practitioner (A/GACNP) Neonatal nurse practitioner (NNP) Pediatric nurse practitioner (PNP)
Nurse midwife	MSN, DNP	Certified nurse midwife (CNM)
Clinical nurse specialist	MSN, DNP	Certification in area of specialization
Other Nursing Roles and Educational Preparation		
Public health nurse	MPH, DNP, DrPH	None
Nurse manager/ leader	MSN, MHA, MBA	None
Clinical nurse leader	MSN	Clinical nurse leader
Nurse doctorate	PhD, DNP	Certification required if DNP is advanced practice role; PhD is research focused

DNA: doctor of nursing in anesthesia; DNP: doctor of nursing practice; DrPH: doctor of public health; MBA: master of business administration; MHA: master of health administration; MSN: master of science in nursing; NCLEX: National Council Licensure Examination

Title VIII of the Public Health Service Act of 1994 authorizes federal support to recruit new nurses into the profession in an attempt to promote career advancement within nursing to improve care delivery and safety. The Affordable Care Act includes several sections that specifically address the role of the APRN. Section 5309 authorizes specific funding to promote nurse retention and career advancement. In addition, several sections of the new law provide specific reimbursement or loan forgiveness to nurses in return for their agreement to establish careers in public health or nursing research and education.[32]

The APRN role is defined by seven core competencies or skillful performance areas. The first core competency of direct clinical practice is central to and informs all of the other areas, as follows:

- Direct clinical practice (central)
- Expert coaching and guidance of patients, families, and other care providers
- Consultation
- Research- and evidence-based practice
- Clinical, professional, and systems leadership
- Collaboration
- Ethical decision making[33]

Although the wording is different, these concepts are similar to those proposed by the Accreditation Council for Graduate Medical Education for physicians (see Chapter 6).

Additional core competencies enhance each specialty area that an APRN pursues. The largest number of APRNs is made up of **nurse practitioners (NPs)**, who may further specialize in primary or acute care of families/individuals across the life span, adult/gerontology, neonatology or pediatrics, women's health, or psychiatric and mental health.

Nurse practitioner (NP)

A registered nurse who has advanced education and certification to carry out expanded healthcare evaluation and decision making regarding patient care; boundaries of independent practice are set by state laws; nurse practitioners are certified in primary care or acute and specialty care.

Each state maintains its own laws and regulations regarding recognition of an APRN, but the general requirements in all states include licensure as an RN and successful completion of a national specialty examination that measures APRN role and population-focused competencies, which include continued competence renewal.

NPs may serve as the routine healthcare provider for children and adults during health and illness or they may serve as a specialist in the acute care setting. Nurse practitioners perform physical examinations; diagnose and treat certain acute and chronic medical conditions; order, perform, and interpret diagnostic studies; prescribe medications and other treatments; provide health maintenance care; and collaborate with physicians as outlined in the rules and regulations of the Nurse Practice Act of the state in which they work.[34] Nurse practitioners specializing in primary care (pediatrics, family, adult) or acute and specialty care (neonatology, critical care, cardiology, palliative care, etc.) are required to be board certified by a national certifying body in addition to being licensed in their state of practice. **Nurse midwives** provide uncomplicated obstetric care, including prenatal, delivery, and postnatal services. **Nurse anesthetists** provide anesthetics to patients in collaboration with surgeons, anesthesiologists, and others. Legislation passed by the U.S. Congress in 1986 made nurse anesthetists the first nursing specialty to be accorded direct reimbursement rights under the Medicare program,[35] and some managed care plans now include APRNs on their lists of primary care providers. Nurse practitioners, nurse midwives, and nurse anesthetists may have varying scopes of prescriptive authority, depending on the state in which they work.

Nurse midwife

A registered nurse who has advanced education and certification to practice uncomplicated obstetrical care, including normal spontaneous vaginal delivery, without direct physician supervision.

Nurse anesthetist

A registered nurse who has advanced education and certification to administer anesthesia without direct physician supervision.

Case managers assist care teams in finding the least costly solution in a lengthy and complex treatment.[36] Patients with permanent or long-term illness or disability develop complex medical and social needs. They often require services from several medical specialties, and social services are necessary to allow them to function at the highest possible level. Nurses, particularly those with post-baccalaureate education and considerable clinical experience, are well positioned to become case managers. Certification is available but not required by law.

Other Advanced Nursing Roles

Case manager

A health professional who advocates for the patient to receive the most appropriate treatment with acceptable quality in the most effective manner and appropriate setting at the best price.

The master's-prepared clinical nurse leader (CNL) assumes accountability for healthcare outcomes for a specific group of clients within a unit or setting through the assimilation and application of research-based information to design, implement, and evaluate client plans of care. The CNL serves as a lateral integrator for the healthcare team and facilitates, coordinates, and oversees the care provided by the healthcare team.[37] The doctor of nursing practice (DNP) degree emphasizes the preparation of leaders for clinical practice, health policy, administration, and clinical research. DNP-prepared nurses work at the highest level of clinical practice with nurse researchers to provide leadership in nursing in a variety of settings,[38] with complementary roles between the DNP and the more research-oriented PhD degree in nursing.[39] Consistent with the IOM report entitled *The Future of Nursing: Leading Change, Advancing Health*, the American Association of Colleges of Nursing has proposed the DNP degree as the minimum requirement for advanced practice nursing by 2015.[40,41]

Nurses are represented in senior leadership, and they make up a significant proportion of middle management. Some are general line managers, supervising

Nurse Executives

large staffs and being accountable for a broad range of expectations. Nurse clinicians with graduate education in the problems of certain patient groups are particularly well prepared for this role in service lines. An acute care nursing unit is a substantial managerial challenge that involves 50 or more employees working 24/7; an annual budget in excess of $3 million; and routine contact with many physicians and most CSS as well as finance, human resources, and environment-of-care management. Nurse executives must blend management and leadership competencies with the core ideology of nursing,[42] drawing on the model developed by the American Organization of Nurse Executives.[43]

Explicit in the ANCC Magnet designation model is a style of leadership that listens, supports, empowers, and shares decision making with nurses based on evidence, benchmarks, and best practices. The principles of Magnet are supported by many HCOs that do not seek the designation but pursue both the empowerment concepts and the shared governance professional model of nursing.[44]

Practice Settings

Nurses practice in the community as well as in HCOs. HCO nursing is far larger, but community nursing is important to improve the health status of communities.

HCO Nursing   Most nurses work in HCOs and specialize both by activity and by patient characteristics, as shown in Exhibit 7.6. Some specializations, such as operating room and critical care nursing, emphasize technical skills. Others, such as extended care of the chronically ill, emphasize comfort and palliative care, but most specializations blend both. All facets of nursing require an understanding of pathophysiology, pharmacology, and health assessment. Unlicensed assistive personnel—nursing assistants, technicians, and unit coordinators—support nurses in most specialties. Nursing assistants and technicians are likely to possess certifications and specialty training for the site and type of patient population being served.

Community Nursing   Community nursing emphasizes prevention and health promotion for the well population. Contacts and encounters are often with groups outside the healthcare framework, providing group and individual counseling and limited personal care in settings where people congregate, such as schools, workplaces, churches, public health departments, and senior citizen centers. Efforts are made to reach populations at particular risk, and financing often includes elements outside the usual health insurance structures. Unlicensed assistive personnel are used less often in this setting. Nursing is only one of several professions that can practice community nursing activities.

Community nursing's advantages lie in the respect for nurses among the target populations and in the nurses' ability to relate the specific topics to a

EXHIBIT 7.6
Nursing
Practice
Specialties in
HCOs

Site	Nature of Activity	Common Subspecialization*
Acute Hospital		
Operating rooms	Collaborate with surgical team	Pediatric, surgical specialty
Birthing suite	Pre- and post-partum care, assist delivery	High-risk obstetrics, neonatology
Intensive care and post-anesthesia care	Demanding, technically complex bedside care	Surgical, cardiovascular, and neonatal
Intermediate care	Less demanding bedside care, patient instruction, and emotional support	Medical, surgical, and pediatric
Emergency services	Wide variation	Trauma, flight
Ambulatory care	Direct care, patient instruction, and emotional support	Surgery, oncology, and cardiology
Primary Care Office	Screening, case management, patient instruction, and limited direct care	By primary care specialty
Rehabilitation	Direct care, patient instruction, and emotional support	Cardiovascular, stroke, and trauma
Long-Term Care Facility	Bedside care, emotional support	Skilled and extended care
Home Care	Bedside care, emotional and family support	Palliative care
End-of-Life Care Hospice Palliative care	Bedside care, emotional and family support	Inpatient, home, and palliative care; pain management

*Other specializations, such as pediatric subspecialties, also are practiced.

broader context of health and disease. Well-run HCOs have moved decisively toward preventive services as a way not only to improve the health status of the communities being served but also to reduce the total cost of care.

Organization

In excellent HCOs, nurse managers lead teams and are accountable for operations scorecards, as indicated in Chapter 5. They work directly with unit medical directors or physician leaders of the service lines, identifying OFIs, participating in PITs, and negotiating improvement goals. They are also supported by a strong nursing organization led by a chief nursing officer (CNO) to ensure credentialing requirements are met, manage nurse training and development, recruit and retain a competent and proficient nursing workforce, implement evidence-based nursing practice standards and functional protocols, and maintain consistent performance of nursing activities. The CNO is a member of senior management and acts as the principal strategic and operational executive to ensure uniform achievement of good nursing practice.

Nursing units with formally negotiated annual goals usually divide their work among several temporary teams assigned to specific patients. In acute inpatient settings, the teams are led by an RN and vary in size and skill levels, depending on patient needs. The shift leader, or charge nurse, of the unit is usually a baccalaureate or higher-educated nurse. The nursing organization design can be modified to fit home care, hospices, and rehabilitation and extended care facilities. Specific policies, procedures, and skills differentiate the various services. Clearly, the procedures for operating rooms are different from those for outpatient psychiatry, but the structure of teams and accountability hierarchy are the same. The staff nurse for chronic care may be an RN or an LPN or, for acute and specialty care units, an RN with a baccalaureate or master's degree. The skill required for outpatient care depends on the role.

The nursing organization in larger HCOs often provides a management structure to support first-line nurse managers, completing the structure described in Exhibit 5.8. The nurse teams have one accountability—to their service line—but two lines of support, from their service line and from the nursing organization, as shown in Exhibit 7.7. This structure is flexible and powerful, and it promotes excellent care. It requires ongoing communication

EXHIBIT 7.7
Nursing Team
Support
Structure

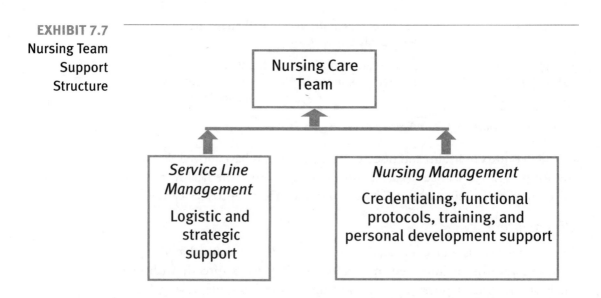

among the professional caregivers; in planning sessions, PITs, and training activities; and when resolving issues.

Measures

The combined developments of evidence-based medicine, electronic information management, and the NOC have made measuring performance of most nursing teams feasible. Formal schemes for measuring nursing care in educational environments[45] and care settings[46] are implemented in excellent hospitals.[46] Exhibit 7.8 shows the kinds of measures that should routinely reported, benchmarked, and used to set goals for the team. The growing body of data from NIC and NOC, using the NANDA paradigm, will provide increasingly valuable answers to core nursing questions about best practice, staffing levels, and training methods. As EHRs make application of the measures more practical, the ability of nursing to identify outcomes and relate them to nursing practice will contribute to evidence-based nursing.

The typical nursing accountability center can measure, set expectations according to comparative norms, and achieve improvements in patient outcomes. Data are collected according to the USA Nursing Management Minimum Data Set (USA NMMDS) uniform standards for the collection of comparable essential patient data.[47] These data then may be reported to the National Database of Nursing Quality Indicators (NDNQI), a repository of information for comparison of nursing-sensitive outcomes.[48] The NDNQI collects data endorsed by the National Quality Forum's nursing-sensitive core performance measures.[49] Examples of nursing performance measures are shown in Exhibit 7.8.

The rich measurement set depends heavily on information systems. As the systems are installed, obvious avenues of improvement appear and are explored. Initially, these are at the level of a single process; integrated and service line opportunities appear later. The process of identifying and addressing these opportunities appears to take several years in most organizations. A third, more rewarding and more challenging phase is beginning where medicine, nursing, and CSSs collaborate toward a goal of cost-effective care.

Managerial Issues

Leadership of high-performing HCOs should pursue two critical strategies. One is to keep nursing work attractive so that the long-term needs of the nation's aging population can be met. The elements of this strategy include deliberate promotion of nursing to school-age students, deliberate recruitment of diverse groups (i.e., post–high school, second degree, mid-career, men, ethnic and racial minorities), and maintenance of rewarding work environments that encourage all nurses to stay in nursing. The second strategy is to improve nurses' effectiveness, using the clinical team concept to amplify each professional nurse's contribution to patient care. The CNO and senior

EXHIBIT 7.8
Nursing Per-
formance
Measures

Dimension	Inpatient Examples	Outpatient Examples (Home Care Program)	Community Nursing Examples
Demand	Number and acuity of patients, percent emergencies	Scheduled home visits, delay for visit	Enrollment in programs, percent eligibles attracted
Costs	Nursing hours per patient day, medical supplies	Payroll costs, home supplies, travel costs	Faculty cost, facility cost, promotional cost
Human resources	Skills mix, education and certification, nurse engagement, turnover vacancies	Skill mix, satisfaction, turnover vacancies	Skill mix, satisfaction, turnover vacancies
Output/ productivity	Discharges, cost/ discharge, cost/member month	Visits, visits/ patient, patients/visiting nurse, costs/patient month	Number of presentations, attendance, cost/ member
Outcomes quality	NDNQI, (incidence of urinary tract infections, ventilator-associated pneumonia, falls, prevalence of restraint, pressure ulcer)	Daily living scores, hospitalizations, transfers to long-term care	Percentage members smoking, percentage seeking prenatal care, count of child trauma
Process quality	NDNQI (incidence of complete care plans, medication errors, presurgery patient education, pain assessement)	Percentage visits late or missed, errors in equipment, supplies	Member awareness, curriculum evaluation, facility evaluation
Patient satisfaction	HCAHPS scores (several questions), number of complaints	Percentage "very satisfied," family satisfaction	Audience evaluation, member satisfaction
Physician satisfaction	Referring and attending physicians "very satisfied," complaints	Percentage referring physicians "very satisfied," complaints	Physician awareness, satisfaction, complaints

HCAHPS: Hospital Consumer Assessment of Healthcare Providers and Systems; NDNQI: National Database of Nursing Quality Indicators management team have a number of vehicles to complete each task. It is noteworthy that Magnet-designated hospitals and other hospitals that follow similar principles generally do not have nursing shortages. They recruit, develop, support, and reward their nursing personnel at all levels in ways that make nursing satisfying work. They "seek and destroy" work elements that are unnecessarily frustrating. They use many kinds of training and support so that nurses gain skills and use them effectively.

Recruitment and Retention

A medium-sized HCO employs several hundred professional nurses, most of whom work at tasks that are both physically and emotionally demanding. There continues to be national concern about projected shortages of nurses.[50] Although the total numbers of younger entrants are growing,[51] baccalaureate nursing school enrollments have slowed and are not keeping pace with the demand despite calls for a more educated nursing workforce.[52]

Efforts to maintain a sufficient cadre of qualified nurses begin with a deliberate effort to reduce turnover and increase work satisfaction.[53,54] Excellent HCOs keep turnover below 10 percent.[55] Many HCOs have much higher staff nurse turnover, sometimes exceeding 50 percent per year. Low turnover has multiple, complementary advantages. Retention is less expensive than recruitment; hiring adds several thousand dollars to first-year costs.[56] More important, the retained nurse's experience will pay off in better patient quality[57] and patient satisfaction.[58] Perhaps most important, the satisfaction of current staff is quickly sensed by potential recruits, and a reputation as a good place to work is a powerful asset. The starting point for the solution is involving nurses in decisions and empowering patient care teams so they can make changes that are needed to improve care.[59]

Compensation is now comparable with that of professional opportunities such as teaching and pharmacy. Although neither of those jobs combines the hours, physical demands, and critical responsibilities of a staff nurse, increased pay is not likely to solve the recruitment problem. Empowering the teams is more promising. It requires both adequate training and personal support. Functional protocols not only standardize processes and equipment usage but they allow team members to rely on each other. New team members need extensive education and assistance in mastering the processes and equipment commonly used on their unit. The Joint Commission has recommended that hospitals institute nurse residency programs to transition new graduates into practice settings.[60] Assigning each new nurse a successful senior mentor has been successful. Huddles, brief team conversations about patient needs, help team members understand not only what to do but what to look for, what patient signals are important, and how to respond quickly when necessary. Team strength behind implementation of the IPOC improves outcomes and patient satisfaction.

The nurse manager or charge nurse is a critical player. She or he must be fully trained in transformational management and the skills needed to run the unit, empowered (her or his questions promptly and effectively answered), and strongly supported by higher-level leaders. High-performing HCOs invest substantially in training nurse leaders. Personal evaluations of staff nurses identify training opportunities. Promising candidates for promotion are identified early and prepared for promotion through deliberate succession planning activities. Ongoing monitoring by senior nurse managers identifies personal growth opportunities; human resources provides programs to exploit them.

The teams are extensively supported, by both the nursing organization and the logistic and strategic units, but they themselves are important management units. Maintaining them involves sustaining the transformational culture, leading the goal-setting negotiations, and handling the staffing and scheduling of team members.

Evidence exists that nurse satisfaction is related to outcomes measures of patient care. In 2014, about 7 percent of U.S. HCOs were designated by ANCC's Magnet Recognition Program for administering exceptional patient care, for providing good nursing practice environments, and for their ability to attract and retain nurses.[61] However, researchers have found mixed results on the relationship of Magnet designation and patient outcomes, work environments, and staffing levels[62] and determined that a Magnet-designation strategy may not be advantageous in rural areas or where there is an inadequate supply of RNs.[63] While Magnet recognition is certainly consistent with the documented solution, it is neither essential nor foolproof.

Improving Nursing's Effectiveness

The tools that leading hospitals use to achieve excellent outcomes are consistent with the operating and cultural foundations described in chapters 1 through 3, emphasizing a transformational culture with effective clinical and other support services, service excellence, and continuous improvement. The following is a checklist that a CNO or chief operating officer might use to review progress toward the critical tasks.

1. *Culture.* A healthy work environment and a culture of respect are established by the mission, vision, and values and supported by training and incentives. Management must "listen" to learn how nurses actually perceive the culture. Listening (see Chapter 15) includes surveying, rounding, forums, open-door policies, and other activities that generate a thorough and timely understanding of nurses' needs.

2. *Staffing.* Nationally, RN staffing has increased on general care units, and the use of LPNs and agency or temporary nurses has declined.[64] The organization must ensure that nurses are rarely or never forced into either dangerously low staffing or excessive overtime situations. It should also offer flexibility in assignment of

patients. A sophisticated program of workload analysis; shift-by-shift monitoring of need; scheduling; and, in units with high census variability, a trained pool of additional personnel is necessary to staff nursing teams effectively. Management must install and maintain the program and monitor it with measures of both staffing and outcomes. In cases where staffing is inadequate, management must be prepared to divert or defer patients.

3. *Communication.* Much nursing time is wasted in rework associated with lost orders or test results. Computerized order entry systems substantially reduce this waste. Similarly, pharmaceutical management systems reduce errors and speed drug distribution, resulting in improved patient safety. Management should provide order entry and pharmacy systems and move with deliberate speed to fully digitalized records.

4. *Ongoing education and credentialing.* Each level of nursing—technician through advanced practice—can improve and expand its contribution through specific clinical education programs and credentialing. Similarly, nurse managers can be trained and coached in the details of their work. Management should invest in more than five days of training per associate per year.

5. *Clinical protocols.* Practice guidelines of all kinds improve quality and promote effective collaboration in clinical teams. They must be kept up-to-date. Management is responsible for an ongoing, effective process to review and revise protocols. The review process should routinely include nurses and use frontline knowledge in the revision.

6. *Transforming the patient care environment.* Studies have shown that nurses spend only 31 percent to 44 percent of their time in direct patient care activities.[65] Changes to the nurse work environment could increase the amount of time available for direct patient care by removing obstacles to the efficient performance of routine nursing tasks.[66] Although the EHR has improved aspects of patient care, bedside nurses spend four hours per day documenting patient information and completing detailed forms seldom viewed by others.[67] Implementation of patient-centered design, systemwide-integrated technology, streamlined documentation and forms completion, seamless workplace environments, and vendor partnerships may positively affect care delivery and allow nurses to spend more time caring for patients.[68]

Excellent nurses and excellent patient care are central to the mission and performance of excellent HCOs. Nurses are powerful patient advocates, and their interventions optimize clinical effectiveness. Excellent HCOs recognize, empower, and reward nurses for their major contributions to patient care.

Additional Resources

American Nurses Association (ANA). 2009. *Nursing Administration: Scope and Standards of Practice.* Silver Spring, MD: ANA.

_____. 2010. *Nursing's Social Policy Statement: The Essence of the Profession,* 3rd ed. Silver Spring, MD: ANA.

Buppert, C. 2015. *Nurse Practitioner's Business Practice and Legal Guide,* 5th ed. Burlington, MA: Jones & Bartlett Learning.

Dunham-Taylor, J., and J. Z. Pinczuk. 2014. *Financial Management for Nurse Managers: Merging the Heart with the Dollar,* 3rd ed. Burlington, MA: Jones and Bartlett Learning.

Finkler, S. A., C. Jones, and C. T. Kovner. 2012. *Financial Management for Nurse Managers and Executives,* 4th ed. Philadelphia, PA: W. B. Saunders.

Institute of Medicine. 2014. *Dying in America: Improving Quality and Honoring Individual Preferences Near the End of Life.* Washington, DC: National Academies Press.

_____. 2010. *The Future of Nursing: Leading Change, Advancing Health.* Washington, DC: National Academies Press.

———. 2004. *Keeping Patients Safe: Transforming the Work Environment of Nurses.* Washington, DC: National Academies Press.

Lindberg, C., S. Nash, and C. Lindberg. 2008. *On the Edge: Nursing in the Age of Complexity.* Bordentown, NJ: Plexus Press.

National Quality Forum (NQF). 2004. *National Voluntary Consensus Standards for Nursing-Sensitive Care: An Initial Performance Measure Set.* Washington, DC: NQF.

Powell, S. K., and H. A. Tahan. 2009. *Case Management: A Practical Guide for Education and Practice,* 3rd ed. New York: Lippincott Williams & Wilkins.

Sullivan, E. J. 2012. *Effective Leadership and Management in Nursing,* 8th ed. Upper Saddle River, NJ: Pearson-Prentice Hall.

Notes

1. Gallup. 2013. "Honesty and Ethics Rating of Clergy Slides to New Low." [Online information; retrieved 6/5/14/.] www.gallup.com/poll/166298/honesty-ethics-rating-clergy-slides-new-low.aspx.

2. Florence Nightingale, quoted in V. Henderson. 1966. *The Nature of Nursing,* 1. New York: MacMillan.

3. Abrams, S. E. 2007. "Nursing the Community: A Look Back at the 1984 Dialog Between Virginia A. Henderson and Sherry L. Shamansky." *Public Health Nursing* 24 (4): 382–86.

4. American Nurses Association (ANA). 2010. *Nursing's Social Policy Statement: The Essence of the Profession,* 3rd ed. Silver Spring, MD: ANA; American Nurses Association (ANA). 2010. *Nursing: Scope and Standards of Practice,* 2nd ed. Silver Spring, MD: ANA; International Council of Nurses. 2014. "Definition of Nursing." [Online information; retrieved 6/05/2014.] www.icn.ch/about-icn/icn-definition-of-nursing/.

5. Institute of Medicine, Committee on Quality of Health Care in America. 2001. *Crossing the Quality Chasm: A New Health System for the 21st Century,* edited by L. T. Kohn, J. M. Corrigan, and M. S. Donaldson. Washington, DC: National Academies Press.

6. NANDA International. 2014. Home page. [Online information; retrieved 6/05/14.] www.nanda.org.

7. Bulechek, G. M., H. K. Butcher, J. M. M. Dochterman, and C. Wagner. 2012. *Nursing Interventions Classification,* 6th ed. St. Louis, MO: Mosby.

8. Moorhead, S., M. Johnson, M. L. Maas, and E. Swanson. 2012. *Nursing Outcomes Classification,* 5th ed. St. Louis, MO: Mosby.

9. Donaldson, N., S. Shapiro, M. Scott, M. Foley, and J. Spetz. 2009. "Leading Successful Rapid Response Teams: A Multisite Implementation Evaluation." *Journal of Nursing Administration* 39 (4): 176–81.

10. Muller-Staub, M. 2009. "Evaluation of the Implementation of Nursing Diagnoses, Interventions, and Outcomes." *International Journal of Nursing Terminologies & Classifications* 20 (1): 9–15.

11. American Society for Healthcare Risk Management. 2013. "Disclosure of Unanticipated Events in 2013." [Online information: retrieved 8/10/14.] www.ashrm.org/search?q=unanticipated+outcome&site=ASHRM&client=default_FE&submit=Search; see also Joint Commission. 2014. *Comprehensive Accreditation Manual.* Oakbrook Terrace, IL: Joint Commission.

12. Henriksen, K., E. Dayton, M. A. Keyes, P. Carayon, and R. Hughes. 2008. "Understanding Adverse Events: A Human Factors Framework." *Patient Safety and Quality: An Evidence-Based Handbook for Nurses,* edited by R. G. Hughes. AHRQ Publication No. 08-0043. [Online information; retrieved 8/10/14.] www.ahrq.gov/professionals/clinicians-providers/resources/nursing/resources/nurseshdbk/nurseshdbk.pdf.

13. De Meester, K., M. Verspuy, K. G. Monsieurs, and P. Van Bogaert. 2013. "SBAR Improves Nurse-Physician Communication and Reduces Unexpected Death: A Pre and Post Intervention Study." *Resuscitation* 84 (9): 1192–96.

14. Wakefield, B. J., M. A. Blegen, T. Uden-Holman, T. Vaughn, E. Chrischilles, and D. S. Wakefield. 2001. "Organizational Culture, Continuous Quality Improvement, and Medication Administration Error Reporting." *Journal of Medical Quality* 16 (4): 128–34.

15. Thomas, R. K. 2014. *Marketing Health Services,* 3rd ed. Chicago: Health Administration Press.

16. White, K. R., P. J. Coyne, and U. B. Patel. 2001. "Are Nurses Adequately Prepared for End-of-Life Care?" *Journal of Nursing Scholarship* 33 (2): 147–51.

17. Porter-O'Grady, T., and S. Finnigan. 1984. *Shared Governance for Nursing.* Rockville, MD: Aspen Systems.

18. Porter-O'Grady, T. 1992. *Implementing Shared Governance.* St. Louis, MO: Mosby.

19. Clavelle, J. T., Porter-O'Grady, T., and K. Drenkard. 2013. "Structural Empowerment and the Nursing Practice Environment in Magnet Organizations." *Journal of Nursing Administration* 43 (11): 566–73.

20. Griffith, J. R. 2008. "Finding the Frontier of Hospital Management." *Journal of Healthcare Management* 54 (1): 57–72.

21. American Nurses Association. 2012. Home page. [Online information; retrieved 6/5/14.] www.nursingworld.org.

22. Nelson, R. 2008. "California's Ratio Law, Four Years Later." *American Journal of Nursing* 108 (3): 25–26.

23. Sochalski, J., R. T. Konetzka, J. Zhu, and K. Volpp. 2008. "Will Mandated Minimum Nurse Staffing Ratios Lead to Better Patient Outcomes?" *Medical Care* 46 (6): 606–13.

24. Chapman, S. A., J. Spetz, J. A. Seago, J. Kaiser, C. Dower, and C. Herrera. 2009. "How Have Mandated Nurse Staffing Ratios Affected Hospitals? Perspectives from California Hospital Leaders." *Journal of Healthcare Management* 54 (5): 321–35.

25. Sullivan, E. J. 2012. *Effective Leadership and Management in Nursing,* 8th ed. Upper Saddle River, NJ: Prentice Hall.

26. Havens, D. S., and L. H. Aiken. 1999. "Shaping Systems to Promote Desired Outcomes: The Magnet Hospital Model." *Journal of Nursing Administration* 29 (2): 14–20.

27. Institute of Medicine. 2010. *The Future of Nursing: Leading Change, Advancing Health.* Washington, DC: National Academies Press.

28. Health Resources and Services Administration. 2013. "The U.S. Nursing Workforce: Trends in Supply and Education." [Online information; retrieved 10/3/13.] http://bhpr.hrsa.gov/healthworkforce/supplydemand/nursing/nursingworkforce/nursingworkforcefullreport.pdf.

29. Pittman, P., C.-N. S. Herrera, K. Horton, P. A. Thompson, J. M. Ware, and M. Terry. 2013. "Healthcare Employers' Policies on Nurse Education." *Journal of Health Administration* 58 (6): 399–411.

30. Rambur, B., B. McIntosh, M. V. Palumbo, and K. Reinier. 2005. "Education as a Determinant of Career Retention and Job Satisfaction Among Registered Nurses." *Journal of Nursing Scholarship* 37 (2): 185–92.

31. National Council of State Boards of Nursing. 2008. "Consensus Model for APRN Regulation: Licensure, Accreditation, Certification & Education." [Online information; retrieved 12/6/13.] www.ncsbn.org/Consensus_Model_for_APRN_Regulation_July_2008.pdf.

32. American Nurses Association. 2013. "Health Care Reform and the APRN." [Online article; retrieved 12/6/13.] www.nursingworld.org/EspeciallyForYou/AdvancedPracticeNurses/Health-Care-Reform-and-the-APRN.

33. Hamric, A. B. 2014. *Advanced Practice Nursing: An Integrative Approach,* 5th ed., edited by A. B. Hamric, C. M. Hanson, M. F. Tracy, and E. T. O'Grady. St. Louis, MO: Elsevier Saunders.

34. American Academy of Nurse Practitioners. 2014. Home page. [Online information; retrieved 6/05/14.] www.aanp.org.

35. American Association of Nurse Anesthetists. 2014. Home page. [Online information; retrieved 6/05/14.] www.aana.com.

36. Park, E., and D. L. Huber. 2009. "Case Management Workforce in the United States." *Journal of Nursing Scholarship* 41 (2): 175–83.

37. Begun, J. W., J. Tornabeni, and K. R. White. 2006. "Opportunities for Improving Patient Care Through Lateral Integration: The Clinical Nurse Leader." *Journal of Healthcare Management* 51 (1): 19–25.

38. Acorn, S., K. Lamarche, and M. Edwards. 2009. "Practice Doctorates in Nursing: Developing Nursing Leaders." *Nursing Leadership* 22 (2): 85–91.

39. Dracup, K., L. Cronenwett, A. I. Meleis, and P. E. Benner. 2005. "Reflections on the Doctorate of Nursing Practice." *Nursing Outlook* 53 (4): 177–82.

40. Lancaster, J., and G. P. Bednash. 2008. "AACN Commentary on 'Professional Polarities in Nursing' Response to the Article by Elaine S. Scott and Brenda L. Cleary." *Nursing Outlook* 56: 50–51.

41. American Association of Colleges of Nursing. 2004. "AACN Position Statement on the Practice Doctorate in Nursing." [Online information; retrieved 7/23/14.] www.aacn.nche.edu/DNP/DNPPositionStatement.htm; American Association of Colleges of Nursing. 2014. "DNP Talking Points." [Online information; retrieved 2/6/15.] www.aacn.nche.edu/dnp/about/talking-points.

42. Jennings, B. M., C. C. Scalzi, J. D. Rodgers III, and A. Keane. 2007. "Differentiating Nursing Leadership and Management Competencies." *Nursing Outlook* 55: 169–75.

43. American Organization of Nurse Executives. 2011. "The AONE Nurse Executive Competencies." [Online information; retrieved 7/23/14.] www.aone.org/resources/leadership%20tools/nursecomp.shtml.

44. Porter-O'Grady, T. 2008. *Interdisciplinary Shared Governance: Integrating Practice, Transforming Health Care,* 2nd ed. Boston: Jones & Bartlett.

45. Canham, D., C.-L. Mao, M. Yoder, P. Connolly, and E. Dietz. 2008. "The Omaha System and Quality Measurement in Academic Nurse-Managed Centers: Ten Steps for Implementation." *Journal of Nursing Education* 47 (3): 105–11.

46. Hendrix, S. E. 2009. "An Experience with Implementation of NIC and NOC in a Clinical Information System." *CIN: Computers, Informatics, Nursing* 27 (1): 7–11.

47. USA NMMDS. 2014. "USA NMMDS." [Online information: retrieved 8/31/14.] www.nursing.umn.edu/icnp/usa-nmmds/; Huber, D., L. Schumacher, and C. Delaney. 1997. "Nursing Management Minimum Data Set (NMMDS)." *Journal of Nursing Administration* 27 (4): 42–48.

48. Press Ganey. 2014. "Press Ganey Acquires National Database of Nursing Quality Indicators (NDNQI)." [Online information; retrieved 8/31/14.] http://press ganey.com/pressRoom/2014/06/10/press-ganey-acquires-national-database-of-nursing-quality-indicators-%28ndnqi-%29.

49. National Database of Nursing Quality Indicators. 2014. "About NDNQI." [Online information; retrieved 8/31/14.] www.nursingquality.org/FAQ#faq-about.

50. Buerhaus, P. I. 2008. "Current and Future State of the U.S. Nursing Workforce." *Journal of the American Medical Association* 300 (20): 2422–24.

51. Auerbach, D. I., P. I. Buerhaus, and D. O. Staiger. 2011. "Registered Nurse Supply Grows Faster than Projected Amid Surge in New Entrants Ages 23–26." *Health Affairs* 33: 81474–80.

52. American Association of Colleges of Nursing. 2014. "AACN Finds Slow Enrollment Growth at Schools of Nursing." [Online information; retrieved 8/31/14.] www.aacn.nche.edu/news/articles/2014/slow-enrollment.

53. Griffith (2008, 62).

54. Upenieks, V. 2005. "Recruitment and Retention Strategies: A Magnet Hospital Prevention Model." *Medsurg Nursing* (Suppl.): 21–27.

55. Needleman, J., P. I. Buerhaus, S. Mattke, M. Stewart, and K. Zelevinsky. 2001. "Nurse Staffing and Patient Outcomes in Hospitals." Final Report, U.S. Department of Health and Human Services, Health Resources and Services Administration, Contract No. 230-99-0021. Boston: Harvard School of Public Health.

56. PricewaterhouseCoopers Research Institute. 2007. "What Works: Healing the Healthcare Staffing Shortage," 1. [Online information; retrieved 7/22/14.] www.pwc.com/us/en/healthcare/publications/what-works-healing-the-healthcare-staffing-shortage.jhtml.

57. Aiken, L. H., J. P. Cimiotti, D. M. Sloane, H. L. Smith, L. Flynn, and D. F. Neff. 2011. "Effects of Nurse Staffing and Nurse Education on Patient Deaths in Hospitals with Different Nurse Work Environments." *Medical Care* 49 (12): 1047–53.

58. Snide, J., and R. Nailon. 2013. "Nursing Staff Innovations Results in Improved Patient Satisfaction." *American Journal of Nursing* 113 (10): 42–50.

59. Houser, J. A., L. B. Erkenbrack, L. C. Handberry, F. D. Ricker, and L. E. Stroup. 2012. "Involving Nurses in Decisions: Improving Both Nurse and Patient Outcomes." *Journal of Nursing Administration* 42 (7–8): 375–82; Twigg, D., and K. McCullough. 2014. "Nurse Retention: A Review of Strategies to Create and Enhance Positive Practice Environments in Clinical Settings." *International Journal of Nursing Studies* 51 (1): 85–92.

60. Chappell, K. 2014. "The Value of RN Residency and Fellowship Programs for Magnet® Hospitals." *JONA: Journal of Nursing Administration* 44 (6): 313–14.

61. American Nurses Credentialing Center. 2014. "Growth of the Program." [Online information; retrieved 7/23/14.] www.nursecredentialing.org/Magnet/ProgramOverview/HistoryoftheMagnetProgram/GrowthoftheProgram.

62. Goode, C. J., M. A. Blegen, S. H. Park, T. Vaughn, and J. Spetz. 2011. "Comparison of Patient Outcomes in Magnet® and Non-Magnet Hospitals." *JONA: Journal of Nursing Administration* 41 (12): 517–23; Trinkoff, A., M. Johantgen, C. Storr, K. Han, Y. Liang, A. P. Gurses, and S. Hopkinson. 2010. "A Comparison of Working Conditions Among Nurses in Magnet and Non-Magnet Hospitals." *JONA: Journal of Nursing Administration* 40 (7/8): 309–15; Kelly, L. A., M. D. McHugh, and L. H. Aiken. 2011. "Nurse Outcomes in Magnet® and Non-Magnet Hospitals." *JONA: Journal of Nursing Administration* 41 (10): 428–33.

63. Abraham, J., B. Jerome-D'Emilia, and J. W. Begun. 2011. "The Diffusion of Magnet Hospital Recognition." *Health Care Management Review* 36 (4): 306–14.

64. Staggs, V. S., and J. He. 2013. "Recent Trends in Hospital Nurse Staffing in the United States." *JONA: Journal of Nursing Administration* 43 (7/8): 388–93.

65. Tucker, A. L., and S. J. Spear. 2006. "Operational Failures and Interruptions in Hospital Nursing." *Health Services Research* 41: 643–62.

66. Hendrich, A., M. P. Chow, and W. S. Goshert. 2009. "A Proclamation for Change: Transforming the Hospital Patient Care Environment." *Journal of Nursing Administration* 39 (6): 266–75.

67. Penoyer, D. A., K. H. Cortelyou-Ward, A. M. Noblin, T. Bullard, S. Talbert, J. Wilson, B. Schafthauser, and J. G. Briscoe. 2014. "Use of Electronic Health Record Documentation by Healthcare Workers in an Acute Care Hospital System." *Journal of Healthcare Management* 59 (2): 130–46.

68. Hendrich, Chow, and Goshert (2009, 274).

8 CLINICAL SUPPORT SERVICES

1. *Supporting evidence-based patient care:*
   - Provide prompt, comprehensive, reliable support for every patient.
   - Reach benchmark for safety and reliability of clinical support services (CSS) activities.
   - Eliminate underuse and overuse of CSS.
   - Keep pace with best practice protocols.

2. *Providing comprehensive service:*
   - Coordinate multiple clinical support needs.
   - Support computerized order entry and results reporting.
   - Provide convenient consultation for physicians and nurses.
   - Manage the complex patient with multiple diseases or conditions.

3. *Recruiting and retaining qualified CSS professionals:*
   - Make the organization the best place to work.
   - Reward performance improvement.
   - Provide continuing education.

4. *Outsourcing and contracting for CSS:*
   - Keep CSS costs and service comparable to those of the competition.
   - Devise relationships that benefit both customer and associate stakeholders.
   - Understand and capture benefits of scale in CSS.

Questions for Discussion

These questions are about applying the chapter content. It's often helpful to discuss them with classmates or mentors, gaining different perspectives on the issues.

1. Consider a pharmacy that serves a large HCO and is measured by the six dimensions in Exhibit 8.6.
   - How will goals be established for next year?
   - Should some measures have higher priorities?
   - What support should pharmacy expect from senior HCO leadership?
   - Would the HCO offer a bonus for goal achievement?

- Are the answers to these questions different if the pharmacy associates are employed by the hospital or serve on a contract with a national pharmacy vendor?

2. The emergence of service lines has substantially changed the accountability of CSS personnel. Many professionals have dual reporting—to the service line and to the CSS (e.g., respiratory therapists assigned to a cardiovascular service line). How should the organization resolve the following issues?
   - How the HCO establishes functional protocols for the CSS services
   - When the CSS associate feels a specific patient's order is inappropriate
   - When caregiving team members are concerned about the CSS service to a specific patient
   - When caregiving team members are concerned about the CSS service in general

3. Under the dual reporting described in Question 2, how should the organization resolve the following issues?
   - Who reviews the credentials of new CSS associates
   - How a CSS associate assigned to a service line can get promoted
   - When caregiving team members are concerned about the service of a specific CSS associate
   - When CSS associates are concerned that caregiving teams are ordering services inappropriately (i.e., the wrong services, too many, or too few)
   - How the CSS associate's bonus is determined (Is it based on the service line team alone, or on the goals achieved by the CSS as well?)

4. A small HCO in a well-managed healthcare system can consider three ways to obtain a CSS. It can "stand alone," hiring its own professionals. It can "outsource," buying service from a local provider. It can "affiliate," arranging for training, procedures, and supervision through its system. What's the best solution? How should the HCO decide what to do? Who should be involved in the decision? What should the system senior management do to support the best solutions for all the system HCOs?

5. Technology advances rapidly in many CSSs. To keep up, investments must be made in learning, training, and equipment. How does an HCO keep all its CSSs up-to-date? What are the mechanisms that identify investment opportunities? What is the mechanism to evaluate those opportunities?

Purpose

Twenty-first-century caregiving requires services from dozens of specialized professionals providing important clinical information (diagnostic services) or specific interventions (therapeutic services). Laboratory testing, imaging, endoscopic procedures, cardiac, and other invasive vessel procedures are common diagnostic services. Drug selection and administration, surgery, anesthesia, obstetric delivery, and physical therapy are common therapeutic services. Many patients also require behavioral, spiritual, and psychological services such as social service, pastoral care, and health education. Challenging ethical dilemmas arise in patient care, and HCOs provide resources to deal with them. These clinical support services (CSSs) are provided through centralized support units or by professionals assigned to a service line accountability center. Most, but not all, CSSs are ordered by an attending physician. They are needed at several sites—outpatient offices, the acute care hospital, long-term care facilities, and home. A serious illness may require several hundred diagnostic, therapeutic, and consultative services from the CSSs listed in Exhibit 8.1.

The purpose of any CSS is

to provide its specialized services at a level that fully meets patients' and caregivers' needs.

The purpose of the HCO is to assist each CSS in achieving its purpose and

to provide each patient with exactly the set of services needed and integrate those services into an excellent interprofessional plan of care.

These two purposes are different, but they are both possible under a common mission, vision, and values. The differences establish the relationship between the CSS and the HCO, giving each critical functions. When the functions are understood, there are several alternatives for affiliation between the CSS team and the HCO. Employment is the most common, but contracts, joint ventures, and corporate subsidiaries are also possible.

An HCO's profile of clinical support services must be consistent with its mission and strategic plan. This means that the size and scope of each CSS must be defined by the HCO, and the annual goals must be negotiated with the CSS and ultimately approved by the HCO governing board. At the same time, each CSS professional has multiple options to pursue his or her career. To make that negotiation attractive to the CSS professionals, the HCO must make itself the preferred place to practice—the "best place to give care."

EXHIBIT 8.1
Clinical Support
Services in a
Large HCO

Diagnostic Services	Therapeutic Services
Audiology	*Anesthesia*
Cardiopulmonary	Pain management
Electrocardiology	Surgical and obstetric anesthesia
Pulmonary function	*Blood bank and transfusion services*
Invasive cardiology	*Nursing*
Clinical laboratory	Birthing suite
Chemistry	Surgery and post-anesthesia care
Hematology	Wound, ostomy, and continence care
Histopathology	*Optometry*
Bacteriology and virology	*Orthotics*
Autopsy and morgue	*Palliative and hospice care*
Consultative services	*Pharmacy*
Ethics committee	Dispensing and counseling
Institutional review board	Intravenous admixture
Diagnostic imaging	*Radiation oncology*
Radiography	*Rehabilitation services*
Computerized tomography	Physical therapy
Positron emission tomography	Respiratory therapy
Radioisotope studies	Speech pathology
Magnetic resonance imaging	Occupational therapy
Ultrasound	
Electroencephalography	*Social and Counseling Services*
Electromyography	
Telemedicine	Community support groups
	Grief counseling
	Pastoral care
	Psychological care
	Social service

Functions

It is obvious from Exhibit 8.1 that CSSs have different characteristics, yet similarities emerge at one level of abstraction above these differences. The managers of social service and radiation oncology, for example, share common functions, which are identified in Exhibit 8.2.

Providing Excellent Care

Both diagnostic and treatment CSSs are integral parts of healthcare. They must individually and collectively meet the Institute of Medicine goal of safe, effective, patient-centered, timely, efficient, and equitable care. They do that with the following processes:

1. *Patient management protocols.* These are adopted by protocol-selection committees on which CSS members participate. They control effectiveness because they

specify when CSSs are required, optional, or not recommended. As a result, they also control the demand for service, placing the sizing of the CSS as an HCO function.

2. *Functional protocols.* Virtually all CSS activities are learned processes that are formalized and scripted as functional protocols. The protocols must be designed to achieve benchmark safety, effectiveness, patient comfort, and efficiency. Each CSS profession designs, tests, and maintains the processes it uses. Many functional protocols must be carefully integrated with other care activities. The CSS identifies and validates performance measures based on the functional protocols. The HCO includes the measures and continuous improvement in its contract.

3. *Scheduling systems.* It is important not only to provide each patient with timely service but also to maintain an orderly workflow within the CSS. Sophisticated scheduling systems achieve this by managing the demand stream. The best scheduling systems integrate all CSSs to minimize the length of the patient care event.

4. *Training.* Each CSS must rely on a mix of professional and nonprofessional associates. Maximizing the contribution of each associate is important to improve safety, patient-centeredness, and costs. It is achieved by careful training and transformational supervision. The HCO shares the training duties, providing training in supervision and continuous improvement, cultural and linguistic competence, and other issues shared by several CSSs. The CSS provides training for its functional protocols, but it often collaborates with human resources management to implement and evaluate the training.

Throughout all the functions, the HCO role can be summarized as providing coordination and support. It maintains the scheduling system (see the Maintaining Patient Relationships section below). It uses process improvement teams (PITs) and planning committees to negotiate protocols and resolve questions that caregivers and CSSs face. These questions range from coordination and availability of services (Will imaging have full service 24/7? What arrangements are made for inpatient meals delayed by testing?) to coverage of uninsured patients (Who pays the rehabilitation costs for a trauma patient without insurance?) to privileges for a specific CSS assigned to various associate groups (Will images taken in outpatient offices be included in the electronic health record, and which ones will be read by the imagist?).

Maintaining Patient Relationships

All CSSs have both patient and caregiver customers. Caregivers order the services; patients receive them; caregivers receive notice of results. Although the clinical laboratory works principally with specimens and the pharmacy supplies many drugs through nursing, most CSSs require intimate patient contact. Given an excellent care function, the issues in satisfying patients are scheduling, amenities, and identifying unusual needs.

The scheduling issues are demanding. Many patients need prompt attention for both safety and caregiving efficiency. CSS delays often add to

Function	CSS Role	HCO Role
Providing excellent care	Provide safe, effective, patient-centered, timely, efficient, and equitable patient services. Select, use, maintain, and teach functional protocols. Participate in patient management protocol selection and development.	Assist in designing work processes and training programs. Ensure appropriate voice in patient management protocol–selection committees.
Maintaining patient relationships	Schedule patients effectively. Train associates in identifying patient needs and using techniques to improve acceptability of care. Maintain cultural and linguistic competence. Provide for uninsured patients.	Maintain a central scheduling system. Provide associate sensitivity training. Provide translators and cultural competence training. Recognize burden of un- or underinsured patients and health disparities.
Maintaining consultative relationships	Assist caregivers with protocol administration. Consult on questionable cases. Provide training to other professions on advances in their CSSs.	Support CSS involvement in PITs and planning activities. Incorporate consultation and training into contract. Resolve rules for nonprofessional administration of CSS services.
Planning and managing operations	Negotiate appropriate long-term relationship. Negotiate goals for operational scorecard dimensions. Maintain regulatory compliance.	Negotiate appropriate long-term relationship. Establish compensation, contribution from HCO's annual strategic goals. Provide resources for regulatory compliance; ensure compliance reporting.
Promoting continuous improvement	Benchmark, identify OFIs, establish and participate in PITs.	Negotiate, support, and reward improvement.

CSS: clinical support service; OFI: opportunity for improvement; PIT: process improvement team the total length of stay and increase the cost per case. The CSS needs a manageable workflow. Its associates need planned schedules, but they also need to have work to do. Idle time drives up the cost per test and reduces their skills.

Sophisticated scheduling systems allow CSSs to balance workflow to their teams while meeting patient needs, including emergencies. The concept for the scheduling system is shown in Exhibit 8.3. Unless volumes of work are large (the laboratory and pharmacy, for example), a CSS that simply accepts patients as they come will have periodic idle times and overflow demand. The first wastes financial resources, and the second endangers safety and effectiveness. Sophisticated scheduling systems can substantially reduce both problems. The secret is to identify a set of patients who do not have emergency needs and are willing and able to come on call. Nonemergency patients already in the HCO are an example. As Exhibit 8.3 shows, emergency patients get immediate care. On-call patients get a fixed future date, but they also can be called sooner. Scheduled patients get a fixed future date. At a given level of emergency allowance, overall efficiency will increase and overall delays will decrease by calling in patients.

Sophisticated computerized scheduling systems are available for major support services and for admission and occupancy management.[1] These programs keep records, print notices, send telephone or e-mail reminder messages

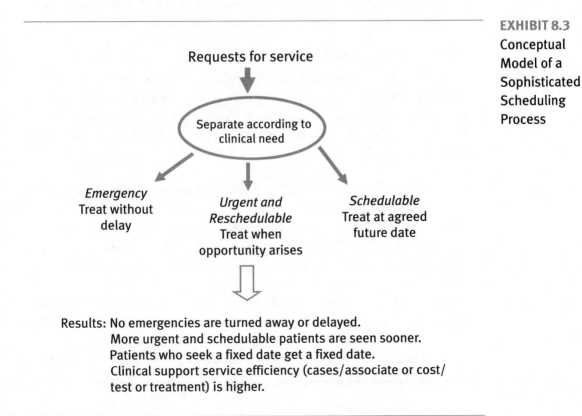

EXHIBIT 8.3
Conceptual Model of a Sophisticated Scheduling Process

Requests for service

Separate according to clinical need

Emergency
Treat without delay

Urgent and Reschedulable
Treat when opportunity arises

Schedulable
Treat at agreed future date

Results: No emergencies are turned away or delayed.
More urgent and schedulable patients are seen sooner.
Patients who seek a fixed date get a fixed date.
Clinical support service efficiency (cases/associate or cost/test or treatment) is higher.

for appointments, and provide real-time prompts to caregiving associates. They automatically monitor cancellations, overloads, work levels, and efficiency. They are integrated with ordering and reporting systems so that the entire process of obtaining a CSS is automatic from the point of the doctor's decision to order it. Most scheduling systems can also be operated in a simulation mode to analyze the costs and benefits of alternative strategies. Simulation outputs are useful in both short- and long-term planning to evaluate potential improvements in demand categorization, resource availability, and scheduling rules.

The scheduling system requires each CSS to establish available hours. The hours should be based principally on efficiency considerations. CSSs should be open only when sufficient demand is expected to support efficiency and skill in the minimum team. Arrangements must be made to call in associates for life-threatening emergencies.

The HCO provides logistic services for many CSSs. These include knowledge management, training and other human resources management, environmental services, accounting and financial services, and internal consulting. They also include sensitivity training for cultural competence, translators, and assistance with patients who present unusual circumstances. The CSS is the customer and final monitor of these services. It should alert its HCO management contact about any failure and expect prompt response. The HCO's ability to provide reliable, high-quality logistic service should be an attraction for a closer relationship.

Maintaining Consultative Relationships

CSSs must view caregivers and interprofessional teams as customers and recognize that caregivers often have alternative sources. Although a few CSSs can work directly with patients, most require physician or advanced practice nurse orders. To complete the orders, CSSs must meet several different aspects of caregiving needs.

- *Comprehensive.* The CSS's level of service must match the requirements of the patient management protocols.
- *Accurate and effective.* Errors in diagnostic tests create unnecessary costs and dangers for patients. Caregivers need to be confident in CSS results.
- *Prompt.* Delays in CSS prolong the care process, reducing efficiency. They also erode patient satisfaction.
- *Supportive of patient needs.* The patients' overall response to the care, both clinically and in terms of satisfaction, is often influenced by the CSS.

In addition to patient-related considerations, CSS must support several needs of the caregiving team:

- *Consultative advice.* Each CSS is an expert resource. Caregivers need to rely on CSS expertise when questions arise about individual patients.

- *Protocol development*. Many questions that emerge from adopting guidelines require CSS participation to answer. Most protocols must be agreed to by the CSS involved.
- *Training*. CSS advances can change how care is given. Many procedures originated in CSS but have moved to general usage; caregivers must often be trained to do them. Others have complex implications for other parts of care, and caregivers must be trained to understand those interactions.
- *Assistance with uninsured patients*. The plans must be worked out in advance and specified in the contract with the HCO (see the Planning and Managing Operations section).

The caregiver needs are met by CSS availability, participation in PITs and planning committees, and support of training activities. Those items must be negotiated in the CSS–HCO contract.

Behind several of these issues lies an unfortunate consequence of the payment system. The CSSs have various relationships to payment. Some, such as social service and bereavement counseling, are almost never billed separately. Others, such as outpatient imaging and laboratory, can have dual physician and hospital payments. The physician portions of these payments are not limited by regulation to CSS professionals. Primary care or specialist physicians who use imaging equipment in their office can collect for each image from most insurance plans. Alternatively or in addition, the physician can order an image from the HCO's imaging service. The payment to the HCO is substantially larger, but it goes to the radiologist and the HCO and not to the primary physician. There are three critical patient care questions here:

1. Is the imaging necessary?
2. Is the radiologist's consultation necessary?
3. Which path is better—the one at the office or the one at the HCO?

The patient care questions are confounded by a fourth, which creates serious conflict of interest: Who gets the money? The problem is not limited to imaging. In one form or another it affects any CSS for which there is direct payment, although it has essentially been solved in pharmacy. Technology improvements change the patient care answers. An imaging consultation that was important in 2014 may not be in the patient management protocol in 2016.

Bundled payments, which Medicare and many private insurance companies are adopting, will improve solutions to these questions because they will force all three parties—the referring physician, the CSS, and the HCO—to negotiate a more cost-effective approach. In the meantime, the HCO plays a major role, negotiating the specific solutions in each protocol and service line. The key to the negotiations is commitment to a mission of excellent care and evidence-based medicine. The patient management protocol should specify when tests or treatments are appropriate and allow completion by the lowest-cost associate who can do the test or treatment safely. That associate must have adequate training and support in case difficulties arise. The principles—evidence-based medicine and commitment to the mission—and the negotiating process must both be included in the contract between the HCO and CSS. The principles must be scrupulously implemented by the HCO, but at the same time, the HCO must assure the CSS associates of a competitive income opportunity. Patient satisfaction, primary caregiver satisfaction, outcomes quality, and process quality measures are all critical in maintaining excellence.

Planning and Managing Operations

Almost any CSS can be envisioned as a small retail business. In fact, many are operated exactly that way. The HCO's strategy is to bring these businesses under one organization. It will ask for commitment to mission and to evidence-based medicine and management. It will enforce these requests by asking for explicit measures of performance, benchmarking, and continuous improvement. It will make its proposal attractive by offering a large, reliable book of business, a record of capability in meeting operating needs, and a culture that is appealing as a place to work. In addition, the HCO must show that it will offer competitive compensation. This concept is a difficult one, given the healthcare financing. It does not mean "As much as you can earn someplace else," because the HCO will expect care limited to appropriateness standards and assigned to the lowest capable level of worker. It does mean "As much as you could earn someplace else given that you accept our commitment to mission and evidence-based medicine."

Excellent HCOs implement that approach to CSS management using a three-part strategy. First, the CSS must be carefully sized to realistic market needs, and the HCO must control the size. Second, the HCO must implement its transformational culture to make the work attractive to professional and nonprofessional associates. Third, the HCO must implement evidence-based management in all the logistic and strategic services the CSS needs. The contract must be competitive in the CSS associates' eyes.

Planning and Sizing the CSS

CSS planning is based on the community epidemiologic planning approach described in Chapter 3. For CSSs drawing directly from the community, populations are age-specific community censuses, the incidence rate is the occurrence of disease in the general population, and the market share is the institution's anticipated share of the particular market, as shown in Equation 1.

Equation 1

$$\text{Demand for a service} = \left\{ \begin{array}{c} \text{Forecast} \\ \text{population} \\ \text{at risk} \end{array} \right\} \times \left\{ \begin{array}{c} \text{Incidence} \\ \text{rate} \end{array} \right\} \times \left\{ \begin{array}{c} \text{Average} \\ \text{use per} \\ \text{incidence} \end{array} \right\} \times \left\{ \begin{array}{c} \text{Market} \\ \text{share} \end{array} \right\}$$

For example, the demand for postoperative physical therapy (POPT):

$$\text{Demand for POPT} = \left\{\begin{array}{c}\text{Forecast}\\\text{procedures}\\\text{requiring}\\\text{POPT}\end{array}\right\} \times \left\{\begin{array}{c}\text{Percent of}\\\text{patients}\\\text{referred}\\\text{for PT}\end{array}\right\} \times \left\{\begin{array}{c}\text{PT visits}\\\text{per patient}\\\text{referred}\end{array}\right\} \times \left\{\begin{array}{c}\text{HCO's}\\\text{market}\\\text{share}\end{array}\right\}$$

or for breast examinations, where average use per incident is 1:

$$\left\{\begin{array}{c}\text{Demand for}\\\text{breast}\\\text{examination}\end{array}\right\} = \left\{\begin{array}{c}\text{Forecast}\\\text{age-specific}\\\text{female}\\\text{population}\end{array}\right\} \times \left\{\begin{array}{c}\text{Age-specific}\\\text{incidence}\\\text{rate}\end{array}\right\} \times 1 \times \left\{\begin{array}{c}\text{HCO's}\\\text{market}\\\text{share}\end{array}\right\}$$

The equation can be specified or aggregated as desired. It might apply to MRI (magnetic resonance imaging) demand by type of procedure, cardiovascular surgeries, births, or any condition for which incidence rates are known.

CSS demand that arises from many different diseases is calculated from general rates of admissions or outpatient visits. Many CSS demands can be estimated from the history of use per patient and forecasts of the number of patients using Equation 2. The equation can be specified or aggregated as needed to obtain reliable results.

Equation 2

$$\text{Demand for widely used CSS} = \left\{\begin{array}{c}\text{Forecast}\\\text{patient}\\\text{encounters}\end{array}\right\} \times \left\{\begin{array}{c}\text{Number of}\\\text{services}\\\text{per encounter}\end{array}\right\}$$

For example:

$$\left\{\begin{array}{c}\text{Inpatient}\\\text{pharmacy}\\\text{demand}\end{array}\right\} = \left\{\begin{array}{c}\text{Forecast}\\\text{inpatient}\\\text{admissions}\end{array}\right\} \times \left\{\begin{array}{c}\text{Number of}\\\text{prescriptions}\\\text{per admission}\end{array}\right\}$$

The equations must be forecast several years into the future and translated into a business plan for the CSS that projects staff requirements by skill level, supply and facility requirements, expected costs, and unit costs. The unit costs can be compared to benchmarks, competitive data, and income forecasts. Annual volumes can be compared to quality minimums. The business plan is presented to both the CSS associates and referring care teams involved for their comments. The plan is presented to the governing board with management's recommendation and both sets of comments. It is adjusted as needed in the annual goal-setting process.

The planning process implements the HCO's mission for quality and cost-effectiveness. The service will be started, continued, or expanded when both cost and quality comparisons are favorable. The service should be discontinued, outsourced, or reorganized whenever quality is threatened or cost is not competitive.

Meeting CSS Support Needs

The HCO's offer to the CSS is that it will thrive under closer affiliation. That requires the HCO to provide a full range of logistic and support services and an attractive work environment. Closer affiliation usually means greater capital investment by the HCO.

The CSS associates work side by side with the caregiving teams, and they share the same logistic support and strategic support. The support must be better than the CSS could acquire elsewhere. CSS associates, like all other associates, must feel that the HCO is "a great place to give care." The transformational culture is sustained by three elements:

1. *Responsive listening by senior management.* Rounds should include CSSs, and CSS associates should feel empowered.
2. *Training for CSS managers.* Just as head nurses and logistic support managers are trained to be responsive listeners and to encourage empowerment, CSS managers should be trained. Because of the small size of many CSSs, coaches and mentors come from other CSSs.
3. *Celebration and rewards.* CSSs should participate in celebration of goals that require collaboration as well as in achievements within their CSS. Their compensation should include bonus opportunities that are comparable to those of other associates.

Building an Effective Contractual Relationship

The HCO has a number of alternative contractual arrangements that it can tailor to a specific CSS. Alternative structures, generally ordered in terms of increasing HCO control and increasing HCO capital investment, include the following:

- *Long-term contract with a separately owned corporation.* An independent corporation owns facilities, employs associates, and sells services to the HCO. The contract should specify as clearly as possible the obligations and intentions of both parties. Quality, patient satisfaction, and efficiency standards can be included, with agreement on measures and benchmarks. The HCO can control professional privileges. Hours of coverage, requirements for teaching, and participation on PITs should be specified. It is difficult to incorporate standards for effectiveness or to prevent the contractor from competing as an independent organization.
- *Joint venture corporation.* The HCO gains partial strategic control and can include explicit reserved powers or supermajority rules that gain control of size, location, clinical privileges, and management appointments. The corporation can

purchase services from the HCO. The principal advantages relate to capital. The joint venture allows CSS professionals to have equity and income compensation. It also permits a for-profit corporation to provide some of the equity capital, relieving the HCO of debt or lease financing.

- *Joint operations.* The HCO owns and operates the facility, including hiring of nonprofessional associates, and can exercise control of privileges, giving it control of size, amenities, and capital investment. Professional guidance is provided by contract with one or several physician corporations.
- *Unified operations.* The HCO owns and operates the facility and employs all professional and nonprofessional associates. This model gives the HCO maximum control, but it must still attract and retain qualified professionals.

Unified operations are the most common solution, particularly among smaller CSSs, and the trend is clearly toward increased HCO control. Revisions to the insurance payment system may encourage even more HCO control. Given the great importance of fixed costs in efficiency, the sizing function is crucial. Services that are missing or too small pose a threat of lost market share to competitors. Those that are too large draw insufficient demand to meet quality and cost standards.

Maintaining Regulatory Compliance

In addition to general standards of the Centers for Medicare & Medicaid Services (CMS) and The Joint Commission, CSSs may have additional and more specific regulatory requirements that may be government mandated or voluntary. CSS leadership must be knowledgeable about regulatory requirements and design and implement policies and procedures accordingly. In addition, ongoing education and training for changing standards is expected.

For example, clinical laboratories must comply with the Clinical Laboratory Improvement Amendments (CLIA) regulated by CMS.[2] Moreover, clinical laboratories may elect to participate in accreditation by the College of American Pathologists (CAP), the gold standard for clinical laboratory quality and performance improvement,[3] or receive accreditation from the American Association of Blood Banks (AABB) for blood banking and transfusion services.[4]

Radiation oncology must comply with the federal Nuclear Regulatory Commission; pharmacy must comply with federal regulations of the Drug Enforcement Administration and the Food and Drug Administration; and dietary must comply with state and local health department regulations that govern the proper and safe handling of food and sanitation, to name a few examples. Each CSS also has continuing education requirements for the many professionals who are represented in specialty areas.

The HCO leadership is responsible for providing resources to support regulatory compliance and also to report compliance to the governing board and other appropriate organizations. Many large HCOs have individual regulatory compliance officers for CSSs.

Promoting Continuous Improvement

The evidence-based model of measures, benchmarks, opportunities for improvement (OFIs), improved goals, and rewards fits well within each CSS. The model, with annual goal setting, should be routine in all CSSs whether the HCO operates the CSS or contracts with a separate corporation. Setting annual operating goals and identifying and justifying new capital investment should be interrelated. Capital is required for improving and expanding facilities, replacing outmoded equipment, and starting new programs. CSSs are a major user of capital. Where capital is supplied by the contractor, the HCO should have the right to approve investments.

Setting Annual Goals

A unit that has been diligent in the preceding year will be able to formulate next year's budget quickly, drawing in large part on work that has already been done in continuous improvement. Quality, costs, patient satisfaction, and associate satisfaction must be based on benchmarks; the management of a CSS that cannot meet benchmarks can usually be replaced by competitors with proven records.

Well-run organizations have clearly defined budget process roles for the CSS, the budget manager (a technical support person or office attached to finance), and the HCO manager. The CSS manager and team are expected to do the following:

- Review the demand forecasts prepared by the budget manager, extending them to the specific levels required in the department and suggesting modifications based on their knowledge of the local situation.
- Identify changes in the scope of services and the operating budget that arise from changes in demand, patient management protocol development, and continuous improvement. Minor changes are incorporated in the operating budget. Major ones are addressed in the capital and new programs budget (discussed below).
- Propose goals for quality and satisfaction, using benchmark and available competitor data.
- Propose goals for staffing, labor productivity, and supplies consistent with demand forecasts, quality improvements, and other constraints.
- Identify OFIs and initiatives that should be developed during the coming year.

The budget manager (see Chapter 13) is expected to do the following:

- Assemble historical data on achievement of last year's budget.
- Prepare forecasts of major CSS demand measures.

- Prepare benchmark and competitor data.
- Promulgate the budget guidelines for changes in total expenditures, profit, and capital investment approved by the finance committee of the board.
- Circulate wage-increase guidelines from human resources and supplies-price guidelines from materials management.
- Assist in calculations and prepare trial budgets until a satisfactory proposal for the board has been reached.

The HCO manager for the CSS is expected to do the following:

- Ensure that the proposed goals do not impair quality or satisfaction in other units.
- Assist the CSS, and encourage steady but realistic improvement.
- Coordinate interdepartmental issues that arise from the budgeting process.
- Meet the budget guidelines set by the governing board or the senior management team.
- Resolve conflicting needs between CSSs.
- Evaluate the progress of the CSS to assist in the distribution of incentives.
- Assist the CSS in pursuing OFIs and implementing them during the coming year.

Implementing Improvements

An important part of the HCO manager's job is facilitating PITs and implementing improvements that often involve several different CSSs and patient care teams. These improvements are likely to be the most rewarding opportunities. For example, costs of pharmaceuticals have been rising rapidly. A pharmacy might pursue a number of internal initiatives to keep departmental cost increases at a minimum, but control of demand and much of drug safety rests with the medical and nursing staffs. The pharmacy section of Exhibit 8.4 shows some initiatives a pharmacy might support. The strategy for pharmacy addresses four areas: price and inventory, formulary, protocols, and prescribing habits. Three of the four require collaboration with the medical and nursing staffs. Initiatives in each area might continue for several years. The diagnostic imaging section of Exhibit 8.4 also shows a set of initiatives. Only the first is wholly within the CSS's control. As the exhibit suggests, improvement initiatives take a number of different forms, leading to PITs with different charges, memberships, and timetables.

Negotiating Goals

CSS operational goals must contribute to the HCO's annual strategic goals and maintain competitive excellence. In addition, they must respond to longer-term changes. Shifts in patient management, driven by evidence-based medicine and changes in technology, will force many CSSs to make major

EXHIBIT 8.4
Improvement
Initiatives in
Two CSSs

Issue	Initiative	Measures	Approach
Pharmacy			
Price and inventory management	Purchasing agreement Inventory management system	Unit cost versus wholesale Inventory turns/year	PIT within pharmacy
Formulary management	Generic drug program Automatic stop orders on common drugs Extra controls for very expensive drugs	Ratio of generic to proprietary Drug cost per case Average costs per dose for specific drugs	PITs working with service lines
Patient management protocols	Alternative therapies and prevention Avoid unnecessary drug use and cost	Drug cost per specific treatment episodes	Protocol review committees
Prescribing habits	Protocol compliance Physician education, counseling	Drug costs per capita Drug cost per specific treatment groups	Counseling with service lines
Diagnostic Imaging			
Reduce retakes	Improve functional protocols and associate training	Count of retakes	PIT within imaging
Improve patient scheduling and results reporting delays	Evaluate and install departmental information system	Patient delays for service Hours from exam to report	PIT with service lines and other CSSs
Inappropriate exams	Final product protocols, physician education	Disease-specific exams per patient	Protocol review committees and service line counseling

CSS: clinical support service; PIT: process improvement team

revisions. Even the well-managed CSS that invests heavily in improvement initiatives may encounter difficulty as medical care changes. The demand for cancer therapies may shift radically if effective new drugs are discovered. The balance between heart surgery and heart catheterization has shifted more than once, as new catheter-oriented stents evolved simultaneously with minimally invasive cardiac surgery. The HCO manager's role includes negotiation of both annual goals and long-term forecasts. The negotiation process has several important characteristics:

- The goal of the negotiations is the optimization of patient needs as a whole, as reflected in competitive needs and external benchmarks. Actions that endanger the HCO's competitive position must be avoided at any cost.
- Competitive financial goals must be met for all parties. HCOs or CSSs that cannot meet those goals must be restructured by consolidation or revision of the mission.
- Each CSS must maximize its own opportunities and defend its own needs, emphasizing quality, patient satisfaction, caregiver satisfaction, and associate satisfaction.
- The negotiating team should include physicians and CSS personnel who can implement agreed-on improvements.
- Negotiations:
  - Examine solutions between related CSSs and with outsourcing and external collaboration.
  - Assure the CSS of a fair hearing.
  - Include rewards for CSS managers and associates who contribute to an effective solution.

A strong strategic plan is essential. If the strategic plan and the facilities, information, and recruitment plans derived from that plan are inadequate, it becomes impossible for the CSS to reach competitive levels on all dimensions. Thus, if a CSS falls short of its constraints, the first questions address the effectiveness of CSS operation, and the second questions address the size and scope of the CSS itself, including issues of outsourcing or eliminating the service. Finally, attention turns to the strategy of the organization as a whole. Repeated and widespread failures in meeting CSS constraints are evidence of an organization or facility that is undersized or underfinanced for market needs. Affiliation with another organization or closure must be considered.

Preparing New Program and Capital Budget Requests

CSS managers are responsible for identifying opportunities and developing **programmatic proposals**—specific proposals for new or replacement capital equipment or major revisions to service—as well as for the annual budget. Technological improvements, aging equipment, changing demand, and revisions in the scope of service can require capital investment and result in major shifts in performance. These must be justified in terms of the HCO's mission. The best investments are those that contribute most to the HCO's mission and stakeholders' expectations. All capital

Programmatic proposals
Proposals for new or replacement capital equipment or major revisions of service.

requests are subject to a competitive review process that places them in rank order and to board action on the basis of the rank order. The review process and board actions are discussed further in Chapter 14.

For example, an imaging department may encounter declining demand for inpatient radiographs, increasing demand for convenient ambulatory radiographs and ultrasound, and increasing demand for magnetic and emission tomography. Substantial capital is required to remove equipment no longer needed, purchase new equipment, and recruit and train staff for the expanded operations. The imaging department and the HCO manager prepare detailed business plans for these changes, documenting both the capital and operating cost changes as well as changes in other performance measures, such as quality of care, patient satisfaction, and referring physician satisfaction. Internal consulting helps develop the factual basis for the proposal; marketing provides advice on location, hours, and other issues; human resources assists with the training; and finance assists with calculations of cost and return on investment. The benefits—contributions to mission—are identified by imaging, with assistance from the performance improvement council (PIC), clinical customers, internal consulting, and marketing.

The proposal, which might suggest changes that cost several million dollars, advances to competitive review when the imaging department is ready. Competitive review compares the proposal against similar requests from other units, ending with a rank-ordered list submitted to the governing board. The criterion for ranking is long-run mission achievement: What is best for the HCO's stakeholders? The benefits the CSS claims in the proposal are related to its operational performance measures. If the proposal is accepted, imaging is expected to adopt and achieve those goals. Many benefits occur outside the CSS, making the collaborative approach to proposal development essential. The proposal is both strengthened and validated in the process, reducing challenges during competitive review.

Quality-Related Benefits   All benefits, including quality benefits, must be compared to the treatment alternative that would prevail if the proposal were not adopted.[5] Although many technological advances are described as improvements in outcomes quality or contribution to patients' health and well-being, the reality is that most proposals involve only convenience and competitive advantage. A service that supplements another one that is available ten minutes away has a quality value equal to ten minutes of travel, even if the service is lifesaving. (It may have a much higher patient satisfaction value.)

If, in fact, the proposal changes the number of people in the community who will achieve a more favorable outcome, its contribution can be analyzed using the epidemiologic planning model.

$$\text{Contribution} = \left\{ \begin{array}{c} \text{Demand} \\ \text{for a} \\ \text{service} \end{array} \right\} \times \left\{ \begin{array}{c} \text{Probability that} \\ \text{service will} \\ \text{improve outcome} \end{array} \right\} \times \left\{ \begin{array}{c} \text{Value of} \\ \text{improvement} \end{array} \right\}$$

The demand term is estimated by the epidemiologic planning model. The probability of improved outcome comes from clinical literature and is a foundation of evidence-based medicine. Quality benefits can theoretically be scaled by a variety of techniques, including forced-choice surveys and Delphi analysis. Most situations will not be difficult to rank. If a new clinical approach substantially prolongs life, and many competitors are adopting it, it will score well and be adopted. Scales exist for the value of human life, ability to work, ability to care for self, added years of healthy life, and similar major contributions.[6] Review committees should use a consistent scale for valuing clinical contribution and recognize the limitations of the scale.

If a process improvement reduces the need for care, dollar estimates are not challenging. For example, if a new diagnostic process with a demand of 1,000 tests per year will reduce length of stay by one day for one-third of those on whom it is used, and a day of stay is worth a marginal cost of $400, the contribution of the process is about $133,000 per year: *Cost-Related Benefits*

$$\text{Contribution} = 1{,}000 \times .333 \times \$400 = \$133{,}200$$

A case can be made for higher values. From an insurer's perspective, the cost per day is the paid price, probably twice the marginal cost. Patients and society might place an even higher price, adding earnings from earlier return to work.

Because of fixed costs and marketing implications, cost and demand are interrelated. First, CSS costs after adoption of the proposal must be competitive with other sources of equivalent services. If they are not, the proposal is inadequate to ensure long-run survival. The CSS must find a way to deliver services competitively. If they are, a benefit is return on investment—the savings a proposal generates expressed as a return on its capital investment over the years of the life of the project or the capital equipment.

Return-on-investment calculations are usually prepared with the assistance of internal consulting and finance. The focus is on changes in cash flows. The contribution can be expressed as return on investment:

$$\left\{ \begin{array}{l} \text{Return on} \\ \text{investment} \end{array} \right\} = \{\text{Contribution}\} \div \{\text{Invested capital}\}$$

The value of cash in future years is less than the value of immediate cash. Return on investment can be calculated for multiyear cash flow streams, allowing comparison of diverse projects. It is also possible to discount cash flow in future years with an assumed rate of interest, creating a net present value of cash flows. Care must be taken to estimate all costs and demands accurately, including hidden ones, and to be sure the claims for savings can truly be met. The proposed costs will be incorporated as an operating budget reduction if the project is implemented. Some cost improvements occur outside the CSS, in which case another unit must agree to them. For example, an improved diagnostic test may reduce drug costs or length of stay. In this case, the cost savings must be traced to the unit where they will occur, and that unit must agree to actual goal changes.

Market Share Improvements   Many proposals improve market share or forestall a loss of market share. A claim that a specific capability will attract or protect market share is a justification for capital investment. The value depends on the magnitude of the shift and the fixed cost involved. Replacing equipment that is critical to continued operations is an obvious, high-priority example. If a modern laboratory must have an automated, multichannel blood chemistry analyzer, and the existing one is no longer reliable, the proposal to replace it will not generate much debate. In less obvious cases, the justification is based on the return on investment. Applications are often complicated. Under global and capitation payments, change in cash flow must be calculated at the level of payment involved. The proposal may be a service that has become generally accepted as part of the protocol for a specific disease or procedure.

The justification must be based on service for the care episode, rather than the operation of the CSS. The budget for the patient management protocol or the service line becomes the critical document, rather than that of the CSS. If it reflects competitive cost and quality, the proposal is worth further consideration. For example, a special laboratory for in vitro fertilization is a CSS for a women's service line. It can be justified only as a complete service, including evidence of sufficient actual demand, medical staff recruitment, all costs for couples seeking the service, payments allowed by various insurers, and evidence of competitive rates of successful fertilization. As a result, these kinds of proposals are usually considered strategic, and ad hoc teams are established to evaluate them.

Defending Capital Proposals

The HCO manager of the CSS and the internal consulting representative are proper advocates of the proposal in the evaluation process. Their job is to prepare the analysis and the justification in the most favorable light. As advocates, they should be prepared to answer questions and make modifications as the proposal progresses. They must also be prepared to accept rejection. By the same token, it is senior management's obligation to see that they do not overstep the bounds of honesty, that others accept their role as advocate, that all projects get a fair and judicious hearing, and that the benefits claimed are translated to actual performance when the project is complete.

The feedback to the CSS comes in two ways—through evaluation of its proposals and through participation in the evaluation of others' proposals. Over time, the CSS learns to identify winning proposals earlier, making the process less onerous.

People

Team Members

Many CSS professionals have extensive formal education, licensure, and requirements for continuing education. The education includes mastery of relevant theory and supervised practice so that the student learns the processes, patient indications and contraindications for them, expected outcomes, and the rules governing process design. Although they are in various stages of implementation, the professions of pharmacy,[7] physical therapy,[8] occupational therapy,[9] and nurse anesthesia[10] have adopted practice doctorate degrees as the first professional "entry to practice" credential. To reduce costs, unlicensed aides or technicians perform many of the actual CSS procedures under supervision. The staffing of most CSS units consists of one or two levels of formally educated professionals and one or more levels of technical personnel, allowing each professional to serve a larger volume of patients. Three managerial issues arise:

1. Maintenance of clinical competence and skill for qualified professionals
2. Education and supervision of nonprofessional personnel
3. Resolution of work assignments between professional and nonprofessional personnel

The first is met by a credentialing process that verifies entry and continuing formal education and a continued record of effective practice, as for medicine and nursing. The process is usually assigned to human resources management. The second is addressed in the HCO's educational programs. The training is usually designed and conducted by the CSS professionals and human resources. The third, resolution of interprofessional and intraprofessional work assignments, must bring in advice from customer stakeholders. It is the responsibility of the HCO manager and is discussed in the Managerial Issues section below.

CSS Management

The manager of each support service is usually an experienced leader in the healthcare profession associated with the service. Many larger CSSs have nonphysician managers along with designated medical directors. Some services—operating rooms and delivery rooms—use specialized nurse managers. These managers collaborate closely with their physician counterparts. Pharmacists, respiratory therapists, and medical social workers have less direct medical involvement, probably because they serve a broad array of specialties.

Beyond their professional training, CSS managers need supervisory skills, including skills in personnel selection, management of committees, continuous improvement concepts, knowledge management, and servant leadership. Managers of the larger CSSs often have master's degrees in healthcare management or in their specialty. Learning effective leadership styles requires more than coursework. Well-managed organizations reinforce good practice with ongoing training, exposure to best practices, coaching, and assistance from internal consulting.

The HCO Manager

Each CSS must be accountable to the HCO governing board. That accountability is through the *HCO manager* (actual titles vary), who is usually a member of the senior management team or someone who reports to a senior manager. The HCO manager has several duties, many of which are described under the CSS functions section above:

1. Responsive listening—rounding frequently, talking with associates in the CSS at all levels and addressing their needs, talking with caregivers who use the CSS
2. Communicating—explaining strategic guidelines, other relevant board decisions, OFIs and matters of interest that arise from various surveillance activities, PIC actions, and the work of PITs that potentially affect the CSS
3. Supporting PITs that need to understand and interact with the CSS processes, and ensuring representation on all PITs that directly affect the CSS
4. Negotiating the annual operational goals—relating the CSS's improvement possibilities to the needs of other units, and identifying and resolving issues of coordinating services and improvement activities
5. Supporting and coordinating capital and new program requests with clinical units and other CSSs
6. Maintaining the succession plan for the CSS
7. Arranging the resolution of interprofessional and intraprofessional work requirements
8. Maintaining the agenda for contract renewal or restructuring of the relationship between the CSS and the HCO

The agenda for contract renewal recognizes that there are alternative opportunities to provide many CSSs. Even fully employed CSSs should be reviewed periodically, and contractual relationships should have explicit revision or renewal dates. The HCO manager should monitor both the array of alternatives and the improvement opportunities offered. Although the normal expectation is to continue the relationship, the HCO's stakeholders are entitled to the best available arrangement. Review of alternatives may lead to a new supplier for the CSS; more commonly it identifies OFIs that can and should be addressed under the existing relationship.

Organization

The organization shown in Exhibit 8.5 is built around CSS teams of professional and nonprofessional associates focused by location or function. As the

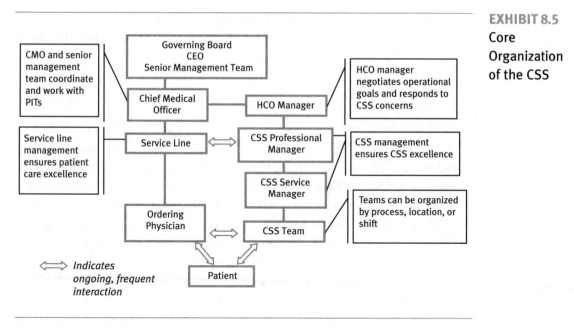

EXHIBIT 8.5
Core
Organization
of the CSS

CMO: chief medical officer; CSS: clinical support service; PIT: process improvement team

exhibit shows, each CSS team has multiple accountability—to its patients, its customers (i.e., the care teams depending on its services), and the HCO. Both CSS and service line associates have operational goals. Frequent and open interchange occurs among the CSS team, the patient, and the physician and also between the CSS managers and the service line managers. HCO managers and senior management are accountable for both goal sets. They work to achieve the goals and improvements by responsive listening, monitoring performance, and using PITs to address all issues of integration and coordination.

CSSs vary widely in size and activity. Most CSSs provide care in both outpatient and inpatient settings. The smallest have only one or two professionals. In some situations, the CSS may be a single person or a single team. The larger CSSs, such as the clinical laboratory, imaging, and pharmacy, can have more than 100 associates working in a dozen or more teams with several subspecialties at several sites. This volume and diversity provide the HCO with a competitive advantage: the ability to meet a superior set of operational goals.

HCO–CSS Relationships

Most small CSSs are employed by the HCO. The larger CSSs with physician leadership often form local medical groups and contract or joint venture with the HCO. Several moderate-sized companies provide imaging and pathology services, contracting with several HCOs in a geographic region. At least one company provides extensive pharmacy support. Contracts generally identify the scope of services to be offered and whether those services are exclusive, commitments for space and equipment, and the management of patient-related information. In addition, they should address the operational scorecard measures to be used, the sources of benchmarks, the goal-setting process, the duties for education and continuous improvement, and the incentive arrangements.

Measures

Exhibit 8.6 summarizes the measures for each of the six operational dimensions: demand, cost, human resources, productivity, quality, and customer satisfaction. With rare exceptions, these measures are appropriate for any CSS. Many of the measures are retrievable from ongoing data collection efforts, such as patient and associate surveys, accounting, and electronic medical records. Very small CSSs have sample size problems. Monthly reporting may not be reliable, but even the smallest CSS should have measures, benchmarks, OFIs, and annual improvement goals. Qualitative data—impressions, examples, and evidence from competitors or best practices—are also important.

Large, complex CSSs have a substantial measurement set, befitting their status as multimillion-dollar enterprises. The HCO manager's focus should be on the aggregate performance, which should be routinely compared with benchmark and competitor values. CSS managers normally operate an internal performance improvement program, and they are rewarded financially for their success. Part of the HCO's support can include educational programs, PITs to address problems of coordination, and the knowledge management system.

Demand and output measures are increasingly available from electronic order systems and patient records. Cost accounting is supported by the transaction accounting system, which is described in Chapter 13. Equipment records are useful for major items; they typically record uses, load factors (time operated divided by time available), service times, and failures. These records are useful in managing maintenance and determining replacement.

Patient, physician, and associate satisfaction data are determined from HCO-wide surveys. Care must be taken to avoid incorrect inferences from small samples. Internal consulting provides statistical analysis (see Chapter 14).

Patient outcomes quality measures are important but limited. Most CSSs contribute to outcomes successes but cannot be accountable for them because too many other activities are required. For the patient to thrive, all the care activities must be correct. CSS outcomes failures can often be tracked and systematically reduced. Anesthesia, for example, can cause fatalities. Over decades, the anesthesiology profession has studied its failures, improved its processes, and reduced its mortality by several orders of magnitude. It contributes to all successful surgeries but cannot make the surgery a success. Most CSS quality measures are intermediate outcome or process compliance measures. In intermediate outcomes, follow-up inspection or a similar assessment reveals if the CSS activity was or was not correctly performed and did or did

Dimension	Measures	Applications
Demand	Requests for service	Used to forecast staff and other resource needs Specified by time, location, kind of service, and urgency of demand
	Market share	Used to track competitive success Specify by competitor and service, if available
Costs	Fixed/variable, direct and indirect costs	Used to analyze and improve work processes
	Physical units of resources	Resource use is specified by time, location, and kind of service
	Age and repair records of equipment	Equipment records trigger maintenance and replacement
Human resources	Retention, absenteeism, injuries, satisfaction, recruitment, and training statistics	Used to ensure "a great place to give care" Specified by worker group
Output and productivity	Units of demand met and not met	Used to identify service failures Used to benchmark efficiency
	Cost per unit of output	Specified by time, location, and kind of service
	Physical units consumed per unit of output	
Quality	Process compliance scores	Used to ensure compliance with functional protocols
	Unexpected event counts	Specified by time, location, and kind of service Unexpected events are investigated 100 percent
Patient satisfaction	Overall satisfaction and specifics of service	Used to ensure favorable patient reaction Specified by time, location, and kind of service
Physician satisfaction	Overall satisfaction and specifics of service	Used to ensure favorable referring physician satisfaction Physician, patient group categories

EXHIBIT 8.6
Performance
Measures for
the CSS

not yield the right information for further treatment. In process compliance, the inspection shows that the functional protocol was or was not followed. The two approaches provide in-depth understanding that identifies root causes of OFIs and facilitates their correction. Pathology laboratories have pursued these measures successfully, allowing them to ensure the accuracy of their diagnostic reports. CAP maintains libraries of measures, values, and education programs[11] and insists on statistically controlled intermediate outcomes for accreditation.[12]

Managerial Issues

Clinical excellence depends on the caregiving team of physicians, nurses, and their associates and on the information and treatment provided by the CSS. The several dozen CSSs reflect the breadth of patient need. An HCO with an excellence in care mission must ensure that each of these services is effectively delivered. Its senior management team does that by systematically pursuing eight questions for each CSS:

1. Do we offer the service, or do we refer patients who need it?
2. How big should our service be?
3. What are the standards of performance and benchmarks our service must meet?
4. What is the form of affiliation that best meets our needs?
5. Does the CSS have the coordination it needs with other HCO units?
6. Are CSS activities correctly assigned to professional and nonprofessional associates?
7. What are the continuous improvement goals the affiliates should meet?
8. What are the longer-term trends and implications for our affiliates?

These questions view the CSS as a semiautonomous unit. They extend the concepts of evidence-based management and transformational management to support an array of relationships from wholly owned to strategic partnership with the CSS.

Should the HCO Offer the Service?

An HCO should offer every CSS that its patients need and that can be provided safely and economically. Safety and economy depend on patient volume. When volume is too low, associates cannot maintain their skills and unit costs mount. The expected volume should be assessed by the epidemiologic planning model. In general, an HCO would refer patients needing CSSs that it cannot offer at acceptable quality and cost. Shared CSS arrangements, even with competing HCOs, may be appropriate. Networks within healthcare systems also help meet the safety and cost thresholds. The experience of similar HCOs is a useful guide.

How Big Should the CSS Be?

The forecast of CSS demand from the epidemiologic planning model indicates the necessary size of the CSS. That forecast must be monitored annually. Shifts in technology, health insurance coverage, and population demographics change the forecast. It is quite possible that a given CSS must be expanded, repositioned, downsized, or closed. The HCO's commitment to excellence in care mandates that it, not the CSS, determines the size and affiliation.

What Are the Standards of Performance?

The standards of performance are determined by benchmarks and minimums for the operational performance measures, particularly those for quality, customer satisfaction, and associate satisfaction. Many CSSs have accreditation standards, either within The Joint Commission standards or through an independent organization. These are minimum standards that should, in general, be fully met. While exceptions may be appropriate, they should receive detailed review and in most cases a plan for correction. (Some accreditation standards may be for the benefit of the service provider, rather than the patient. The clearest challenge to these standards is convincing evidence that patient safety and satisfaction can be met without them.)

Benchmark remains the goal for CSSs, as for all activities. A multiyear plan to reach benchmark may be appropriate. Continued operation below benchmark raises a serious question: If an alternative provider offers service at benchmark, why should the alternative be denied the HCO's customer and physician stakeholders? In other words, if this CSS team cannot make benchmark but another supplier can, the HCO is obligated to transfer to the successful supplier.

The ethical principles of nonmaleficence and beneficence suggest a strong obligation. The ethical principle of justice suggests the current supplier deserves a chance to correct the situation. Among other considerations, changing suppliers has a cost in itself. Abruptly terminating a relationship may cause other associates to question the HCO's trustworthiness, eroding a critical component of the transformational culture. At least one analyst places patient concerns uppermost. Davenport insists that every patient's right must prevail over associate concerns.[13]

What Form of Affiliation Best Meets the HCO's Needs?

The major possibilities for formal CSS affiliation are described in the Building an Effective Contractual Relationship section above. The best possibility is the one that offers long-term performance closest to benchmark. The criterion is easy to identify but difficult to meet. The preferred solution is probably ownership; the HCO has ultimate control of employment, privileging, capital, protocol selection, training, location, and operating performance measures. Alternatives might be selected to facilitate associate incentives, to reduce capital costs, or to take advantage of skills developed through horizontal integration.

A small number of commercial companies have offered CSS management services. Unlike the record in environmental services, where outsourcing is the rule (see Chapter 12), it appears that few have captured substantial market share. Successful models include pharmacy services, some imaging services, and long-term acute care provision.

A growing option for extending the CSS function to distant affiliates is **telemedicine,** or telehealth.[14] This type of affiliation may best meet the needs of patients and communities at a distance from tertiary or quaternary care. The diagnostic service or remote monitoring function is conducted at the affiliate location and transmitted to the HCO to be interpreted by a specialist, thus improving timeliness, access to specialty care, and clinical outcomes.[15]

Telemedicine
The use of medical information exchanged from one site to another via electronic communications to improve a patient's clinical health status.

Does the CSS Have the Coordination It Needs?

CSSs are, by definition, *part* of excellent care. Integrating their services into an excellent whole is sometimes a challenge. Patients' needs and various CSSs interact. Certain drugs affect laboratory values; certain procedures require fasting; patient allergies and sensitivities require procedure modification. Changes in a patient management protocol must be incorporated into CSS procedures. CSS performance can be improved with access to parts of the patient record. An affiliation agreement may call for services, such as training, information exchange, and environmental services from the HCO. Failures in meeting these needs impair the CSS's ability to meet its goals and can be catastrophic.

The management role is clear and independent of the contractual model. The HCO manager is expected to round frequently, be available for issues that arise, and provide a constructive response to all requests. The CSS can rely on its HCO manager to understand and represent its interests. It can expect to be invited to any committee or PIT that is addressing an issue of concern. These integrating and coordinating activities are essential for the CSS to achieve its goals and thus must be completed regardless of structure.

CSS associates work side by side with other HCO associates. The HCO's culture of empowerment should extend to the CSS associates. Thus, part of an affiliated CSS's operating scorecard is its associate satisfaction. The HCO manager should be alert and responsive to potential tensions. CSS managers should be trained in supervision, provided with coaches, and included in multi-rater or 360-degree evaluations to assist them in implementing a transformational culture.

Are CSS Activities Correctly Assigned to Professional and Nonprofessional Associates?

Medical technology tends to begin with specialized professionals; as it ages, it moves to less specialized and nonprofessional caregivers. Images, once solely interpreted by radiologists; electrocardiograms, once solely under cardiologists' purview; and "conscious sedation," once undertaken solely by anesthesiologists, are examples where a specific CSS has moved to much broader use. The transition to broader use is not always smooth, and the payment structure, which tends to lag the technology, complicates the transition. The criterion for the level of skill and training necessary to provide a given test or treatment is straightforward: It should normally be assigned to the lowest-cost associate who is capable of maintaining quality and patient satisfaction standards.

Applying the criteria is sometimes challenging. Should the treating specialists be allowed to read images in their specialty, or must the interpretations be validated by a radiologist? With new forms of anesthesia such as conscious sedation, must an anesthesiologist be present? Can a nurse interpret an EKG (electrocardiogram)? Definitive studies are rare.[16] Standards of practice, a less rigorous level of evidence, are acceptable. If orthopedists and cardiologists elsewhere are privileged to act on their own interpretation of images, they should be allowed to do that in our HCO. Transfers to nonprofessionals must be interpreted with care. If a technician can prepare an echocardiogram at the Johns Hopkins Hospital, the task can be assigned to technicians at other HCOs if they are trained and monitored as the Hopkins technician is trained and monitored.

The process to resolve these issues should be assigned to medical staff protocol committees and PITs that can assemble evidence and recommend the safe but cost-effective solution. The committees and PITs must be guided to work from evidence rather than authority. Often, the solution is to permit lower-skilled associates to proceed in uncomplicated cases, review the evidence emerging, and broaden their assignment as their record of success grows.

What Are the Continuous Improvement Goals?

One of the contributions of continuous improvement is its ability to adjust to changing conditions over time, avoiding a major disruption caused by falling behind the rest of the world. Negotiating annual goals ties each unit to the larger economy and supports a review of the relation of the unit to its environment, including technology, regulation, customers, competitors, and associates. Problems that could become disabling can be identified and corrected well before catastrophe strikes. The annual strategic goals, benchmarks, and deliberate review of best practices and competitor practices stimulate and sustain this process. As a result, the HCO keeps control of CSS activities. It has assurance that the CSS is operating in the best interests of the HCO stakeholders. Even where a CSS operates almost autonomously, the HCO manager maintains comparative performance data and the contract calls for negotiated goals. Knowing that contract renewal is likely but not automatic makes negotiation realistic.

What Are the Long-Term Trends?

Similarly, the HCO is in control of much of the potential demand for any CSS and is charged with identifying long-term trends. It has the obligation to pursue promptly the implications of these trends. Most problems are easier to solve with advance warning; surprises in the business world are rarely good news.

Many of the most valuable goals require collaboration among several CSSs and service lines. The OFIs are likely to appear in the annual strategic review process or in the deliberations of the PIC, where multiple perspectives can be integrated and overall performance benchmarked. Identifying and pursuing these goals is an important part of the jobs of senior management and the HCO manager. Pursuit usually means extensive discussion with the units likely to be involved, seeking the most effective, least disruptive path to change. In some cases, it can mean extensive revision or termination of relationships with a CSS. The rule for managing those events returns to the ethical balance between rights of patients and rights of associates. Patients must come first, but contractual rights should be upheld. Thus, any contract needs termination clauses, and they set the stage for effective negotiation. Termination should be rare; negotiation should be continual.

Additional Resources

Brunt, B. A. 2008. *Evidence-Based Competency Management for the Operating Room,* 2nd ed. Marblehead, MA: HCPro.

Madsen, W. C., and K. Gillespie. 2014. *Collaborative Helping: A Strengths Framework for Home-Based Services.* New York: Wiley.

Moseley III, G. B. 2013. *Managing Legal Compliance in the Health Care Industry.* Burlington, MA: Jones & Bartlett Learning.

Papp, J. 2014. *Quality Management in the Imaging Sciences,* 5th ed. St. Louis, MO: Mosby.

Notes

1. Cerner Corporation. 2014. "Hospitals and Health Systems." [Online information; retrieved 7/9/14.] www.cerner.com/solutions/Hospitals_and_Health_Systems/.
2. Centers for Medicare & Medicaid Services. 2014. "Clinical Laboratory Improvement Amendments (CLIA)." [Online information; retrieved 7/9/14.] www.cms.gov/Regulations-and-Guidance/Legislation/CLIA/index.html?redirect=/clia/03_interpretive_guidelines_for_laboratories.asp.
3. College of American Pathologists. 2014. "Accreditation." [Online information; retrieved 2/10/15.] www.cap.org/web/home/lab/accreditation?_afrLoop=10876906244427#%40%3F_afrLoop%3D10876906244427%26_adf.ctrl-state%3D12xqyccfne_4.
4. American Association of Blood Banks. 2014. "Standards and Accreditation." [Online information; retrieved 7/9/14.] www.aabb.org/sa/Pages/default.aspx.

5. Iezzoni, L. 2012. *Risk Adjustment for Measuring Health Care Outcomes,* 4th ed. Chicago: Health Administration Press.

6. Arnold, D., A. Girling, A. Stevens, and R. Lilford. 2009. "Comparison of Direct and Indirect Methods of Estimating Health State Utilities for Resource Allocation: Review and Empirical Analysis." *British Medical Journal* 339 (7717): 385–88.

7. American Association of Colleges of Pharmacy. 2014. "About AACP." [Online information; retrieved 7/9/14.] www.aacp.org/about/Pages/default.aspx.

8. American Physical Therapy Association. 2014. Home page. [Online information; retrieved 7/9/14.] www.apta.org.

9. American Occupational Therapy Association. 2014. "FAQ on OT Education and Career Planning." [Online information; retrieved 7/9/14.] www.aota.org/Education-Careers/Considering-OT-Career/FAQs/Planning.aspx.

10. American Association of Nurse Anesthetists. 2007. "AANA Announces Support of Doctorate for Entry into Nurse Anesthesia Practice by 2025." [Online information; retrieved 7/9/14.] www.aana.com/newsandjournal/News/Pages/092007-AANA-Announces-Support-of-Doctorate-for-Entry-into-Nurse-Anesthesia-Practice-by-2025.aspx.

11. College of American Pathologists. Home page. [Online information; retrieved 7/9/14.] www.cap.org/apps/cap.portal?_nfpb=true&_pageLabel=home.

12. College of American Pathologists, Commission on Laboratory Accreditation. 2012. "2012 CAP Accreditation Checklist Edition." [Online information; retrieved 7/9/14.] www.cap.org/apps/cap.portal?_nfpb=true&cntvwrPtlt_action Override=%2Fportlets%2FcontentViewer%2Fshow&_windowLabel=cntvwrPtlt&c ntvwrPtlt{actionForm.contentReference}=laboratory_accreditation%2Fealert%2Fe-alert_2012_checklists.html&_state=maximized&_pageLabel=cntvwr.

13. Davenport, J. 1997. "Ethical Principles in Clinical Practice." *Permanente Journal* 1 (1).

14. McCann, E. 2013. "Telehealth Sees Explosive Growth." *HIMSS Healthcare IT News.* [Online information; retrieved 7/9/14.] www.healthcareitnews.com/news/telehealth-sees-explosive-growth.

15. American Telemedicine Association. 2013. "Telemedicine's Impact on Healthcare Cost and Quality."[Online information; retrieved 7/9/14.] www.americantelemed.org/docs/default-source/policy/examples-of-research-outcomes---telemedicine%27s-impact-on-healthcare-cost-and-quality.pdf.

16. Schilling, D., A. Rosenbaum, S. Schweizer, H. Richter, and B. Rumstadt. 2009. "Sedation with Propofol for Interventional Endoscopy by Trained Nurses in High-Risk Octogenarians: A Prospective, Randomized, Controlled Study." *Endoscopy* 41 (4): 295–98.

POPULATION HEALTH

Critical Issues in Population Health

1. *Maintaining the HCO's core contribution to population health:*
   - Deliver clinical excellence in the HCO's personal health services.
   - Support excellence in all personal health services.

2. *Expanding the HCO mission, vision, and values, and understanding the commitment to population health:*
   - Identify strategic differences between *excellence in care* and *population health*.
   - Change the strategic plans to reflect the population health mission.
   - Understand the financial implications of population health.

3. *Improving primary care and management of chronic diseases:*
   - Create the patient-centered medical home.
   - Integrate post-acute care.
   - Deliver palliative and end-of-life care.

4. *Building effective prevention as a platform for healthy populations:*
   - Assess the health needs of the community.
   - Promote effective prevention strategies.

5. *Building effective coalitions with other agencies:*
   - Establish population health measures and goals.
   - Collaborate with other agencies to reach population health goals.

Questions for Discussion

These questions are about applying the chapter content. It's often helpful to discuss them with classmates or mentors, gaining different perspectives on the issues.

1. A large, not-for-profit HCO begins its move from an "excellence in care" mission by a review of comprehensive personal health services, as shown in Exhibit 9.1. How would you organize a systematic evaluation of community needs and opportunities? What task forces, what tasks are they charged with, and who are their members? What data sources? What consultants?

2. Your HCO, like many, assists some community groups with specific health goals rather than support a community coalition with broad goals, such as those shown in Exhibit 9.4. What arguments would you prepare to address the governing board:

   a. To support developing a community coalition and broad population health goals?

   b. To support continuing the current policy instead of developing a community coalition?

3. The local library holds a monthly town-hall meeting attended by more than 100 residents, recorded for the web, and covered in several local news media outlets. You are asked to present a program that advocates for population health improvements. What would you emphasize?

4. The president of the local not-for-profit hospice wants to have lunch. She is concerned that your hospital HCO is not referring as many patients as it should. Should you invite her to lunch? If so, what should you do to prepare? If not, does her interest require any other action?

5. Your HCO has developed contractual affiliations with several primary care physician groups and is integrating them as a primary care service line. Several of the physician leaders approach you, saying that they would like to move toward implementing the patient-centered medical home concept. Make a checklist of questions you need to think about before you respond.

Purpose

The purpose of HCO participation in population health management is

to use the HCO as a vehicle to improve the health status of its community.

Population health envisions sustaining all members of the community at their highest possible level of functioning, both for their individual happiness and for the collective community benefit. Achieving the vision helps individuals aspire to the best possible quality of life. It helps the community as a whole with lower healthcare costs and a larger, stronger workforce. Achieving the vision involves changes in many sectors of the community, at the least education, the workplace, safety, environment, and healthcare.[1] Success in population health is measured by residents' ability to lead a productive life, their life expectancy, the incidence of preventable disease and premature death, and disease prevention indicators such as immunization rates and the availability of support services.[2]

HCOs' most important contribution to population health is excellence in individual patient care. Delivery of safe, effective, patient-centered, timely, efficient, and equitable care is one foundation of population health, and it is carried out only by HCOs. HCOs face important limitations in moving from an individual patient focus to a community focus. Their patients are often only a subset of the community. Their financing pays principally for care rather than prevention. (Lower healthcare costs for the community mean lower revenue to HCOs.) HCOs have many resources committed to specialized treatment, including facilities and highly trained caregivers who cannot easily convert to other activities. HCO efforts to implement the population health mission must recognize the limitations and deal with them effectively.

Only not-for-profit HCOs would commit to a population health mission. It is not consistent with the market forces driving profit maximization. They would make the commitment because it is in their stakeholders' long-run interests. Many leading not-for-profit HCOs are already committed to population health (see Exhibit 1.7). *Population health* is different from *excellence in care*, moving from process to outcome as a corporate focus. The Affordable Care Act (ACA) encourages HCOs to do so. The ACA rewards eliminating unnecessary admissions. It requires a community benefit review every three years as part of the IRS Form 990 Schedule H Community Benefit Calculations in order to retain tax exemption for the nonprofit HCO.[3]

In broad perspective, the concept of population health has solid empirical support. Substantial income gains arose historically from improving population health, first by an increase in the food supply and the conquest of infectious disease, particularly through water purification,[4] and later by immunization and improved acute care.[5] Several advanced countries maintain health that is superior to that in the United States, with substantially less expenditure on acute care.[6] In detail, however, moving from the current U.S. system to the ideal is challenging. Prevailing attitudes, organization structures, financing, and employment all must change. Inherent conflicts of interest exist: If I am a cancer treatment specialist, prevention of cancer may reduce my future income. For an HCO, strong programs of population health mean less revenue, most seriously in areas such as oncology, cardiovascular care, and the neonatal intensive care unit.

The United States has not historically supported the elements of Exhibit 9.1 equally.[7,8] Three interrelated issues have shaped a system that emphasizes acute care, often at the expense of more cost-effective alternatives:

1. *Availability of healthcare financing.* Hospitalization, the initial focus of health insurance, is still the most widely available and most generously funded type of care.[9] Ambulatory, rehabilitation, hospice, and home care coverage have become more prevalent, but payment levels tend to be low. In continuing care, Medicaid remains the substantial payer, subject to severe funding problems and restricted to low-income families. Private continuing care insurance, although available, is not widely used. Many of the patients most in need of the expanded services in Exhibit 9.1 are uninsured. Chronic disease is more prevalent among people with lower income, increasing the chances that those with need will be unable to finance care.

2. *Provider compensation.* The way insurance pays for care and the amount offered affect the income of provider organizations. Hospitals and physicians are compensated separately and are paid on the basis of treatments given rather than health achieved. Payment per treatment creates a dysfunctional reward for additional treatment. It does not reward efforts to sustain the patient's health, and it rewards prolonged, repetitive, and unnecessary care.[10] Primary care and chronic disease management are rewarded at much lower prices than specialty care, to the point where chronic disease management is only about 60 percent effective[11,12] and a serious shortage of primary caregivers has emerged.[13] Public health departments, which might address preventive and health maintenance needs, have been chronically underfunded.[14] Continuing and palliative care have also been less generously funded than acute care.

3. *Organizational responses.* The result of the financing and compensation structure is a vast array of largely unconnected provider organizations. In most communities, doctors' offices, home care programs, and hospices tend to be small, private, for-profit corporations with missions that address single levels of personal healthcare (Exhibit 9.1). Long-term care facilities not affiliated with hospitals are usually owned by multibillion-dollar, national, for-profit corporations or small, local, for-profit corporations, but both struggle to provide effective care at available levels of funding.[15] The median size of the 5,500 U.S. hospices was 150 admissions per year in 2012. About 63 percent are for-profit.[16]

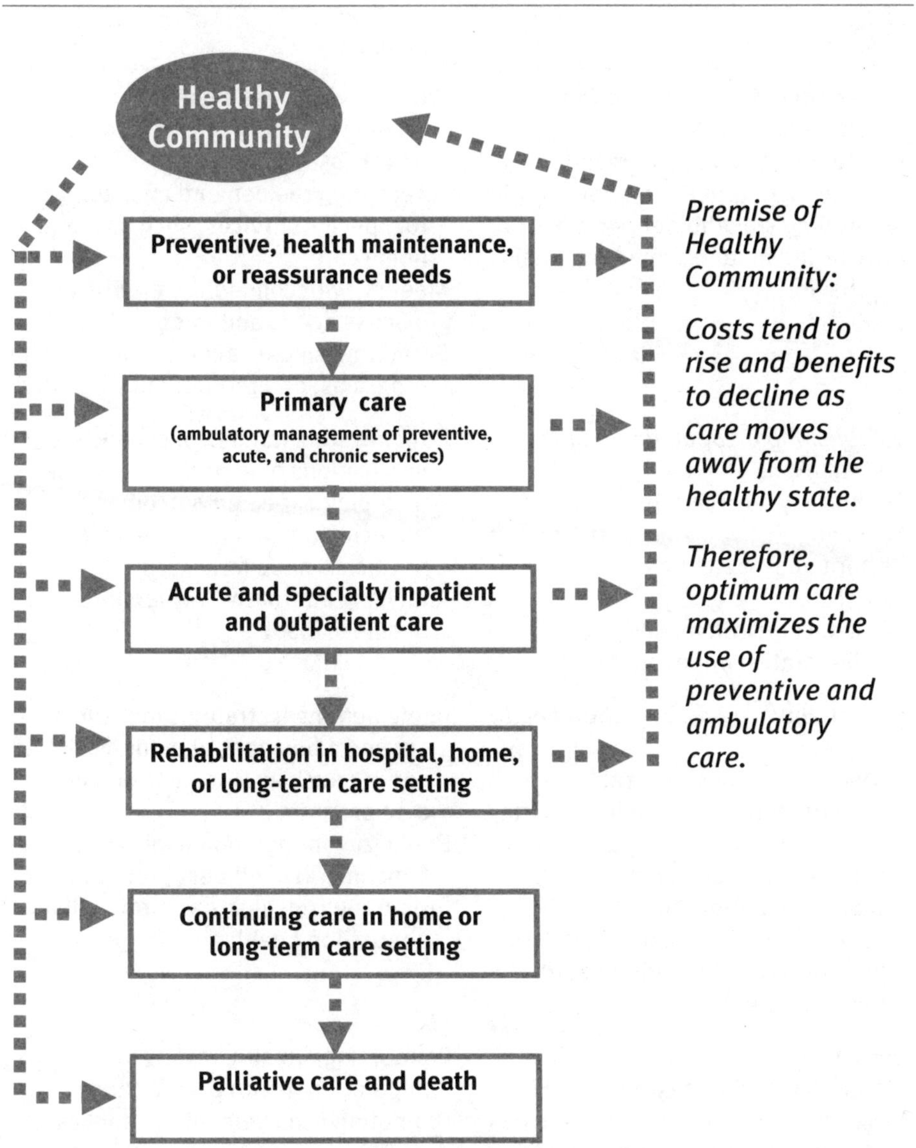

EXHIBIT 9.1
A Conceptual
Model of
Personal
Services for
Population
Health

Healthy
Community

Preventive, health maintenance,
or reassurance needs

↓

Primary care
(ambulatory management of preventive,
acute, and chronic services)

↓

Acute and specialty inpatient
and outpatient care

↓

Rehabilitation in hospital, home,
or long-term care setting

↓

Continuing care in home or
long-term care setting

↓

Palliative care and death

*Premise of
Healthy
Community:*

*Costs tend to
rise and benefits
to decline as
care moves
away from the
healthy state.*

*Therefore,
optimum care
maximizes the
use of
preventive and
ambulatory
care.*

Many healthcare experts feel that the imbalances of the current U.S. system fail to promote population health.[17,18] The critics believe that more attention to health promotion, prevention, and chronic disease management will result in a healthier population with lower healthcare expenditures per capita and a higher earning capacity.[19,20,21]

Functions

The functions required to implement a population health mission are shown in Exhibit 9.2. They are framed in a way that allows a traditional HCO to

EXHIBIT 9.2
Functions That
Implement a
Population
Health Mission

Function	Examples
Understanding and promoting population health Forecasting need and demand Identifying intervention opportunities Identifying stakeholder positions Advocating for and promoting health behavior	Working with health department and others to identify important local health issues Forecasting the demand and supply for specific services, such as nursing home care Meeting with community groups to discuss needs and roles Promoting smoking cessation, exercise programs, and reproductive health
Establishing a population health strategy Community advocacy group Mission Performance measures Financing Market, competitive, and collaborative opportunities	Building stakeholder consensus around implications of expanded mission Developing expected outcomes, financial forecasts, and revised physician-need forecasts Analyzing alternative ownerships and business models
Operationalizing a population health strategy Service operations: patient recruitment, care planning, staffing, training, budget and finance, continuous improvement Building an integrated network: collaboration with existing units; promotion of population health opportunities	Implementing a strategic measures set and a business plan for a specific service such as a hospice or a home care program Publicizing population health measures, benchmarks, and best practices Promoting consensus around realistic population health goals
Improving performance Identifying community health OFIs Developing collaborative approaches Building local understanding and contribution Strengthening public commitment	Conducting ongoing review of population health performance Promoting achievements of advocacy group Celebrating goals attained Lobbying for changes in regulation and reimbursement

OFI: opportunity for improvement

move stepwise into population health, expanding via individual services and levels or by developing a comprehensive response. The functions are applicable to *each* of the levels in Exhibit 9.1 as well as to *all* of those levels. The needs assessment function—understanding and promoting population health—is a contribution to the HCO's strategic planning in itself. Pursued for all levels, it provides a breadth of perspective that protects acute care services from unexpected difficulties. It also identifies an agenda of response opportunities. The remaining functions—identifying, implementing, and improving response strategies—can be applied to single-purpose activities or to a comprehensive population health program.

Understanding and Promoting Population Health

This function is a focused expansion of the HCO's general boundary spanning and forecasting, which measures community need for each component of service. The function (1) provides quantitative forecasts for specific services at each level of Exhibit 9.1, (2) identifies the provider and customer stakeholders who currently provide the service, and (3) provides information on opportunities that can be used to identify and prioritize program revisions.

The three components collectively create a **community needs assessment**. The needs assessment is best done comprehensively because the need for specific services is interrelated. A focus on a single level of Exhibit 9.1 can be seriously misleading. For example, the demand for hospital care is interrelated with primary care, home care, and hospice care. Once developed, the community needs assessment identifies opportunities in population health in sufficient detail to plan specific responses. It also serves as the foundation for a program to educate stakeholders and promote interest in improvement.

Community needs assessment
A process for identifying and quantifying opportunities for improvement in a community.

Mercy Health System, serving Janesville, Wisconsin, has prepared a 60-slide community needs assessment and a multi-page action plan for each of the three counties it serves. It has supplemented public sources with county population surveys and focus groups, allowing it to identify perceived needs as well as actual use of services. The assessments are designed for public consumption. They address Purpose, Data Collection Methods, Demographics, General Health Status, Behavioral Risk Factors, Maternal & Child Health, Mental Health, and Health Resource Availability. The action plans identify Objective, Strategies, Measure of Success, Timeline, and Partners. The plan for Janesville and Walworth County is particularly thoroughly developed, following the Community Health Improvement Plan and Process required of county health departments in Wisconsin. A countywide steering committee uses multiple work groups to establish the action plan.[22]

Forecasting Need and Demand

Population health services, like all healthcare services, should be sized to meet expected demand and designed to respond to stakeholder desires, using the epidemiologic planning model introduced in Chapter 2 and the marketing approach and techniques described in Chapter 15. The model can be used to forecast incidence, prevalence, and demand for all personal healthcare services.

Incidence and prevalence are closely related in acute care, but they are different in chronic care. The prevalence of a disease or condition is an important indicator of need, but it is rarely the same as the demand for services because care can be approached in alternate ways and is influenced by availability of service and the patient's financial resources. All three measures can be benchmarked. There is wide variation across the United States in the incidence and prevalence of disease and in the cost of care.

The model forecasts these measures for diseases and conditions that can be prevented, ameliorated, or managed by community health programs, including many mental illnesses. It can also be used to forecast numbers and characteristics of disease-free people by preventable risk factors, such as obesity or child safety. The full array of population health services is surprisingly large and diverse. Prevention and health maintenance services are available for many different population subgroups. The Centers for Disease Control and Prevention (CDC) Task Force on Community Preventive Services has identified 17 major prevention and health maintenance topics and has listed and evaluated more than 200 interventions.[23]

Specific risks or conditions can be grouped in various ways to facilitate planning decisions. Exhibit 9.3 shows groupings according to the level of prevention, the populations served, and the programs or organizations that provide service. These groupings are important in designing responses.

1. The level of prevention is often key to the cost-effectiveness of a specific action and an important factor in prioritizing opportunities. Primary prevention is usually the most cost-effective, not only because the interventions (primarily vaccines and behavioral education) are relatively low cost but also because the diseases prevented are often high cost and life-curtailing. Secondary prevention is more problematic. Screening for existing disease has been a popular hospital activity, but its cost-effectiveness depends on keeping the cost per case screened low. All positive results must be pursued, but many of these are false, wasting expensive resources. The key to cost-effectiveness usually lies in targeting high-risk groups, where false positives are less frequent.[24] Tertiary prevention must focus on a specific disease group, but it can be cost-effective when the risks of death and disability are high.[25]

2. The population served is useful in program design—programs can be tailored by age and interest group and promoted through appropriate vehicles, as in high school–based programs for adolescents and primary care office programs for chronic disease populations or women in childbearing years. The ability to focus both the marketing and care delivery is a major factor in program design. Advertising and care delivered to people who do not need it are a waste.

3. The service program, or kind of intervention, is useful in identifying existing sources of care and potential collaborators. Existing provider organizations can contribute important specialized knowledge and market contacts. Both are useful, making collaboration the strategy of choice in designing responses.

Prevention Level	Examples of Risks	Examples of Prevention Activity
Primary: Maintenance of health	Obesity	Dietary and exercise management
	Environmental hazards	Lead and asbestos removal Childproofing Community control of environmental hazards
	Smoking and substance abuse	Alcohol use laws Smoking cessation
Primary: Prevention of specific disease	Infectious diseases	Immunization, infection control
	Trauma	Seatbelts, helmets, alcohol management, domestic violence
	Prematurity and birth defects	Prenatal care
	Ischemic heart disease and stroke	Aspirin, anticoagulants
Secondary: Early-stage identification and elimination of disease	Cancer	Screening and early treatment
	Diabetes	Screening and dietary management
	Developmental defects	Drug and lifestyle management, remedial childcare
	Hypertension	Screening and blood pressure management
Tertiary: Reduction of the impact of chronic disease	Post-acute cardiovascular or stroke care, arthritis, trauma	Drug and lifestyle management Rehabilitation Home care and telemedicine

Population at Risk	Examples of Risks	Examples of Prevention Activity
High school students	Safe driving	Driver training
	Substance abuse	Alcohol law enforcement
	Sexual and reproductive activity	Classroom education, counseling services
Young families	Family planning, child safety, domestic abuse, health maintenance, disease screening	Maternal and reproductive health services, counseling, exercise programs, well-baby services
Elderly	Functional losses, chronic diseases, terminal illness	Home safety, rehabilitation programs, disease management, palliative care

EXHIBIT 9.3
Grouping of Disease and Prevention Forecasts, by Prevention Level, Population at Risk, and Service Program

(continued)

EXHIBIT 9.3
Grouping of
Disease and
Prevention
Forecasts, by
Prevention
Level,
Population at
Risk, and
Service
Program
(continued)

Service Program	Examples of Risks	Examples of Prevention Site
Primary care	Acute disease, chronic disease, early detection, maternal and child health management	Primary care office, industrial clinic, school clinic, retail store
Post-acute recovery	Postoperative rehabilitation	Hospital, rehabilitation center, nursing home
Continuing care	Diminished functional status, terminal illness	Home care program, nursing home, palliative care, hospice

In addition to their role in planning interventions, quantitative forecasts are used to set goals and evaluate results. Success of many primary prevention programs is measured by reduction in incidence. Incidences of early and late detection are used to evaluate secondary prevention. Prevalence of patients by functional status is used to evaluate tertiary prevention. The forecasts are also useful in promoting community awareness and understanding. The Center for Health Care Strategies, a group dedicated to improving the health of chronically ill and otherwise disadvantaged people, offers a web-based return-on-investment model that allows comparison of alternative strategies.[26]

Identifying Intervention Opportunities

The second step in developing the needs assessment is to identify the current providers of various services. Few community health needs are totally ignored. Much more commonly, an existing organization offers some service. Preventive services are offered by HCOs, schools, public health departments, and faith organizations. Primary care is offered by schools, workplaces, retailers, and physicians' offices. Community clinics, many of which are federally qualified health centers, now serve nearly 20 million Americans. Most of the clinic's clientele are disadvantaged, or as the National Association of Community Health Centers (NACHC) puts it, "medically disenfranchised." The 1,200 NACHC clinics have documented improved quality and effectiveness of care.[27] Rehabilitation is offered through hospitals, rehabilitation centers, home care programs, and nursing homes. Continuing and palliative care are offered through home care, hospice, and nursing home programs. As the examples in Exhibit 9.3 suggest, these services vary greatly by ownership, audience, approach, and resources. They often vary as well in quality and effectiveness. Comparing current services to prevalence and demand identifies unmet needs and opportunities for improved service. The epidemiologic planning model, plus an inventory of current services, generates an opportunity for improvement (OFI) list that can be publicized, prioritized, and discussed by various stakeholders.

The inventory must go beyond a simple tally of available services. Deliberate efforts must be made to ensure that programs are meeting community demand and standards for quality, effectiveness, patient satisfaction, and efficiency. Special attention is often necessary for disadvantaged populations.

1. *Unmet demand can be identified from surveys of waiting times for service.* Oversupply can be identified from occupancy information and financial performance. Best practices from similar communities can be used to evaluate both, although a comprehensive approach is necessary. The best practice in many of these activities is neither the most nor the least demand, but it contributes most to a comprehensive measure like mortality or cost per capita.

2. *Safety and quality of patient care apply to all levels.* The Centers for Medicare & Medicaid Services (CMS) offers quality assessment systems and data for nursing homes, home health agencies, hospitals, and kidney dialysis facilities.[28] Data are drawn from Medicare and Medicaid patients, but these are large proportions of the total patient load for these services. Hospitals expand the CMS data set with additional measures required by The Joint Commission. These values are not made public, but they can be released if the hospitals agree. Hospices are also accredited by The Joint Commission, although no set of specific measures is in place.[29] Various standards for primary prevention activity are available, and the CDC *Community Guide* links to them.[30] In those areas where measurement systems exist, the goal should be to make them public and use them for continuous improvement. In other areas, evidence of commitment to quality, such as maintenance of accreditation standards, should be recognized.

3. *Economy and efficiency are critical.* The nonacute programs in Exhibit 9.1 are generally underfunded. An economy-oriented business approach—careful program design, selective location, and continuous improvement of cost per case—is essential. This approach goes beyond efficiency. It continuously tests customer satisfaction against economy, seeking to eliminate all costs not essential to sustaining market share. It is substantially different from approaches to acute care, which has much richer financial support.

4. *Effectiveness criteria are also essential.* The community health concept is cost-effective only if less costly levels of care substitute for higher-cost interventions. Cost-effectiveness has been limited principally because the services are provided to persons who did not need them. For example, a home care program can be used to avoid costly days of acute hospital use, but it can also be used to substitute for less costly self-care and family support.[31] To meet cost-effectiveness criteria, the program must encourage the former and strongly discourage the latter. This problem is universal in community care. Even primary prevention, usually the benchmark of cost-effectiveness, can be ineffective if the cost of the intervention, including its adverse effects, exceeds the cost of care for the disease. The vaccine for human papilloma virus has been challenged as not cost-effective. The evidence suggests that it is effective only if limited to a carefully defined population.[32]

A substantial consensus on how to implement cost-effective programs is now available on many elements of community health. Prevention criteria are provided by the CDC *Community Guide*. The CDC's Task Force on Community Preventive Services categorizes more than 200 preventive interventions as "Recommended," "Insufficient Evidence," and "Not Recommended." The two categories of recommendation are further divided into "Strong Evidence" and "Sufficient Evidence."[33] The National Guideline Clearinghouse contains criteria for many of the remaining levels of Exhibit 9.1. Primary care guidelines are available for specific risks and age categories. Acute and rehabilitation criteria are offered by disease and condition. Disease-specific guidelines are also offered for home and palliative care.[34] The Clearinghouse does not include guidelines for continuing nursing home care, and the demand is known to be dependent on factors such as housing and family support as well as the effectiveness of preceding levels of healthcare. The CMS PACE program OASIS-B measures address issues of effectiveness of continuing care that can identify opportunities to manage continuing care.[35]

Identifying Stakeholder Positions

In most communities, both customer and provider stakeholders have highly focused needs. Many customer stakeholders are seeking a solution to a specific problem that afflicts them or their families. Employers are seeking healthier workers and lower health insurance costs. Many provider HCOs offer a limited service that contributes to a single level of Exhibit 9.1. Building collaboration between these groups is frequently the key to community health success. Collaboration creates three important opportunities. Partners can bring established contacts to important target markets. Partners can bring valuable knowledge and experience in specialized procedures. Partners can share resources for a larger total and more efficient scale of operations. The list of potential collaborators is long. In most communities it includes the following:

- *Government agencies in public health, welfare, education, environment, and justice.* These agencies are frequently in touch with high-risk and disadvantaged populations.
- *Employers.* Many have a financial stake in success through reduced insurance premiums.
- *Faith-based organizations.* These organizations are a source of volunteers and can be effective at marketing community health programs.
- *Civic and cultural organizations,* such as United Way, homeless shelters, and the YMCA.
- *Other HCOs,* including competitors in acute care and potential competitors in other levels of care, under both for-profit and not-for-profit organizations.

Extensive listening is the foundation of collaborative activity. High-performing HCOs pursue an ongoing listening and relationship-building strategy that supports collaborative community health. Their programs have several elements:

1. *Routine surveillance of public information and reports from interested groups and organizations.* Virtually all government information is public. Many nongovernmental organizations involved in health promotion maintain extensive public information in print and on the web.
2. *Personal contacts* with leadership of important organizations.
3. *Monitoring of consumer interests* through focus groups and surveys.
4. *Creation or support of community-wide groups sharing health goals.* These may be permanent and official (receiving recognition and financial support from established corporations or government agencies) or ad hoc at varying degrees of formality to address specific topics of interest. HCOs often subsidize these efforts with in-kind support, such as meeting space and computer linkage. They participate in funding recognized entities.
5. *Establishment and maintenance of contractual relationships.* Hospitals have ongoing contractual relationships with primary care physicians, nursing homes, rehabilitation services, home care agencies, and hospices. The HCO's acute services are frequently essential to the success of these programs. These relationships can be the foundation for expanded and improved activities and can include substantial HCO capital and operating investment.
6. *Service on other boards and committees by HCO managers and trustees and recognition in HCO board membership or on planning committees and process improvement teams with relevant charges.* HCO associates are often willing to volunteer similar services to other community health organizations.

Advocacy and Promotion

An HCO with a population health mission should join and encourage the voices promoting health, assisting in publicizing needs, promoting individual and collective response, and devising solutions. A communications plan for a community includes the following:[36]

1. Clear definitions of services and terminology
2. A summary of the needs assessment, available on the web and promoted through a collaborative network, including local media
3. Efforts to reach specialized customer stakeholder interests segmented by age, gender, disease risk, and expressed interest:
   - Reports, factual summaries, and reference materials
   - Speaker bureaus and planned communication to customer stakeholder segments

- Advertising and other promotion to increase customer awareness of individual services

4. Efforts to reach provider stakeholders with reliable information about demand, need, existing programs, and proposed programs

The sites that provide community health activities are all valuable avenues for communication. People who enter them often have specific needs and typically have a receptive bias toward community health concepts. The contact opens an opportunity to expand their understanding. Thus, the promotion strategy, like the implementation strategy, emphasizes collaboration.

The actions of HCOs are important reinforcement for community health concepts. High-performing HCOs do not allow smoking on site. Their emphasis on patient safety is extended to the safety of their associates and guests. They provide and promote cost-effective prevention for patients and families. They provide exercise opportunities, healthy meals, and counseling to their associates. They explicitly recognize patient autonomy, and they encourage the use of advance directives and designated patient advocates. They tailor their benefit programs to promote prevention and meet important health needs. SSM Health Care went beyond Exhibit 9.1 to eliminate bottled water[37]

because of the environmental impact of making, transporting and disposing of the bottles. The effort supports the stance of the Franciscan Sisters of Mary, the congregation that sponsors SSM Health Care, to "respect, appreciate and live in harmony with creation and direct our actions to preserve the earth."

. . . "This effort means that more than half a million bottles of water will be eliminated at SSM's facilities each year," says Sister Mary Jean Ryan, FSM, President and CEO of SSM Health Care. One of the biggest problems with bottled water is that it takes fossil fuels to produce the bottles, and then more fossil fuels are used to transport the bottles to their final destination. "Eliminating bottled water is a contribution we can make as a system to protect our fragile environment," says Sister Mary Jean.

Actions like these have both real and symbolic value.

Establishing a Population Health Strategy

As indicated in chapters 2 and 3, any activity of an HCO must have a leadership structure, an explicit purpose contributing to the larger mission, performance measures, financing, and a set of goals. If an HCO establishes a wholly owned patient care venture, these elements are implemented as in other wholly owned care. If it is a collaborative venture, the leadership structure provides a mechanism to monitor the relationship, establish future goals, and resolve difficulties. Strategies in community health are no exception, although they more commonly follow the collaborative approach. In targeted strategies, the elements are established in a two-party contract. These are also common in acute care—for example, in joint venture services lines. At the present time, most HCOs that address community health issues appear to focus on single-issue campaigns rather than a global approach.[38,39] HCOs in a variety of settings have moved to more comprehensive programs, using a variety of collaborative approaches.[40] Successful comprehensive community health strategies use a general community advocacy group to create a leadership structure.

Establishing a Community Advocacy Group

Potential partners exist for most specific community health activities. One could envision a network of two-party contracts, but the list of potential collaborators is long, and effective solutions for many targets require several parties. The more comprehensive ventures in population health begin early to develop an advocacy group broadly representative of the various interests. The group is designed to bring together diverse interests and viewpoints for the general benefit, building a network of civic engagement on community health. It usually begins with informal visits between individuals, expands to discussion sessions, and in many communities evolves to a formally appointed commission or board with a regular agenda and established relationships with major stakeholders. The initial discussions of stakeholder positions undertaken as part of the needs assessment provide the starting point. The needs assessment provides the focus.

Many communities already have advocacy groups. Several states have established programs to encourage such groups. The federally sponsored Healthy People Consortium has 350 national membership organizations and 250 state health, mental health, substance abuse, and environmental agencies.[41] Many of the members have local offices or representatives. The National Civic League provides publications, definitions of measures, and other resources to support the development of advocacy groups.[42] The Kansas University Work Group for Community Health and Development offers the multipart Community Tool Box of guides, measures, best practices, and examples that it claims is "the largest and most comprehensive resource of its kind in the world."[43]

Once formed, the advocacy group operates as a governing board would to build consensus on strategy. It assumes independent authority and elects its leadership.[44] It also facilitates contracts between various stakeholders to implement the strategy.[45] An HCO that provides high-quality acute care can add materially to an existing community group. Its role in acute care makes it central to many customer markets. New mothers, patients with chronic disease, patients recovering from acute care, and terminal patients are important examples. The HCO also has substantial resources—including strategic planning and needs assessment, facilities, and expertise—that can be contributed to a collective effort.

Exhibit 9.4 describes the goals of a comprehensive community health program (located in Kearney, Nebraska) with 20 years' history. Today, it boasts more than 150 organizational stakeholders and over 1,000 volunteers. It has developed a complex structure with a governing board, many active committees, and ten coalitions focusing on various goals.[46] The program

EXHIBIT 9.4
Community Health Goal Attainment: The Record of Buffalo County, Nebraska

2010 GOALS: HAS BUFFALO COUNTY ATTAINED THESE GOALS?

LEAD LEVELS IN CHILDREN—Moving Toward Target

AIR QUALITY GOAL:
Smoke-Free Nebraska—Goal Attained
Worksite Wellness—Moving Toward Target

ACCESS TO HEALTHCARE:
Health Insurance for Buffalo County Adults—Moving Away From Target
Heath Insurance for Minority Adults—Moving Away From Target
Health Disparities—Moving Away From Target

SAFETY:
Youth Seat Belt Use—Goal Attained (*Want to monitor as a 2020 Indicator)
Fall Prevention in Older Adults—Goal Attained (*Want to monitor as a 2020 Indicator)

AFFORDABLE HOUSING—Unknown

TRANSPORTATION—Moving Away From Target (*Change in 2010)

STRESS ON THE FAMILY UNIT

SUBSTANCE ABUSE:
Youth Tobacco Use—Goal Attained (*Want to monitor as a 2020 Indicator)
Adult Tobacco Use—Moving Toward Target
Youth Alcohol Use—Goal Attained (*Want to monitor as a 2020 Indicator)
Adult Alcohol Use—Data not available to determine goal attainment
Youth Marijuana Use—Moving Toward Target
Youth Access to Illegal Drugs on School Property—Moving Toward Target

MENTAL HEALTH:
Youth Depression—Goal Not Attained
Youth Suicide—Moving Toward Target
Adult Depression—Moving Toward Target

OBESITY/OVERWEIGHT:
Youth Overweight/Obesity—Goal Not Attained
Adult Overweight/Obesity—Goal Not Attained
Overweight & Obesity—Goal Not Attained

HEALTH & SPIRITUALITY—Goal Attained

INFANT MORTALITY
Infant Mortality—Moving Toward Target
Post Neonatal Infant Mortality—Moving Toward Target

Source: Buffalo County Community Partners, Kearney, NE. www.bcchp.org/wp-content/uploads/2010/08/2010-Goals-Attainment-Report.pdf.

is notable for its quantitative measurement and deliberate goal setting. Its governing board of 21 people includes individuals from local public health, education, city government, business, and the faith community. Its goals are established by the board. Every goal has measures of achievement. Trends are posted regularly from a variety of sources. The 2010 goals are the second set. Exhibit 9.4 indicates that only five of the 26 goals were "attained." Five were "not attained" and five were "moving away from target." Eleven are "moving toward target." While this record might appear discouraging, (1) Buffalo County has clearly identified its population health needs and developed strategies to address them, and (2) there is hard evidence of positive progress on two-thirds of their goals. That is a great deal more than most counties can say.

Establishing the Purpose of Collaboration

The intent of the collaboration is generally stated as a *purpose* in two-party relationships and as a *mission* in more comprehensive ones. The terminology helps illustrate the independence of the community advocacy group. The most effective groups are independent of the HCO or any other specific member. The purposes they adopt can go well beyond personal health services to more fundamental needs in environment, employment, or education. Health may be important on the list of needs, but far from first. Such a perspective may be necessary to make substantial inroads on many serious health problems.[47]

An HCO's participation in an advocacy group recognizes a concordance between its mission and the group's. Important, sensitive issues are involved in the decision to participate. These relate to the prioritization of resource use between competing elements of a comprehensive community health program and commitments in acute care. The collaborative mission must be carefully implemented to preserve existing relationships. The HCO's mission statement must go beyond excellence in acute care. Wording of mission, like that of North Mississippi Medical Center—"to continuously improve the health of the people of our region"—is an unequivocal commitment that does not interfere with the HCO's ability to deliver quality acute care. Mercy Health System's "provide exceptional healthcare services resulting in healing in the broadest sense" balances traditional with expanded commitment.[48] The goal is to gain understanding and acceptance of the broader mission from all stakeholders and commitment from as many as possible.

Support for a community health mission is obtained through the usual visioning exercise, which deliberately asks hundreds of stakeholders to focus on the group's most basic purposes. The stakeholders are gathered in groups and the case for community health presented. The case is not complex:

> A healthy community is happier and more productive because the individuals in it are healthier and more productive. There is a lot more to health than simply acute hospital-oriented care. In general, our community needs to be sure we

prevent disease whenever possible, treat people with disease as effectively and economically as possible, and help people approaching the end of life do so in comfort, with grace, and, if possible, in the presence of their loved ones.

This case has broad appeal. It reflects the professional commitment of most healing professions, the values of most faiths, and what most of us instinctively feel. As stakeholders contemplate the mission, several specific and practical questions are likely to arise, and the HCO spokespersons should be prepared to discuss them:

- *Financial implications for current activities.* Implementing a community health mission requires capital that otherwise could be invested in expanding acute services. How will this trade-off be managed?
  1. Capital decisions for the HCO will continue to be made by its governing board in the overall interests of the community, recognizing both the importance of existing relationships and the HCO's unique role in acute care.
  2. The HCO's capital review process is designed to give all stakeholders an opportunity to comment and to identify the most valuable investments in light of the mission.
  3. The board intends to keep our community competitive with others in all levels of care. The board will support acute care investments that are scientifically sound, efficient in settings like ours, and generally accepted by health insurers.
  4. Our sound financial position allows us to do this, and the board is committed to maintaining that soundness.

     The answer places the question in context, clarifies both the authority and the process of decision making, and states the philosophic position of the board. It ensures that, despite the importance of community health, acute care will not be neglected.

- *Income implications for provider stakeholders.* This question is related to the preceding question, but it often comes from practitioners of high-tech specialties, who in the traditional not-for-profit structure receive access to substantial free capital and trained personnel in the HCO. The answer reiterates the first answer, pointing out the relevant specific opportunities that have been funded recently and noting that the HCO has, in fact, remained competitive with other sites. It also reiterates the HCO's commitment to using its medical staff planning function so that every physician has an opportunity to earn a competitive income. The solution will be successful if the supply of high-tech specialists is kept in balance with clinically justified demand.

- *Justice.* The question is "Should our HCO serve the needy or the insured, paying customer?" although it is rarely so boldly phrased. The issue is the extent to which the HCO is appropriately a vehicle for overcoming society's more general problems of poverty, income distribution, and disadvantaged populations.

The HCO's not-for-profit status is justified in part by its contribution to these problems. The answer for most HCOs is to serve these goals only to the extent external funding permits. That often means a general commitment to offer only services for which payment is typically available and to set a specific limit on the funding to be transferred to uncompensated care.

- *Faith-based restrictions on medical care.* The expanded mission raises several potential areas of ethical conflict in addition to those inherent in acute care. The nonreligious not-for-profit HCO's position emphasizes patient autonomy, the right of each individual to choose his or her care for any reason, including reasons of faith. Religious HCOs operate similarly, but they reserve the right not to provide any treatment or service inconsistent with their faith. Both make an effort to avoid offending those who hold strong convictions. Preventive services, such as reproductive health, are one troublesome area; management of death is another, but less controversial, one. Potentially disturbing positions are implemented by carefully targeted promotion, location, corporate separation, and similar devices designed to isolate those who desire the service from those who find it offensive.

To be convincing, the HCO's answers to these questions must be backed by a record of trust and success. The record of the leading hospitals shows that the stakeholder reservations reflected in the questions can be overcome.

Measuring Performance

Community health service teams should be measured like any other healthcare team, using the operational dimensions of demand, cost, worker satisfaction, efficiency, quality, and customer satisfaction. Examples are shown in Exhibit 9.5. As in both the Buffalo County and Mercy examples, the teams use history, competition, benchmarks, and values to identify OFIs and set goals. They conduct continuous improvement activities like all other teams. They must be committed to "keeping our community competitive," recognizing concerns about impact on the acute care mission.

In addition, individual community health programs are measured strategically in terms of their cost per case and cost per capita. These measures are used in cost–benefit or cost-effectiveness evaluations that provide the scientific evidence supporting the programs. Benefits are usually per capita counts of more serious events avoided (e.g., premature death or disability, preventable disease incidence or treatment incidence, such as hospitalization, absenteeism, and income loss).[49]

Formal evaluation of cost-effectiveness is best left to researchers working at a national level. The CDC's Task Force on Community Preventive Services has documented the process it uses to recommend programs.[50,51] Obtaining local outcomes values is sometimes practical. Cost per case and per capita should be monitored and benchmarked as a check on program effectiveness.

EXHIBIT 9.5 Examples of Operational Measures for Population Health Programs

Program	Need/Demand	Productivity	Quality and Effectiveness
Well-baby care	Incidence from birth data and forecasts Demand from existing programs	Cost/service (e.g., cost of standard vaccine packages) Cost/visit Cost/infant	Percent immunized Incidence of preventable condition reported (e.g., infectious disease, trauma, violence) Incidence of manageable condition reported (e.g., hearing, visual, or functional limitation)
Asthma management	Incidence/prevalence from epidemiologic model or survey Demand from existing programs	Cost/visit Cost/patient-year Cost/capita	Incidence of asthma-related disability from surveys (www.cdc.gov/asthma/questions.htm) Clinical data on asthmatic pulmonary function (outcomes) Clinical data on asthmatic treatment (process)
Home care	Waiting lists or unmet demand Comparison to similar communities Demand from existing programs	Cost/visit Cost/patient-month Cost/capita	Patient, family, and physician satisfaction Adverse events CMS OASIS C measures*
Hospice	Waiting lists or unmet demand Comparison to similar communities Demand from existing programs	Cost/visit Cost/patient-month Cost/capita	Patient, family, and physician satisfaction Hospice referrals as percent of total mortality or disease-specific mortality Hospice-specific quality measures** The *Dartmouth Atlas of Health Care* 2008 Tracking the Care of Patients with Severe Chronic Illness †

Note: All programs will measure associate satisfaction and client satisfaction by survey. Program accounting records will measure resource consumption and counts of volumes, scheduling delays, and percent of capacity used.
*www.cms.hhs.gov/HomeHealthQualityInits/06_OASISC.asp#TopOfPage
†www.dartmouthatlas.org/atlases/atlas_series.shtm
**Information from Kirby, E. G., M. J. Keeffe, and K. M. Nicols. 2007. "A Study of the Effects of Innovative and Efficient Practices on the Performance of Hospice Care Organizations." *Health Care Management Review* 32 (4): 352–59.

Financing

As indicated, the HCO's population health mission must be limited to what can be reasonably financed. Even the largest HCOs cannot ignore the market realities of medical care, including the emphasis on high-tech acute intervention built into both private and government insurance programs. It is arguable that Americans have the healthcare system they want. If they wanted a different emphasis than acute care, high-tech intervention, there is no shortage of models to copy. On the other hand, many believe that the current emphasis is unstable; the cost cannot be allowed to grow as it has in the past. Population health is a major vehicle to control long-term costs. The balance between these competing visions must be maintained by governing board policies. The policies that have proven effective for HCOs are as follows:

- Every service line must be planned and operated in a way that pursues continuous improvement to minimize cost and maximize all revenue consistent with its mission, vision, and values. This means that each service line must justify its contribution and that no individual receives care beyond what is effective.
- Capital investments and deficit coverage can be viewed as community dividends or benefits and funded at the discretion of the HCO board using three broad criteria:
  1. All funded activities should have a potential benefit that reasonably exceeds the support required, even though the benefit may be difficult to measure.
  2. The HCO's total investment cannot exceed prudent levels indicated in the long-range financial plan.
  3. Acute care needs that keep the community competitive with others must take priority because they are the HCO's core mission.

These criteria are designed to ensure continued financial performance of the organization as a whole. They force collective consideration of all needs, including community health; provide a cost–benefit criterion for prioritizing opportunities; and protect long-term stability. To protect the acute care activities, many high-performing HCOs set an upper limit to investment in underfunded services. A few, such as SSM Health Care[52] and Catholic Health Initiatives,[53] mandate a minimum as well.

Promoting Population Health Opportunities

The final step in a community health strategy is the systematic use of the existing marketplace to expand the maximal use of appropriate services. This includes assisting existing organizations to improve and using collaborative opportunities to increase market penetration. Deliberate promotion—*social marketing*[54]—is essential for many community health activities. While people immediately relate "doctor" and "hospital" to "health," none of the other personal health services has the same level of recall. Some of them, particularly palliative care and some preventive activities, carry negative impressions that education and marketing must overcome. Coalitions with specific interest groups are valuable and completely consistent with social marketing concepts. Many groups with targeted missions have attracted the people most interested in their mission—the core ready-to-buy market. They form an invaluable nucleus for promotion. The acute care services should support these groups, using protocols that limit unnecessary services and encourage appropriate referral.

Competing organizations can also be influenced by a well-designed strategy. They can be drawn into joint ventures, or encouraged by market pressures to expand or improve services. A large HCO controls a substantial market share that it can direct to selected providers on the basis of quality and cooperation. (Potential antitrust implications exist in any action taken directly toward competitors. Although enforcement in comprehensive community care would be unusual, consultation with legal counsel is appropriate.)

Operationalizing a Population Health Strategy

Once established, the strategy must be implemented. Three elements are important. Individual teams must be established, trained, supported, and held accountable, a process no different from acute healthcare. Stakeholder support must be maintained and, if possible, increased. This effort must overcome both ignorance and faulty preconceptions that are more widespread in nonacute services. Finally, coalitions—whether with individual organizations or through an advocacy group—must be maintained and encouraged to be effective.

Supporting Caregiving Teams

The functions that community health units must perform are essentially the same as those required of acute service lines and nursing units. From an organizational perspective, the differences between a hospice, a primary care clinic, a health promotion program for teenagers, and an intensive care unit (ICU) lie in the clinical details, not the organization. Clinical, logistic, and strategic support must be provided for community health teams as it is for more traditional ones. The organizational foundations for excellence—transformational management, performance measurement, evidence-based management, and evidence-based care—are the same. They must be put in place and supported by education, repetition, and reward.

High-performing HCOs are well equipped to fill these needs, using the same approaches that support acute care teams.

Building Stakeholder Support

Identifying and understanding collective opportunities and building networks of civic engagement are ongoing challenges. Communities are composed of individuals linked in multiple diverse groups that network their lives. These stakeholder groups are, by nature, advocatory and protectionist, and they are frequently confrontational. Community health is only one area of society where finding the key to collaboration is essential. Education; economic development; and the operating infrastructure of roads, utilities, safety, and justice are others. The solution lies in mechanisms of civic engagement and social connectedness that facilitate coordination and cooperation for mutual benefit.[55] The elements used successfully in many communities are extensions of those used in high-performing traditional healthcare: extensive communication and honest listening, respect for all participants, evidence of the need and the possibility that translates the need to opportunity, continuous improvement, and the willingness to begin with achievable goals and work toward values and benchmarks. These elements are achieved not only by personal leadership but also by identifying and supporting like-thinking partners. Stakeholders become advocates when they are assured that their concerns are met and the benefits are realistic.

For an HCO that is pursuing community health at any level, maintenance of the network of collaborators is an important activity. The advocacy group and individual contracts are the mechanism for identifying, ranking, and pursuing OFIs and for dispute resolution. Each contract should be assigned to an individual manager to monitor, including listening to and negotiating issues that arise. This is no different from monitoring other contracts, such as supplies or joint ventures.

Supporting the Advocacy Group

A successful community advocacy group formalizes the stakeholder participation. It pursues functions that resemble those of the governing board:

1. Establishing the community's health mission, including the scope and roles of contributing groups
2. Maintaining a supportive relationship that allows contributing organizations to identify and achieve specific community health goals
3. Creating an overall strategy, and maintaining financial support
4. Encouraging performance measurement, acceptable quality of care, and comprehensive response to individual patient needs
5. Monitoring general measures of the community health, identifying OFIs, and assisting in response

Community coalitions lack the authority of governing boards, but they can bring stakeholders together, identify collaborative opportunities, encourage contracts between agencies, and draw attention to global measures of community health.

The advocacy group will have an HCO representative who assumes a leadership role with regard to community health. The high-performing HCO has several resources to contribute toward these functions. In addition to a cash contribution, it can offer seasoned governing board members and provide staff support to prepare agendas and manage meetings. It can share the rules and culture that make its own board successful. It can offer its training programs for coalition staff, and it can contribute the time of its senior executives.

Improving Performance

All elements of high-performing HCOs must be subject to continuous improvement. Population health activities are no exception. The cycle of OFI identification, goal setting, process improvement, and celebration of achievement must be built into the model of population health. All the operating units conduct quarterly assessments of progress, identifying and addressing OFIs and preparing for enhanced goals in the coming year. If a community-wide advocacy group exists, the group engages in annual self-assessment and improvement just as the governing board does. The individuals responsible for maintaining the HCO's relationship and the continued success of collaborative ventures also review achievement quarterly, make sure goals are achieved, and work with their partners to identify new goals.

People

Population health teams may be direct caregivers, such as home health, hospice, or immunization clinic associates. They may also be community health advocates, school nurses, occupational health providers, long-term care nurses, or personal health aides. Population health services' caregiving teams must be recruited, trained, and supported like acute care teams. Because of the limited financing, nonacute services of all kinds have operated at lower wage levels than acute care has. Volunteers and family members play an important role.

Providing safe, effective, patient-centered, timely, efficient, and equitable care that uses less skilled individuals requires systematic and careful organizational support. High-performing community health sites implement the following elements:[56]

1. Clear, frequently communicated mission and vision
2. Carefully designed work processes and protocols, providing specific advice on when assistance should be sought and how it can be obtained
3. Training for specific duties in a limited situation, such as a dialysis unit or a nursing home, including indicators of complications and resources to assist when complications occur
4. Measured performance, retraining, celebration, and rewards
5. Frequent and transformational contact, with emphasis on encouragement

This approach is little different from that used in high-performing acute care organizations. Applied with care and diligence, it allows patients, lower-wage employees, volunteers, and family members to support effective care and reduce costs. It has been applied in a variety of community health settings. The following are examples:

- Schoolteachers can be trained to provide instruction on healthy lifestyles, including classroom instruction, individual counseling, and personal modeling of good health habits.[57]
- Volunteers in the faith community can make important contributions. Parish nurses promote healthy behavior and undertake screening.[58] Stephen Ministries and similar activities can support individuals and families in times of stress.[59]
- Volunteers deliver Meals on Wheels,[60] provide transportation, and assist in all levels of care delivery through palliative care and bereavement support.[61]
- Low-wage workers can be trained to undertake important clinical responsibilities in primary and continuing care settings.[62]
- Family members can be trained to manage patients with severe disabilities.[63]

Measures

Operational

Each community health activity should be measured using the operating dimensions for performance measurement. Exhibit 9.5 shows examples for typical specific activities. A number of approaches adapt the dimensions to the needs of preventive and chronic care teams:

1. *Both need and demand should be measured.* Need should be estimated by population subgroup so that unmet needs can be identified as OFIs. For example, need and demand for primary and secondary prevention services are appropriately measured by age group, geographic area, and cultural characteristics. This allows not only identification of unmet need but also a starting point for correction—through the schools for teenagers and through culturally targeted media and civic organizations for cultural groups at higher risk.

   Need is measured by the incidence or prevalence of a specific condition, such as overweight, arrests for driving under influence, pregnancy, and asthma. Statistics for these conditions are drawn from national or regional surveys and databases and are used in the epidemiologic planning model to infer and forecast local values. Effective ambulatory care includes a wide range of needs. Those related to pregnancy, child rearing, and statistically important chronic diseases can be individually forecast. A separate forecast can address other miscellaneous primary care. Home care, hospice, and nursing home care need estimates present unusual problems. The need for these services is influenced not only by disease incidence but also by income, cultural attitudes, and availability of family support. Models for estimating need are available in the literature, but they require household or acute care patient surveys that are expensive to implement.[64,65,66] Occupancy levels, waiting times, and comparisons to similar communities are used as substitutes.

   Waiting times are accepted as indicators of unmet demand for all healthcare services. Specific definitions, such as "the third available routine visit date" are used to reduce random variation. Waiting lists or counts are generally less reliable. They frequently accumulate patients who are not actually demanding service, because their condition has changed or their initial entry was opportunistic.[67]

2. *Resource consumption—quantities and cost of resources used—is handled as for any other team.* Resource conditions often emphasize capacity and occupancy. Facilities for these services must sustain high occupancies to minimize costs.

3. *Human resource status is measured by surveys, turnover rates, absenteeism rates, vacancy rates, and safety as with other healthcare teams.*

4. *Output is measured, as usual, in numbers of clients served and counts of services delivered.* The target population also must be measured. Counts of clients served per 1,000 members of the target population are an important indicator of market penetration. For example, a health behavior program for teenagers would track the number of teenagers participating as a fraction of the number in the community. A hospice program would monitor the number of referrals as a fraction of the number of deaths.

   Productivity is measured as cost per service, cost per case or patient, and cost per capita. Cost per service is a useful test of team efficiency. Cost per case is the product of cost per service times the number of services per client. The number of services introduces an element of effectiveness. Cost per capita is the total cost of the activity divided by the population served. Judgments of program effectiveness or benefit are made at the per capita level. All of these can be benchmarked and used to evaluate OFIs. Quality measurement should include outcomes measures and process measures linked by evidence to those outcomes. The link is often less than fully proven, but the best available indicators should be used.

5. *Customer satisfaction is usually obtained by survey.* Client or patient satisfaction is supplemented by family satisfaction and referring physician satisfaction, where appropriate.

The operation of population health activities should include benchmarking, goal setting, and continuous improvement. Each activity should produce a list of OFIs and their needs to address them. These lists can be compiled by the advocacy group and used to guide future efforts. They can be summarized as indicators of overall progress as part of the strategic population health measures.

Strategic

Strategic measures should monitor the overall contribution of population health programs. A healthy community is one where people lead long, healthy, productive lives. The concept is commonly implemented by measuring the opposites—death, disease, and activity limitation. The model for the strategic evaluation is provided by Healthy People 2020.[68] Population data must be constructed from CDC health statistics, CMS Medicare hospitalization statistics, data from local sources, and ad hoc surveys.

Some states augment the federal data with all hospital admissions and various other health indicators, such as school vaccination records. A uniform crime-reporting system provides data on domestic violence, drug usage, and alcohol-related accidents. Epidemiologic planning models use the public data, often supplementing it with private sources, such as insurance claims, to infer community-level values. The *Dartmouth Atlas* provides data on hospitalizations and per capita expenditures based on Medicare reports for hospital service areas and referral areas. It is updated annually, with a three-year lag.[69] Its measure of Medicare expenditures in the last two years of life is particularly useful as an indicator of chronic disease care effectiveness. Exhibit 9.6 provides a template for available strategic measures. The strategic measures of population health can all be calculated for small civil divisions, such as census tract, postal code area, or township, and aggregated to typical HCO market communities. They can all be benchmarked and trended over time, providing a foundation for a community health needs assessment and an annual review.

In addition to these data, strategic measures of community health should summarize the effort of all the various agencies and organizations involved. If these organizations follow continuous improvement management, they will have operational measures, benchmarks, and OFIs. They will also have conventional financial reports and stakeholder satisfaction data that can support summary statements and OFIs. This data set provides community leaders, including the advocacy group, with a platform of information to set strategy.

Managerial Issues

HCO managers have two roles in population health. First and most important, their professional training gives them a knowledge foundation in the scope and value of community health that few others share. HCO managers have unique insight into the interplay of acute care and other population health services. Second, the managerial skills that have led to high performance in acute care are clearly applicable in other health settings. HCO managers know how to implement transformational evidence-based management. That approach is the documented best practice for acute care, and it appears to be equally powerful across the spectrum of community care. The two roles suggest four recurring issues that managers must address: (1) promoting and teaching the issues and opportunities, (2) extending the transformational culture and evidence-based management to population health activities, (3) expanding and improving primary care and the management of chronic diseases, and (4) maintaining the network of civic engagement.

EXHIBIT 9.6
Population
Health
Scorecard

Dimension	Population Health Examples
Strategic measures of population health	*Measures from government health statistics:* Mortality, by cause, with emphasis on preventable death Natality, with emphasis on neonatal mortality, prematurity, and limitation Infectious disease rates *Measures from Medicare and Medicaid:* Per capita hospitalizations by diagnostic group Incidence of chronic disease Cost of hospitalization Cost of medical care in last two years of life *Measures from government agencies:* Domestic violence Alcohol-related events Heath and immunization of school children *Measures from community surveys:* Health insurance premiums Health insurance coverage Preventable emergency care Premorbid and treatable conditions: obesity, hypertension, depression Unfilled demand for health services
Financial performance	*Financial structure of advocacy group:* Grants and gifts for population health received by advocacy group and member organizations Financial performance of independent, affiliated, and wholly owned organizations supporting population health
Operations of caregiving units	Summary of OFIs from operations at each level of population health, drawn from their operational measures
Market performance and stakeholder satisfaction	Measures of access for disadvantaged groups Measures of acute care readmission rates Measures of cultural competence in healthcare Customer and provider stakeholder satisfaction

OFI: opportunity for improvement

Promoting and Teaching Population Health

Several core issues reflected in Exhibit 9.1 are not well understood by Americans at large:

1. *Prevention is in itself a multicomponent activity.* Primary prevention involves environmental management, immunization, and behavioral elements. It has the highest payoff. Even though environmental management (i.e., air, water, and food supply; contaminants such as lead and mold) requires expensive

collaborative action, it eliminates disease for a lot of people. Thus, primary prevention generally gives the best return on investment.

2. *Many Americans suffer from chronic diseases such as diabetes, high blood pressure, asthma, and mental illness.* While these diseases cannot be cured, they can
be managed. Primary care provides ongoing support to minimize the costs of
chronic disease. The support, which can be carried out in large part by nonphysicians, is a major contribution to community health.

3. *Twenty-first-century acute care is astonishingly expensive.* Emergency visits are
measured in hundreds of dollars, and outpatient treatments often in thousands.
A single hospitalization approaches one-half of an individual's annual income.
Health insurance hides these costs from the users, as it is designed to do. They
cannot be escaped from a community perspective. Although acute care HCOs
provide substantial benefits to the community—health to individuals and income
through their associates—the cost of those benefits must ultimately be weighed
against other social opportunities and the cost of health insurance. The keys to
controlling unnecessary use of acute care are evidence-based medicine, evidence-
based management, and community health.

4. *The proper goal of the healthcare system at the end of life is to maximize comfort for
both patient and family.* This is a different goal from prolonging life, although it
is not automatically inconsistent. Americans generally need to be aware of this
to understand the difference. Community health programs need to help them
implement their understanding.

The first task of HCO managers is to understand these issues. They are
not simple. They are not self-evident, and they are not widely demonstrated
in the United States today. Once grasped, they force a change in perspective
about community health and a new vision of what HCOs can do. As more
Americans understand them, major gains can be made. The spread of these
ideas will be from professionals—the concepts are entirely consistent with
the ethical goals of the healing professions—to other influentials in American
communities. Employers, trustees, public officials, elected representatives,
religious leaders, and teachers can and should master these concepts. HCO
managers must teach them.

Extending Management Concepts to Population Health Care Teams

The activities of population health care teams in prevention, primary care,
rehabilitation, continuing care, and palliative care are all different, and so are
the activities of labor and delivery teams, emergency teams, surgery teams,
and ICU teams. These differences in clinical content do not support any fundamental differences in organization and management.

The keys to high performance are the same across all of healthcare.
Transformational management approaches that actively support worker needs
are one key. Continuous improvement, with its requisite measurement, benchmarking, OFI identification, and goal setting, is the second. Evidence-based

medicine is the third key. The science that identifies and develops high tech-nology also provides the facts to support its appropriate use. The combination of the three can be a definition of *evidence-based healthcare management.* These keys are being used in all high-performing acute care applications. The same keys likely promote effective population health.

The HCO can create primary care, home care, palliative and hospice, and continuing care service lines by service contracts, joint ventures, or acqui-sition. It can offer training services to affiliated organizations. It can encourage its leadership to serve on boards of these organizations.

Expanding and Integrating Primary Care

Primary care is a diverse set of clinical events, including critical primary, second-ary, and tertiary preventive care as well as more routine support for minor illness and trauma. It is the most frequent contact that people have with healthcare by an order of magnitude. (Four out of 5 Americans visit a doctor, a clinic, or an emergency department each year; only 1 in 16 stays overnight in a hospital.[70]) It is, as noted, not done well. Too many patients fail to get the treatment they need when they need it, leading to more serious illness, work loss, and more expensive care. Part of the problem is patient oriented. Lack of financial resources, lack of transportation, cultural and language differences, and the barriers imposed by disease itself make it difficult for some patients to get the care they need. Part of the problem is the diversity and independence of providers. Primary care is provided by a wide variety of practitioners in a wide variety of settings.

Adopting the medical home concept is an important step toward rationalizing primary care. The concept, which has been around for several decades and has had different labels, is that every patient has a single care team that coordinates his or her ongoing care. Under the leadership of the Commonwealth Fund and the National Committee for Quality Assurance, the professional organizations for family practice, internal medicine, pediatrics, and osteopathy adopted standards and guidelines for the *patient-centered med-ical home* in 2008. The standards identify the following key characteristics:[71]

- Ongoing relationship with a personal physician trained in comprehensive care
- Physician-led care team
- "Whole person orientation" emphasizing "care for all stages of life"
- Coordination of care "across all elements of the complex health system"
- Emphasis on quality, safety, and evidence-based medicine
- Use of the electronic medical record and knowledge management sys-tems for care, performance improvement, patient education, and enhanced communication

The community health centers are also committed to the patient-centered medical home. The concept is central to the accountable care organizations supported by the ACA. It does not solve all problems. It is a complex vision to implement.[72] Any HCO committed to the population health mission should work to implement the patient-centered medical home concept. Community health centers for persons who face difficulties finding care are a proven success.

Maintaining the Infrastructure for Population Health

Community health is not solely the responsibility of traditional not-for-profit HCOs; indeed, those HCOs that select an excellence-in-care mission are explicitly limiting their responsibility. For HCOs that accept the obligation, the critical organizational issue is bringing together, coordinating, and if possible expanding a community-wide effort. It is a problem that the United States has not solved well.

The prevailing theory, simply stated, is that government agencies should be responsible for all of those activities best approached in common: environmental control, safety and legal compliance, public health, and public education. The market should handle all activities best left to the individual to decide. The not-for-profit or nongovernmental organization introduces a third vehicle, more flexible than the first and more committed to the common good than the market, to address unresolved concerns.[73] A theoretical case can be made that local government should address community health; convene the advocacy group; compile strategic measures; and lead in identifying, prioritizing, and achieving OFIs. The reality is that local government is understaffed to meet the challenges in its more central responsibilities. Similarly, the market, although deeply invested in health, deals poorly with its externalities. The not-for-profit might be the best vehicle to approach this complex problem.

When the traditional HCO steps into a role to manage population health, it is usually the largest and best-funded organization. That gives it substantial leverage. When it has achieved high performance in its traditional areas, it has built an organizational mechanism that increases its leverage and that can be copied successfully by other service organizations. The core problem that it faces is expanding the community's collective effort to identify and address health problems. The first need is comprehensive personal healthcare. As a result of the stimulus of the ACA, many HCOs are acquiring or building primary care, rehabilitation, and continuing and palliative care organizations. A second approach is to build coalitions for these services, strengthening other organizations as providers by supporting contracts or developing joint ventures. The best combination remains to be seen. Beyond personal healthcare, HCOs must form multiple-agency systems like those in Buffalo County and Janesville, Wisconsin. These systems will require continuing management, but as these (and other) communities have shown, they can be effective.

The key to a coordinated approach to population health lies in the diligent pursuit of the four functions, measuring need and performance, maintaining effective interpersonal relationships, rigorously using performance measures to identify OFIs, and pursuing continuous improvement. Introducing the measurement and improvement activities that have been proven successful in acute care substantially improves population health as a whole.

Additional Resources

Begun, J. W., and J. K. Malcolm. 2014. *Leading Public Health: A Competency Framework*. New York: Springer.

Community Tool Box, a service of the Work Group for Community Health and Development at the University of Kansas. http://ctb.ku.edu/en.

Health Research & Educational Trust. 2014. *The Second Curve of Population Health*. Chicago: Health Research & Educational Trust. www.hpoe.org/pophealthsecondcurve.

Kern, L. M., A. Edwards, and R. Kaushal. 2014. "The Patient-Centered Medical Home, Electronic Health Records, and Quality of Care." *Annals of Internal Medicine* 160 (11): 741–49.

National Committee for Quality Assurance. 2008. *Standards and Guidelines for Physician Practice Connections—Patient-Centered Medical Home (PPC-PCMH)*. [Online information; retrieved 7/1/14.] www.ncqa.org/portals/0/programs/recognition/PCMH_Overview_Apr01.pdf.

Prybil, L., F. D. Scutchfield, R. Killian, A. Kelly, G. Mays, A. Carman, S. Levey, A. McGeorge, and D. W. Fardo. 2014. *Improving Community Health Through Hospital Public Health Collaboration*. Lexington, KY: Commonwealth Center for Governance Studies.

U.S. Department of Health and Human Services. "Healthy People 2020." [Online information; retrieved 7/2/14.] www.healthypeople.gov/2020/default.aspx.

Notes

1. Commission to Build a Healthier America. Home page. [Online information; retrieved 6/30/14.] www.commissiononhealth.org.
2. Kindig, D. A. 2007. "Understanding Population Health Terminology." *Milbank Quarterly* 85 (1): 139–61.
3. U.S. Internal Revenue Service. 2014. Schedule H, Form 990. [Online information; retrieved 6/30/14.] www.irs.gov/uac/About-Schedule-H-Form-990.
4. Fogel, R. W. 2004. *The Escape from Hunger and Premature Death, 1700–2100*. Cambridge, UK: Cambridge University Press.
5. Murphy, K. M., and R. H. Topel. 2006. "The Value of Health and Longevity." *Journal of Political Economy* 114 (5): 871–904.
6. American College of Physicians. 2008. "Position Paper: Achieving a High-Performance Health Care System with Universal Access: What the United States Can Learn from Other Countries." *Annals of Internal Medicine* 148 (1): 55–75.
7. Starr, P. 1982. *The Social Transformation of American Medicine*. New York: Basic Books.
8. Fuchs, V. R. 2008. "Three 'Inconvenient Truths' About Health Care." *New England Journal of Medicine* 359 (17): 1749–51.
9. Catlin, A., C. Cowan, M. Hartman, and S. Heffler. 2008. "National Health Spending in 2006: A Year of Change for Prescription Drugs." *Health Affairs* 27: 1–29, Exhibit 7.

10. Jencks, S. F., M. V. Williams, and E. A. Coleman. 2009. "Rehospitalizations Among Patients in the Medicare Fee-for-Service Program." *New England Journal of Medicine* 360: 1418–28.

11. McGlynn, E. A., S. M. Asch, J. Adams, J. Keesey, J. Hicks, A. DeCristofaro, and E. A. Kerr. 2003. "The Quality of Health Care Delivered to Adults in the United States." *New England Journal of Medicine* 348 (26): 2635–45.

12. Mangione-Smith, R., A. H. DeCristofaro, C. M. Setodji, J. Keesey, D. J. Klein, J. L. Adams, M. A. Schuster, and E. A. McGlynn. 2007. "The Quality of Ambulatory Care Delivered to Children in the United States." *New England Journal of Medicine* 357 (15): 1515–23.

13. Hackbarth, G. M. 2009. "Reforming the Health Care Delivery System." Testimony by the Medicare Payment Advisory Commission.

14. Public health activity has not exceeded 3.2 percent of national health expenditures in 52 years and fell to 2.7 percent in 2012, according to the Centers for Medicare & Medicaid Services. 2014. "National Health Expenditures; Aggregate and per Capita Amounts, Annual Percent Change and Percent Distribution: Selected Calendar Years 1960–2012." [Online information; retrieved 6/30/14.] www.cms.gov/Research-Statistics-Data-and-Systems/Statistics-Trends-and-Reports/National HealthExpendData/Downloads/tables.pdf.

15. Levinson, D. 2008. "Memorandum Report: Trends in Nursing Home Deficiencies and Complaints." OEI-02-08-00140. Office of Inspector General, U.S. Department of Health and Human Services. [Online information; retrieved 6/30/14.] www.oig.hhs.gov/oei/reports/oei-02-08-00140.pdf.

16. National Hospice and Palliative Care Organization. 2013. "Hospice Care in America." [Online information; retrieved 6/30/14.] www.nhpco.org/sites/default/files/public/Statistics_Research/2013_Facts_Figures.pdf.

17. Commonwealth Fund. 2009. *The Path to a High Performance U.S. Health System: A 2020 Vision and the Policies to Pave the Way.* [Online information; retrieved 6/30/14.] www.commonwealthfund.org/publications/fund-reports/2009/feb/the-path-to-a-high-performance-us-health-system.

18. Miller, M. E. 2008. "Report to the Congress: Reforming the Delivery System." Medicare Payment Advisory Commission. [Online information; retrieved 6/30/14.] www.medpac.gov/documents/20080916_Sen%20Fin_testimony%20final.pdf.

19. Examining Community-Institutional Partnerships for Prevention Research Group. 2006. "Building and Sustaining Community-Institutional Partnerships for Prevention Research: Findings from a National Collaborative." *Journal of Urban Health* 83 (6): 989–1003.

20. Kindig, D. A., Y. Asada, and B. Booske. 2008. "A Population Health Framework for Setting National and State Health Goals." *Journal of the American Medical Association* 299 (17): 2081–83.

21. Schroeder, S. A. 2007. "Shattuck Lecture: We Can Do Better—Improving the Health of the American People." *New England Journal of Medicine* 357 (12): 1221–28.

22. Mercy Health System. "Community Needs." [Online information; retrieved 2/10/15.] http://mercyhealthsystem.org/community-needs/.

23. Task Force on Community Preventive Services. 2014. *The Community Guide: What Works to Promote Health.* [Online information; retrieved 6/30/14.] www.thecommunityguide.org/index.html.

24. Rabin, R. C. 2009. "Benefits of Mammogram Under Debate in Britain." *New York Times.* [Online information; retrieved 4/15/09.] www.nytimes.

com/2009/03/31/health/31mamm.html?_r=1&scp=5&sq=breast%20
cancer&st=cse.

25. Raikou, M., and A. McGuire. 2003. "The Economics of Screening and Treatment
in Type 2 Diabetes Mellitus." *Pharmacoeconomics* 21 (8): 543–64.

26. Center for Health Care Strategies. "ROI Forecasting Calculator." [Online information; retrieved 6/30/14.] www.chcsroi.org/Welcome.aspx.

27. National Association of Community Health Centers. 2009. "Chart Book." [Online
information; retrieved 6/30/14.] www.nachc.com/client/documents/Chartbook_
Update_20091.pdf.

28. Centers for Medicare & Medicaid Services. "Quality Initiatives—General Information." [Online information; retrieved 6/30/14.] www.cms.hhs.gov/QualityInitiatives
GenInfo/01_Overview.asp#TopOfPage.

29. Casarett, D. J., J. Teno, and J. Higginson. 2006. "How Should Nations Measure
the Quality of End-of-Life Care for Older Adults? Recommendations for an International Minimum Data Set." *Journal of the American Geriatrics Society* 54 (11):
1765–71.

30. Task Force on Community Preventive Services (2014).

31. Weissert, W., M. Chernew, and R. Hirth. 2003. "Titrating Versus Targeting Home
Care Services to Frail Elderly Clients: An Application of Agency Theory and
Cost-Benefit Analysis to Home Care Policy." *Journal of Aging & Health* 15 (1):
99–123.

32. Kim, J. J., and S. J. Goldie. 2008. "Health and Economic Implications of HPV
Vaccination in the United States." *New England Journal of Medicine* 359: 821–32.

33. Task Force on Community Preventive Services (2014).

34. Agency for Healthcare Research and Quality. 2014. National Guideline Clearinghouse. [Online information; retrieved 7/1/14.] www.guideline.gov.

35. Centers for Medicare & Medicaid Services. "Nursing Home Quality Initiative."
[Online information; retrieved 7/1/14.] www.cms.hhs.gov/NursingHomeQuality
Inits/25_NHQIMDS30.asp#TopOfPage.

36. Butterfoss, F. D. 2007. *Coalitions and Partnerships in Community Health*, 259–61.
San Francisco: Jossey-Bass.

37. SSM Health Care. 2005. News release, March 28. [Online information; retrieved
3/13/09.] www.ssmhc.com/internet/home/ssmcorp.nsf/Documents/B85F28E
32066A3B786257457005E3775?OpenDocument.

38. American Hospital Association. 2014. "Nova Awards." [Online information; retrieved 7/1/14.] www.aha.org/aha/news-center/awards/NOVA.html.

39. *Ibid.*, "Community Connections, Ideas and Innovations for Hospital Leaders."
Chicago: American Hospital Association.

40. *Ibid.*, "Foster McGaw Prize." [Online information; retrieved 7/1/14.] www.aha.
org/aha/news-center/awards/foster/index.html.

41. U.S. Department of Health and Human Services (HHS). 2014. "Healthy
People 2020." [Online information; retrieved 7/1/14.] http://healthypeople.
gov/2020/about/default.aspx.

42. National Civic League. 2014. Home page. [Online information; retrieved
7/1/14.] www.ncl.org/.

43. Kansas University Work Group for Community Health and Development. 2014.
"About the Work Group for Community Health and Development." [Online information; retrieved 7/1/14.] http://communityhealth.ku.edu/about/overview.

44. Griffith, J. R., and K. R. White. 2003. *Thinking Forward: Six Strategies for Highly
Successful Organizations*, chap 4. Chicago: Health Administration Press.

45. Butterfoss (2007).

46. Buffalo County Community Partners. 2008. *2008 Report to the Community.* [Online information; retrieved 5/10/10.] www.bcchp.org/node/28.

47. Lantz, P. M., R. L. Lichtenstein, and H. A. Pollack. 2007. "Health Policy Approaches to Population Health: The Limits of Medicalization." *Health Affairs* 26 (5): 1253–57.

48. Quoted in Griffith, J. R. 2009. "Finding the Frontier of Hospital Management." *Journal of Healthcare Management* 54 (1): 57–73, p. 64.

49. Kindig (2007).

50. Briss, P. A., S. Zaza, M. Pappaioanou, J. Fielding, L. Wright-De Agüero, B. I. Truman, D. P. Hopkins, P. D. Mullen, R. S. Thompson, S. H. Woolf, V. G. Carande-Kulis, L. Anderson, A. R. Hinman, D. V. McQueen, S. M. Teutsch, and J. R. Harris. 2000. "Developing an Evidence-Based Guide to Community Preventive Services—Methods." *American Journal of Preventive Medicine* 18 (1, Suppl.): 35–43.

51. Zaza, S., L. Wright-de Aguero, P. A. Briss, B. I. Truman, D. P. Hopkins, M. H. Hennessy, D. M. Sosin, L. Anderson, V. G. Carande-Kulis, S. M. Teutsch, and M. Pappaioanou. 2000. "Data Collection Instrument and Procedure for Systematic Reviews in the Guide to Community Preventive Services." *American Journal of Preventive Medicine* 18 (1S): 44–74.

52. SSM Health Care. "Preface: Organizational Profile." 2002. [Online information; retrieved 7/2/14.] www.ssmhealth.com/system/exceptional-care/awards/documents/ssm_application_summary.pdf.

53. Griffith and White (2003).

54. Lee, N. R., and P. A. Kotler. 2011. *Social Marketing: Influencing Behaviors for Good,* 4th ed. Los Angeles: Sage.

55. Putnam, R. D. 1995. "Bowling Alone: America's Declining Social Capital." *Journal of Democracy* 6 (1): 65–78.

56. Pfeffer, J. 2006. "Kent Thiry and DaVita: Leadership Challenges in Building and Growing a Great Company." Stanford University Graduate School of Business Case OB-54.

57. Nicklas, T. A., C. C. Johnson, L. S. Webber, and G. S. Berenson. 1997. "School-Based Programs for Health-Risk Reduction." *Annals of the New York Academy of Sciences* 817: 208–24.

58. McGinnis, S. L., and F. M. Zoske. 2008. "The Emerging Role of Faith Community Nurses in Prevention and Management of Chronic Disease." *Policy, Politics, & Nursing Practice* 9 (3): 173–80.

59. Stephen Ministries. 2014. "How to Begin Stephen Ministry in Your Church." [Online information; retrieved 7/2/14.] www.stephenministries.org/stephenministry/default.cfm/928.

60. Meals on Wheels Association of America. 2014. Home page. [Online information; retrieved 7/2/14.] www.mowaa.org/Page.aspx?pid=183.

61. Hospice Foundation of America. 2014. Home page. [Online information; retrieved 7/2/14.] www.hospicefoundation.org/hospiceInfo/volunteer.asp.

62. Proser, M. 2005. "Deserving the Spotlight: Health Centers Provide High-Quality and Cost-Effective Care." *Journal of Ambulatory Care Management* 28 (4): 321–30.

63. Munck, B., B. Fridlund, and J. Martensson. 2008. "Next-of-Kin Caregivers in Palliative Home Care—from Control to Loss of Control." *Journal of Advanced Nursing* 64 (6): 578–86.

64. Lafortune, L., F. Beland, H. Bergman, and J. Ankri. 2009. "Health State Profiles and Service Utilization in Community-Living Elderly." *Medical Care* 47 (3): 286–94.

65. Kadushin, G. 2004. "Home Health Care Utilization: A Review of the Research for Social Work." *Health & Social Work* 29 (3): 219–44.

66. Mara, C. M., and L. K. Olson (eds.). 2008. *Handbook of Long-Term Care Administration and Policy.* Boca Raton, FL: CRC Press.

67. Armstrong, P. W. 2009. "What Do We Know? Limitations of the Two Methods Most Commonly Used to Estimate the Length of the Prospective Wait." *Health Services Management Research* 22 (1): 8–16.

68. HHS (2014).

69. *Ibid.*, 75; Dartmouth Atlas of Health Care. 2014. Home page. [Online information; retrieved 7/2/14.] www.dartmouthatlas.org/.

70. Centers for Disease Control and Prevention. 2014. "Ambulatory Care Use and Physician Office Visits." [Online information; retrieved 7/2/14.] www.cdc.gov/nchs/fastats/physician-visits.htm.

71. National Center for Quality Assurance. 2008. "Standards and Guidelines for Physician Practice Connections®—Patient-Centered Medical Home (PPC-PCMH™)." [Online information; retrieved 7/2/14.] www.ncqa.org/portals/0/programs/recognition/PCMH_Overview_Apr01.pdf.

72. Carrier, E., M. N. Gourevitch, and N. R. Shah. 2009. "Medical Homes: Challenges in Translating Theory into Practice." *Medical Care* 47 (7): 714–22.

73. Gray, B. H., and W. J. McNerney. 1986. "For-Profit Enterprise in Health Care: The Institute of Medicine Study." *New England Journal of Medicine* 314 (23): 1523–28.

III

LOGISTIC AND STRATEGIC SUPPORT

10 KNOWLEDGE MANAGEMENT

Critical Issues in Knowledge Management

1. *Translating knowledge to strategic performance improvement:*
   - Support an evidence-based culture.
   - Relate knowledge improvement to clinical service improvement.
   - Use centralized and contract knowledge management (KM) services.

2. *Maintaining the reliability of information:*
   - Define, standardize, and generate accurate performance measures.
   - Deal with external causes of variation.
   - Deal with random variation.

3. *Promoting effective use of data:*
   - Expand the electronic health record (EHR).
   - Establish certification and meaningful use.
   - Ensure prompt access to reports and records.
   - Provide statistical analysis and forecasting.

4. *Protecting individual privacy, the archive, and the information systems:*
   - Protect patient and associate privacy rights.
   - Guard against failure, misuse, theft, or destruction.

5. *Planning improvement and growth:*
   - Systematically expand the use of knowledge to achieve the HCO's mission.
   - Continuously improve KM services.

Questions for Discussion

These questions are about applying the chapter content. It's often helpful to discuss them with classmates or mentors, gaining different perspectives on the issues.

1. Your HCO is moving from an excellence-in-care to a population health mission. How will the KM planning committee systematically add population health measures to service line and unit scorecards?

2. Your HCO is opening a new clinic using the same EHR and information systems in place at its other clinics. Clerks, nurses, and physicians will all input information to the EHR and several management systems. What should the KM training program for new associates include? How would you accomplish that training economically?

3. When you visit the intensive care unit, the nurse manager asks you to explain to the clinical associates what the risk-adjusted mortality report means. A check on the intranet reveals that the measure is adjusted for the patient's age, sex, diagnosis, and APACHE (Acute Physiologic and Chronic Health Evaluation) score at the time of admission, based on a systemwide database. The monthly mortality rate is reported as adjusted, with a 3 standard deviation confidence limit. What do you say to the associates?

4. The KM planning committee would like to evaluate performance measures—"Does our system have all the right measures in place?" Your large, multiple-site HCO generates about 2,000 different measures each month, supporting several hundred operational scorecards and strategic scorecards for each service line or geographic site. "Are we missing measures that would improve mission achievement?" was the theme of the committee's discussion. You'll be forming a performance improvement team (PIT). You want to explain to the PIT what constitutes a "right measure" or how we identify measures that will improve mission achievement.

5. The HCO's finance committee has set a limit of $100 million per year on new capital investment. Expansion of the EHR will be expensive—at least $40 million per year for three years. The chief information officer has asked you to help develop a case for the investment. What are the next steps?

Purpose

The purpose of knowledge management (KM) is

> to translate the HCO's complete knowledge resource to improvement of its strategic performance.

The complete knowledge resource has four essential parts:

1. The learning from many sources that is in each associate's head.
2. The current communications that drive each associate's agenda of tasks and documentation of their completion. For clinical associates, this is principally the electronic health record (EHR). For all units, it includes the reports of team performance supporting the unit scorecard.
3. The *data warehouse* of protocols, processes, performance information, proposals, and forecasts that guide the completion of tasks and the continuous improvement processes.
4. Assistance to all associates, helping them find, evaluate, and apply knowledge from the data warehouse, publications, and the World Wide Web.

The improvement of strategic performance is a matter of integrating these components in ways that deliver to each associate everything she needs to know, on time and without error. Like teammates, supplies, and equipment, knowledge becomes a foundation of the associate's success. In the continuous improvement world, knowledge means both how to do the job and how to improve the job. Knowledge must be supplied subject to two constraints:

1. The privacy rights of individuals must be protected at all times.
2. The knowledge resource and the KM system must be protected against failure, loss, or misuse and the security of information ensured.

The purpose is inescapably tied to the EHR. The vision for EHRs is of a modernized, interconnected, and vastly improved system of information delivery that supports excellent care across the stages of patient need and across multiple healthcare providers. KM supports the EHR, but also the full scope of evidence-based management—measurement, benchmarking, process improvement, goal setting, and rewards—for all HCO units, not simply the clinical ones.

Functions

The purpose is implemented through the six functions shown in Exhibit 10.1. KM can be considered in two parts: the up-to-the-minute flow of specific

EXHIBIT 10.1
Functions of
Knowledge
Management

Function	Content
Providing prompt and useful access to management information (the data warehouse)	• Captures, stores, and retrieves operational data to support management and clinical decisions • Provides training in the use of electronic systems and consulting service in interpretation and information availability • Provides protocols, processes, training videos, and other materials supporting training programs • Conducts and interprets statistical analysis of performance and other data • Maintains a historical record • Supports ongoing audits to ensure data quality
Providing prompt and useful access to clinical information—the EHR	Records and communicates each patient's integrated care plan in the EHR—including medical condition, needs assessments, medical and nursing diagnoses, treatments, medication, and unexpected events
Ensuring reliability and validity of data	Defines measures and terminology; supports accurate, complete data input; applies appropriate specification and adjustment; and estimates reliability of data
Maintaining communications and software support	Operates a 24/7 electronic and voice communication utility with web access, supports software used in clinical and business functions, and integrates information for multiple applications
Ensuring the appropriate use and security of data	Guards against loss, theft, and inappropriate application
Improving knowledge management services continuously	Establishes a prioritized agenda for progress, incorporates user view, commits a block of capital funds for several years, and supports an annual review of specific projects

EHR: electronic health record

data—such as orders, conditions, and performance—that guides the job to conclusion, and refined and aggregated information that supports continuous improvement. The two parts support two major sets of KM activity: management information and clinical information. Automation has revolutionized the scope, manner, frequency, and speed of both data and information.

Providing Prompt and Useful Access to Management Information

KM captures, aggregates, and refines data from all parts of the HCO, stores it in the data warehouse, and provides it constantly to support current operations and the continuous improvement processes. Many, but not all, data sources for the warehouse are shown in Exhibit 10.2.

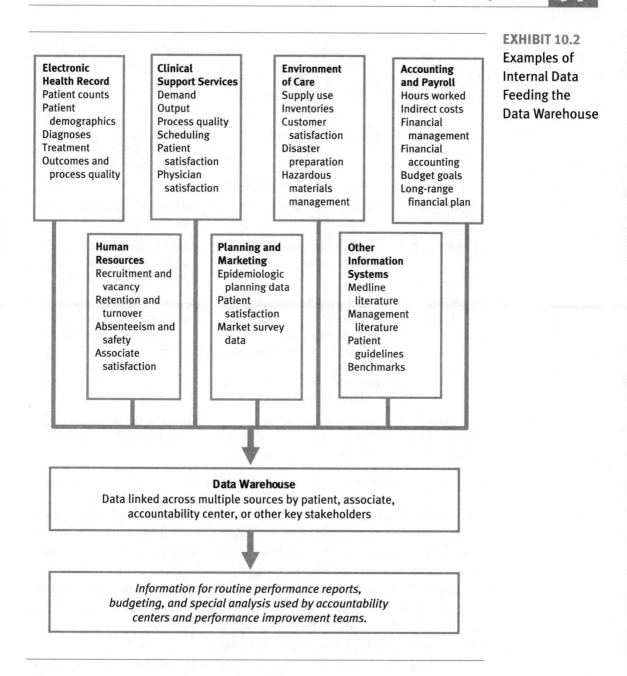

EXHIBIT 10.2
Examples of
Internal Data
Feeding the
Data Warehouse

Electronic Health Record
Patient counts
Patient demographics
Diagnoses
Treatment
Outcomes and process quality

Clinical Support Services
Demand
Output
Process quality
Scheduling
Patient satisfaction
Physician satisfaction

Environment of Care
Supply use
Inventories
Customer satisfaction
Disaster preparation
Hazardous materials management

Accounting and Payroll
Hours worked
Indirect costs
Financial management
Financial accounting
Budget goals
Long-range financial plan

Human Resources
Recruitment and vacancy
Retention and turnover
Absenteeism and safety
Associate satisfaction

Planning and Marketing
Epidemiologic planning data
Patient satisfaction
Market survey data

Other Information Systems
Medline literature
Management literature
Patient guidelines
Benchmarks

Data Warehouse
Data linked across multiple sources by patient, associate, accountability center, or other key stakeholders

Information for routine performance reports, budgeting, and special analysis used by accountability centers and performance improvement teams.

Using the Data Warehouse

The data warehouse and web access facilitate extensive information retrieval and analysis. Examples of important uses of information are shown in Exhibit 10.3. Use of the warehouse is supported by **database management systems**. Database management allows both aggregation and disaggregation, accessing individual fields of data within a record so that different sets of records can be accessed, combined,

Database management system
A system for aggregating and disaggregating electronic data designed to facilitate the recovery and use of data.

EXHIBIT 10.3
Common Uses
of Information
in High-
Performing
HCOs

Application	Data Warehouse Information	World Wide Web Information
Reporting performance	Recent data relative to goals Graphs, statistical process control	—
Identifying OFIs	Drill down to identify potential causes Local benchmarks and comparative performance	Journal articles, collaboratives, and comparative information
Setting goals	Local trends, benchmarks, and forecasts	External benchmarks and best practices
Supporting PITs	Analytic models, simulations, and forecasts	Books and journal articles, regulatory standards, and recommended practices
Reviewing protocols	Reported variances from protocol Drill-down of outcomes to show patient-specific groups Analytic models and simulations	National clearinghouses, commission reports, journal articles, websites, and books
Managing individual patients	Patient management protocols Functional protocols	Journal articles, guidelines, and diagnostic software

OFI: opportunity for improvement; PIT: process improvement team

and analyzed quickly. For example, discharges are routinely disaggregated by age, sex, and diagnosis to create specific outcomes statistics. The patient management protocol can be attached to each diagnosis, allowing counts of process statistics such as the number of patients receiving a recommended treatment. Both outcomes and process statistics can be aggregated into rigorously adjusted measures that permit comparison across varying patient populations. This ability to create "apples to apples" comparison is a critical element of the quality reporting, making benchmarks possible.

The internal data are often integrated with information from external sources. The web is used to verify the latest published work and consensus positions on complex issues.[1] The National Library of Medicine's PubMed has more than 19 million articles from 5,200 journals indexed in its Medline section. Most have abstracts. Other search engines find management literature. Commercial vendors provide direct access to the journals themselves.[2] Alliances and not-for-profit groups, such as the Institute for Healthcare Improvement, The Joint Commission, and Hospitals in Pursuit of Excellence, maintain websites of training materials, benchmarks, and user commentary. All of these external sources become important when processes are studied for improvement. The insights gained by these studies help process improvement teams identify new alternatives.

The "warehouse" is in constant use. KM associates map the data sources and the calculations to automate quality statistics, costs, and other elements of the unit and strategic performance reports. When performance improvement teams (PITs) address performance opportunities for improvement (OFIs), information can be disaggregated to begin an investigation of root causes. Teams use the warehouse routinely to forecast trends, analyze relationships, and model alternative approaches. Automated drill-down allows leaders to track the sources of statistics to the individual patient level.

Henry Ford Health System, a 2009 recipient of the Malcolm Baldrige National Quality Award, summarizes its data management as follows:

> Through a highly integrated corporate data store, which contains clinical, revenue, and cost information from all HFHS business units, we are able to conduct comprehensive analytical program reviews, develop e-dashboards to facilitate performance measurement, analysis and improvement, and provide a repository to enable clinical research. The data store warehouses 21 years of data from HFHS systems such as registration, billing, lab and radiology systems. It is accessible by all HFHS employees through password protected log-ins and is the basis of the System Dashboard (strategic scorecard).[3]

Training and Supporting Users

Success for KM means that the HCO effectively uses information (analogous to meaningful use, described later in the chapter), a more demanding standard than simply providing and explaining the information. Effective use requires a strong user training and support program. Training and support are generally provided in segments, beginning with use of the hardware and software, progressing through common applications, and continuing to analysis and interpretation. A help desk is available for ongoing support.

KM often works with other units to provide a comprehensive training experience. Much of the training is delivered just-in-time. For example, a new associate involved in patient registration (where the identifying information for the medical and billing records is captured) needs training in approaching patients and families, understanding confidentiality and elementary rules about guardianship, using the input screens, and learning the appropriate definitions. Most important, the associate has to know when she needs help and where to get it. (Simple questions become complicated quite easily. What is the correct address for a minor with divorced parents? Who signs the admission form? What do you do if the parents disagree or if one is missing?) Human resources and the associate's manager provide most of this training, but KM is involved at several steps:

1. A video describes the HCO's mission, vision, and values. Additional videos explain the HCO's policies regarding relations with patients and associates, dress, compensation, and benefits. Mastery of these policies can be tested. Learning can be repeated as necessary.
2. A training module teaches completion of electronic forms for data entry. The module can include multiple scenarios that test the associate's understanding.
3. Procedures and support materials for issues such as HIPAA (the Health Insurance Portability and Accountability Act), guardianship, and advance directive can be automated. Mastery of access and key content can be tested.
4. A set of frequently asked questions can be provided for specific areas. Associates can supplement these with files of their own notes.

The electronic training resources provide a relatively inexpensive foundation that documents mastery and builds the associate's confidence. It can be accessed repetitively and complemented by more advanced training, such as proxy patients, role-playing, supervised trial, and mentoring. The combination achieves the goal, which is to create an associate who delights the customer, is loyal to the organization, enters the data completely and correctly, and ensures privacy and security.

Training for more complex tasks is accomplished similarly, by breaking the process down into components. Thus, sophisticated systems can be built. For example, patient diagnosis is made by physicians, captured in standardized words, translated to International Classification of Diseases (ICD) codes by clerical employees, and coded to diagnosis-related groups (DRGs) or ambulatory patient classifications (APCs) by programmed algorithms. Most cases are not difficult to code, but the handling of multiple diagnoses is challenging, important, and commonplace among older patients. The ICD coders have access to code lists with definitions and examples, interpretation of terminology, and training in reviewing the record to catch diagnoses omitted by the physician (a review that can be automated in the EHR). They can specialize in a limited set of diseases. They also have the option of returning electronically to the physician for further clarification. Finally, a blind test can be run to check intercoder consistency and reliability, and audits can be focused on the codes where errors are more likely.

Providing Prompt and Useful Access to Clinical Information — The EHR

Most large HCOs have made substantial progress in implementing the EHR. Commercial vendors supply the software, maintain it, and often provide consultation to support operations. Even incomplete applications have made substantial contributions. Using patient management protocols, accurately tracking medications and other repeated treatments, summarizing patient progress, and identifying unmet needs are all substantially simpler with an EHR. Reporting and analysis of outcomes and process quality measures, a central feature of the unit and strategic scorecards, is only practical because of automation.

The EHR can be used by multiple providers in many settings and geographic areas to coordinate the patient's care. Acute episodes and continuing care of chronic disease now involve dozens or even hundreds of caregivers. Many caregivers never see each other, and they frequently work for different HCOs. They still need to know the following information promptly:

- What is wrong with this patient?
- What are we doing for this patient? What has been done in the past?
- What must we *not* do for this patient (in terms of allergies, advance directives, other important contraindications)?

A huge fraction of the difficulties and delays in patient care occur because a caregiver or caregiving team did not have the answers to these three questions. The traditional paper records were notoriously difficult resources; the EHR is the likely answer.

In 2009, President Barack Obama signed the Health Information Technology for Economic and Clinical Health (HITECH) Act as part of the American Recovery and Reinvestment Act. Administered by the Office of the National Coordinator for Health Information Technology (ONC), HITECH contains specific incentives designed to accelerate the adoption of health information technology (HIT) by the healthcare industry, healthcare providers, consumers, and patients.

The ONC, located in the U.S. Department of Health and Human Services (HHS), is charged "to support the adoption of health information technology and the promotion of nationwide health information exchange to improve health care" and support "nationwide efforts to implement and use the most advanced health information technology and the electronic exchange of health information."[4]

The ONC

- sets the standards and certification criteria that EHRs must meet to assure healthcare professionals and hospitals of what the systems they adopt are able to do;
- specifies minimum functions of EHR;
- directs the State Health Information Exchange Cooperative Agreement Program, which funds states' efforts to rapidly build capacity for exchanging health information across systems within and across states; and
- provides Challenge Grants to states to encourage innovations for health information exchange.[5]

Meaningful use

Measurement thresholds that range from recording patient information as structured data in the EHR to integrating the information across care providers and demonstrating value in exchange for incentive payments from CMS.

Under ONC guidance, the Centers for Medicare & Medicaid Services (CMS) provides incentive payments through the Medicare Shared Savings Program to eligible professionals (licensed independent practitioners) and HCOs that adopt certified EHRs and successfully achieve **meaningful use**, measurement thresholds that range from recording patient information as structured data to exchanging summary care records.[6] Meaningful use refers to the ability to demonstrate not only implementation of the EHR (Stage 1 of the incentive program) but integration of the record (Stage 2) and ability to derive value (Stage 3) from the use of HIT by improving the overall care experience for the patient.

Big data

Large and complex data sets that may be analyzed for patterns.

Engaging patients in shared healthcare decision making is encouraged by meaningful use Stages 2 and 3. Patient-generated health data as a concept is promising, although challenges remain in identifying what and how to integrate **big data** into the patient's EHR and how to maintain privacy,[7] beyond the limited requirements of HIPAA.[8]

Any HCO's EHR should be designed to meet the meaningful use standards and be compatible with the state's information exchange. The commercial vendors that supply the software for the EHR are committed to the national goal and offer support for installation, maintenance, training, and necessary modifications.

Ensuring the Reliability and Validity of Data

Inaccurate data are misleading and potentially dangerous. Effective use of data requires both maximizing accuracy and understanding the level of accuracy achieved. For example, most applications involve comparing two data sets—this record versus this patient's identification, drug ordered versus drug in hand, actual versus goal, this year versus last year, Team A versus Team B. Two errors are always possible—deciding that the two are different when they are the same, or accepting the two as the same when they are different.

In modern HCOs, with thousands of associates making tens of thousands of decisions every day, minimizing both types of error is essential. Four steps are necessary for doing so: (1) Standard definitions must be established, (2) the definitions must be consistently applied as data are captured, (3) statistical specification and adjustment must be included when necessary, and (4) random variation and confidence limits must be estimated. Part of KM is a structure of expert committees, rules, and software to fulfill these steps. The goal is to produce measures that are fully understood and accepted by their users so that the debate can be about the OFIs, not the measures themselves. Like much of evidence-based management, this is an ongoing, heuristic process; measures acceptable last year may need redesign.

Defining Measures and Terminology

A standing committee of the HCO oversees the definitions of measures to ensure appropriate standardization. Nationally accepted definitions are used wherever possible because they facilitate benchmarking and all forms of outside communication. If additional measures are necessary, they are tested in a single or small set of pilot applications and locally standardized to expand their use. The definition includes statistical specification and adjustment. The committee's decisions are incorporated into educational programs and software to ensure consistent application. The committee can audit use of definitions on its own or through internal audit mechanisms.

Sharp HealthCare, a Baldrige Award recipient, identifies the following criteria for accepting a measure:

- Reference in evidence-based literature
- Use by regulatory and public reports
- Availability of competitor data
- Use by other Baldrige Award recipients
- Availability of benchmarks in healthcare and beyond

Sharp evaluates potential benchmarks for comparability and statistical validity, reliability, and specification.[9]

Many complex terms are used on a national or international basis and must be standardized accordingly. Clinical diagnoses, accounting definitions, and hospital statistics are examples. Diagnoses are standardized by ICD, maintained by the World Health Organization.[10] CMS requires ICD coding for payment of claims, and the effort is under way to replace ICD-9-CM (Clinical Modification) with ICD-10.[11] Similarly, accounting and financial terms are standardized by a national panel—the Financial Accounting Standards Board. The American Hospital Association maintains a set of common definitions and statistics for national reporting.[12] The Joint Commission and CMS have agreed on a set of commonly defined quality measures.[13] HIPAA mandates the use of standard definitions for common patient transactions.[14,15] HCOs are legally required to use these standardized measures. It is necessary to standardize not only definitions but also interfacing hardware, software, and data specifications.

Much standardization is accomplished through voluntary trade associations, such as the American National Standards Institute. The National Quality Forum is a nonprofit association dedicated to creating "consensus standards for performance measurement," an essential step toward any external benchmarking.[16] The National Quality Measures Clearinghouse is "a public resource for evidence-based quality measures and measure sets" that "also hosts the HHS Measure Inventory."[17] The Health IT Standards Committee is charged with making recommendations to the ONC on standards, implementation specifications, and certification criteria for the electronic exchange and use of health information.[18]

Consistent Data Capture

Standard definitions must be rigorously applied to each transaction. Both completeness and accuracy are needed. Missing information can be as destructive as errors. The following steps ensure that the information entered into the database is as accurate as possible:

1. *All important information is electronically edited and audited at entry.* Edits are based on a single field of information; the field must contain a particular kind of data, such as certain numbers or letters, or selection from a certain list; these eliminate omissions and keystroke errors. Audits compare two or more fields and flag inconsistency; cross-checks of age, gender, and diagnosis are common examples. Manual audits—reentries by different personnel—can be conducted periodically to assess and maintain the desired accuracy level.

2. *Automated entry is preferable to human entry.* Scanners and devices to retrieve information from electronic archives are superior to their human counterparts. Entry forms, with selections from drop-down lists, are superior to free text.

3. *Retrieval is preferable to reentry.* Information should be captured for electronic processing only once. Subsequent references require reentry of a few fields of identifying information before the complete entry can be recovered.

4. *Training and consultation are used to improve accuracy.* Judgment is often required for entries such as account or ICD codes. Users must be trained to achieve consistency. Managers, accountants, and internal auditors provide advice on difficult questions.

Commercial software is now available for most clinical information-capture operations. It is designed for accurate entry and user convenience, includes extensive edits and audits, and facilitates prompt retrieval and linkage across multiple data sources.

Specification and Adjustment

Specification
A statistical analysis that identifies values for a measure by defined subsets of a population, to allow accurate comparisons for each specified group.

Adjustment
A statistical technique to aggregate values from specified population subsets, allowing comparison of samples from populations with differences in the relative size of subset populations.

Accurate definitions and careful data capture substantially reduce error in data sets. But with human patients being treated by human caregivers, cases are never truly identical; some random variation always remains. As the data are aggregated over time and work sites, questions of comparability arise: How can Population A be made more comparable to Population B? Such questions are answered by **specification**, identifying subsets of the data that show less variation, and **adjustment**, using specification subsets to estimate comparable total populations. Specification and adjustment allow apples-to-apples comparison; they are important in many clinical measures.

Diagnosis is an important basis for specification and adjustment. DRGs and APCs group patients with similar ICD-10 diseases into homogeneous populations. They are used for the Medicare prospective payment system. CMS calculates a severity index for each DRG patient group from its entire database and a severity-weighted cost or length of stay (LOS) for each DRG.

Outcomes other than cost or LOS, such as mortality or recovery rates, are similarly adjusted. The adjustments are usually part of the measure definition. They are also often adjusted for age, gender, and race. Severity adjustment allows at least a crude comparison of costs between HCOs, service lines, or other groupings. There are other possible adjustments for variables beyond the caregiving teams' control. The possibility of an omitted variable should be raised as part of a root cause analysis: "Are there other characteristics, or any other factors outside the unit's control, that we should consider?" Caregivers' response to unprovable quality results is often "These patients are sicker." Thorough adjustment addresses the factors that make patients "sicker." The omitted variable question becomes "We've adjusted for the common patient differences. Can you identify a factor outside our control that we should investigate?"

Reporting Variability and Reliability of Estimates

Few performance measures are exact. In healthcare, the list is limited to simple counts and some accounting information. Commonly used measures, such as laboratory test values, cost per case, LOS, percentage of loyal patients, number of safety incidents, mortality rates, and complication rates are all subject to random variation that can mislead users. Specification and adjustment reduce, but never remove, random variation. Statistical analysis assigns confidence limits around reported values and estimates of the probability that a specific difference is worth investigating. Investigating noise (W. Edwards Deming's *special causes*—meaning factors that are may not recur or cannot be corrected) is a waste of time; when a variation is significant (Deming's *common causes*), an investigating team is likely to be able to find a cause for the difference. The level of significance indicates the probability that a cause can be found.

The variability of a measure is as important as the value, and both should be reported. The usual variability indicators are standard deviation (used to compare two individual values) and standard error (used to compare two samples with several individual values in each). Modern **statistical process control** software calculates both measures, shows trends and significance graphically, and automatically flags significant differences. "Significant at 99 percent" (3 standard deviations, or 3 sigma) is a forecast that 99 times out of 100 a diligent team will find a potentially

Statistical process control
A method of identifying significant changes in measures subject to random variation.

correctable cause. It is commonly used as a guide. All 3 sigma variations are OFIs. Smaller ones can usually be ignored.

Maintaining Communications and Software Support

KM maintains the communications and software for all ongoing HCO activities. Many individual communications, like a patient admission, a supplies order, an invoice, a paycheck, an e-mail, or a voice conversation, occur each day. Smartphones, tablet computers, and laptop devices have changed work patterns on hospital floors. With the growth of telemedicine—to support home and office care at distant sites and to provide instant support in intensive care units—the communications network now includes streaming video and live two-way communication.[19,20]

These communications use various hardware and software platforms. Many require integration across platforms. KM must support all of these transactions, and record many of them. The systems must be convenient and prompt, be available 24/7/365, and have reliability near 100 percent. Communications hardware and software have reached very high standards. The major KM activity is integrating the systems and managing the contracts.

HCOs need a large number of applications to support specific activities. The needs range from general-purpose software, like word processing and spreadsheets, to advanced statistical analysis and modeling, like the epidemiologic planning model and the long-range financial plan, to specific clinical applications like analytic programs for imaging. Training is necessary for most of these applications, which is commonly supplied by the vendor.

KM must ensure that these software packages are supported by the HCO information system, that they are consistent with the definitions and standards, that their data can be integrated, and that they offer appropriate security. The software is licensed, and KM manages the licenses, including negotiating prices. KM associates work with ad hoc task forces or committees to ensure that the apps, the training, and other work processes are aligned. Henry Ford Health System's process is shown in Exhibit 10.4. Step 2 suggests substantial efforts to optimize the software and its use. KM negotiates with both the users and the suppliers to get the best results. The software review process itself is subject to continuous improvement, as indicated in Step 5.

Integrating Data from Multiple Sources

Integrating the wide range of hardware and software platforms has historically been a substantial challenge. Most of the special-purpose software must draw data from several different sources. For example, a caregiver's drug-ordering decision requires data from the patient's record; from a protocol suggesting alternatives; from a pharmacy system that maintains inventory; and from a drug administration system that will audit dosage, contraindications, and drug interactions. The administration system will trigger nurse alerts, enforce

EXHIBIT 10.4
Software
Selection,
Approval, and
Maintenance
System

Step	Activity
1	• Stakeholders identify needs via ongoing assessments • Hardware, software, project requirements are specified
2	• Information Technology (IT) develops solution alternatives in collaboration with stakeholders • Technology partners offer upgrades or innovative approaches
3	• IT steering committees and subcommittees serve as "Investment Review Boards" • Priorities set and funding approved during annual budget planning
4	• IT updates three-year rolling strategic plans • Project plans include necessary resources
5	• Stakeholders evaluate project outcomes • IT steering committees assess effectiveness

Source: Henry Ford Health System. 2009. Malcolm Baldrige National Quality Award Application, p. 24.

patient identification, and record administration. Beyond these communication activities, the data will be integrated to support a variety of analytic applications, such as drug error rates, studies of pharmacy workloads, and audits of diagnostic coding.

The modern solution is standardized definitions and software. Historically, much HCO software was developed independently. These systems—called **legacy systems**—were not designed to integrate with others. Over time, the problem of legacy systems will diminish, but the core issue of meeting the needs of both the within-system user and the external user will remain.

Legacy system
Outdated computer software that lacks the features found in more current versions.

Ensuring the Appropriate Use and Security of Data

The integrated software systems and data warehouse are resources of incalculable value. They and the hardware supporting them are subject to several perils. Physical destruction or loss can result from mislabeling, theft, fire, electrical power disturbances, floods, magnetic interference, and deterioration.[21] Communications can be interrupted by power or equipment failure. Data, software, and hardware can be stolen or sabotaged by outsiders or associates. Clinical, financial, and personal information owned by the individual patient or associate can be stolen or inadvertently exposed. KM is responsible for managing cybersecurity.[22]

Protecting Against Loss, Destruction, or System Failure

The normal protections against loss, destruction, or system failure are physical protection of sites, duplication of both data and hardware, separate geographic locations of originals and duplicates, selection of personnel, and antivirus software. Thus, central hardware sites are safely located and physically protected. Processing hardware is deliberately redundant. Shadow systems maintain duplicate records available within a few seconds. Routine backups are kept in separate, ultra-secure sites. Personnel working in KM are subject to careful selection, bonding, surveillance, and auditing. Outsiders are kept out by passwords and security devices.

The entire KM operation depends on an electricity supply, and some parts have narrow tolerances for voltage and frequency variation. HCOs normally have two separate feeds from the national electric power grid, plus local generators and specifically designed "uninterruptible" power supplies.

A well-managed HCO has a formal plan for maintaining security and a recovery plan for each of the perils. KM is responsible for maintaining this plan, including monitoring effectiveness and conducting periodic drills for specific threats.

Maintaining Confidentiality of Information

KM is responsible for designing and maintaining systems to protect information against unauthorized use. Most data about individual patients and employees are confidential and protected, and the organization is liable for misuse. HIPAA mandates rigorous privacy and confidentiality protocols that protect patient data from unauthorized use.[23,24] KM must identify the confidentiality requirements for each type of data and incorporate controls in operations to ensure that they are met.[25] These usually take the form of verifying patient authorization, requiring user identification, and restricting specific kinds of access to qualified users. Identification cards, passwords, and voice readers are currently used to protect access; biometric identification is expected to grow in the future.

Confidentiality is also important in archiving and retrieval. The data warehouse must be protected from inappropriate use, and reporting must be constructed in ways that prevent inferences about individuals from aggregate data. Centralized archiving and monitoring of data uses and users protect against these dangers. Restrictions on access to identifiable sets of data or certain combinations of data can be built into the archive or the data retrieval system.

The issue of confidentiality is important, but relative. Many healthcare confidentiality problems are similar to other information sources that are now automated, such as driving records, credit records, and income tax files. The manual systems were far from foolproof. The real question is one of benefits of convenient access versus risk of damage.[26] Reasonable steps to reduce the risk are required, backed by ongoing programs to ensure compliance. Properly designed, electronic systems can reduce the chance of misuse or inappropriate access and can also improve appropriate use.

Improving Knowledge Management Services Continuously

KM is a rapidly changing activity. It identifies OFIs from its own measurement and benchmarking system; from regulation; from new technology in the marketplace; and from user requests for expanded service, such as "mHealth," mobile integration of KM activities for hospitals and health systems.[27]

It requires a steady stream of funds for new capital equipment, expanded services, and expanded training and support. Demand for improvement will exceed supply, creating a waiting list that tends to be longer in better-managed organizations. KM improvements are complex. They must be integrated with changes in work processes in other units to yield benefits. Important projects can require several years to complete.[28] As a result, KM requires a sophisticated planning process for continuous improvement,[29] such as the one shown in Exhibit 10.5, managed by a KM planning committee or steering committee. The process generates a KM plan, part of the long-term HCO plans. Successful planning processes have several important characteristics:

- *They are built around explicit collaboration with application units, because KM cannot itself control the results.* Most proposals have four parts:
  1. A KM change (new hardware, software, or information capability) will be installed in some HCO activity other than KM.
  2. The installation will support improved work processes.
  3. The improved work processes will improve operational measures.
  4. Improved operations will create improvements in HCO strategic measures.

       For example, software to improve patient scheduling in outpatient offices will increase the number of patients who can be seen. If marketing and other parts of the primary care service line are effective, the number of outpatients seen and correctly treated will increase. As outpatient visits increase, HCO revenue and profit will increase.

- *They establish project teams with detailed goals, analogous to facility construction projects.*[30] Any KM PIT must include all the caregiving, support, and strategic units using or supplying the data, and any contractors supporting relevant software. A major software selection project is likely to work through a battery of subteams establishing the software vendor, pilot tests, an installation timetable, revised patient management protocols, and an associate training plan. The recommendation will have explicit endorsement by HCO associates or contractors accountable for progress and operational improvement.

- *The project teams are monitored by the KM planning committee.*[31] Larger HCOs will have several project teams operating at once and will need the planning committee as a managing body.

- *Funding is established on a multiyear basis, usually by allocating a portion of the total funds available for new programs and capital to KM projects.* For the foreseeable future, most HCOs will spend a significant fraction of their capital funds on KM improvement. The amounts, the benefits, and the timetables will be built into the long-range financial plan and other planning activities.

- *The governing board's review focuses on two questions: "What are the strategic improvements that justify the investment?" and "How closely do the documented successes from installed projects track the benefits expected?"* These questions put a premium on KM performance and enforce continuous improvement of internal operations.

EXHIBIT 10.5
Knowledge Management Planning Process

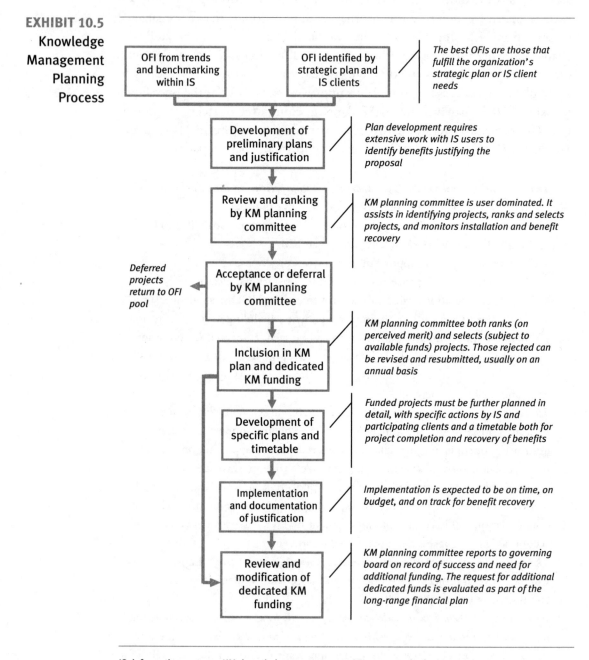

IS: information systems; KM: knowledge management; OFI: opportunity for improvement

The process makes KM a supplier to the other units of the organization. It demands that the KM staff both listen to and work closely with their internal customers. An opportunity that arises internally must be thoroughly studied to develop justifications; that study requires review of its implications for customer work processes.[32] Review by a customer-dominated KM planning committee keeps the department plan and the KM plan focused appropriately on service.

People

KM staff includes numerous professionals in programming, hardware maintenance, statistics, user support, and training. They are led by the chief information officer (CIO) and the KM planning committee and are organized by function.

Chief Information Officer

The role of CIO has emerged with the growth of KM and has grown with the centrality of KM itself. CIOs report to either the CEO or chief operating officer and are part of the senior management team. The CIO role requires mastery of information technology in healthcare and managerial skills. First and foremost, the CIO must see that the KM unit effectively supports the organization. The role also requires leadership and negotiating skills. In many situations, the CIO's role is to convince others of the power of information and encourage them to use it effectively.[33] Like other senior management, the CIO should have a succession plan for the critical personnel in KM and individual development plans for all managers to help them achieve their potential. Many high-performing HCOs are increasing clinical skills in KM units. The chief medical information officer has assumed a prominent role on the KM team.[34,35]

Education for the CIO can follow several routes. Training in computer operations, management engineering, or medical records administration provides a useful beginning,[36,37] but an advanced degree in management engineering, business, or health administration is valuable. Many CIOs in larger facilities have doctoral-level preparation. Experience in healthcare information systems is clearly essential. Consulting experience is also common in CIO backgrounds. A professional organization—the Healthcare Information and Management Systems Society (HIMSS)—provides continuing education and professional certification.[38]

KM Planning Committee

KM planning and oversight transcend all HCO functional boundaries. The KM planning committee must deal with issues similar to those faced by the governing board.[39] The charge to the committee includes the following:

- Participating in the development of the KM plan, resolving the strategic priorities, and recommending the plan to the governing board
- Ranking KM investment opportunities and recommending a rank-ordered list of proposals to the governing board
- Assisting KM clients in identifying and meeting KM opportunities
- Supporting the definitions and standards committee
- Monitoring performance of the division and suggesting possible improvements

The KM planning committee routinely comprises key personnel from major departments, particularly finance, internal consulting, medicine, nursing, and clinical support services. The CIO is always a member and may chair the committee. Members of the governing board may serve on the committee. The team uses a variety of task forces and subcommittees, expanding participation in component activities but using its authority to coordinate.[40]

Organization

KM organization must establish accountability for each of its five functions. Glandon, Smaltz, and Slovensky suggest that KM be divided into subsections for Strategy, including systems design, standard definitions, and operating policies; Design and Transition, which emphasizes technical operations; and Operations, which emphasizes associate support.[41] In Exhibit 10.6, we have expanded their perspective to emphasize the importance of customer service. Many of the operations are highly technical; specialists in operations for various support services and service lines are common. A highly flexible,

EXHIBIT 10.6
Accountability Structure for the Communications Function

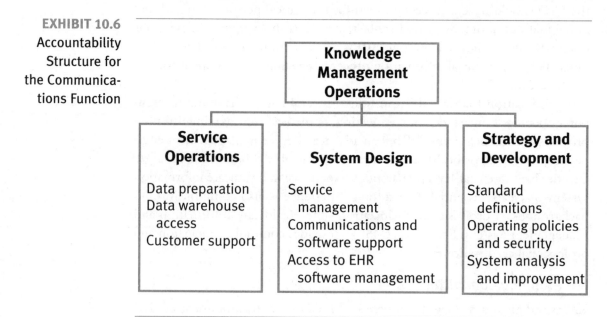

EHR: electronic health record

integrated and empowered culture is essential, but the KM team members must understand their scorecard goals and collaborate to meet them.

Measures

Performance measures for KM should cover the full set of six dimensions shown in Exhibit 10.7. Benchmarks, customer needs, competitive outsourcing alternatives, and the experience of consultants are used to guide negotiations over annual goals. Most of the measures in Exhibit 10.7 are derived from standard cost accounts, automated operating logs, activities of the KM units, and the details of the improvement portfolio. Many can be automated and obtained at low cost. Some require special surveys of line managers. Consultant evaluations can be used to identify goals. A large number of specific activity measures can be devised to supplement the list in Exhibit 10.7. The KM planning committee has an important role in the goal-setting negotiations.

Managerial Issues

Properly implemented KM has become a central component of any excellent HCO's strategy and an essential foundation for every HCO clinical or support team. Capable associates in all fields now expect KM services to be available; recruitment and retention will be difficult if they are lacking. The KM products—information and knowledge—implement the concept of evidence-based decision making and a learning culture. The mission-critical issues, where hands-on monitoring and support by the senior management team and the KM leadership are essential, are as follows:

- Ensure effective day-to-day communications.
- Expand implementation of the EHR and invest in big data clinical analytics.[42]
- Promote the integration of information from multiple sources to guide operations improvement.
- Maintain progress of the KM plan components toward excellence in care and improvement of the strategic scorecard.

The keys to achieving these lie in the KM planning committee, the effective delivery and coordination of KM services, and the appropriate use of consultants and contract suppliers.

Exploiting the KM Planning Committee

KM is a dynamic activity, a moving target where no HCO can say, "It's finished." That makes the portfolio of projects under the KM planning committee the key to future success. As with the governing board, the committee

EXHIBIT 10.7
Measures of
Knowledge
Management
Performance

Dimension	KM Function	Measure
Demand	Reliability and validity of data	New measure requests, response time "Hits" on data warehouse materials Counts of measures in place
	Data communications	System users System peak users
	Information retrieval	Counts of measures, benchmarks in use Counts of service requests Counts of trainees
	Appropriate use and security	Passwords issued Protection systems enabled
	KM planning and improvement	Projects managed
Costs and resources	All	Units and costs of resources Capital expenditure Machine capacity
Human resources	All	Associate satisfaction, retention, absenteeism, and work loss days
Output and productivity	All	Counts of services completed Productivity measures divide cost incurred by counts of service completed
Quality	Reliability and validity of data	Counts of measures benchmarked Statistical tests of reliability, sensitivity Audit scores
	Data communications	Response delay Systems uptime Audit scores Unexpected events
	Information retrieval	Trainee mastery scores
	Appropriate use and security	Audit scores System attacks Consultant ratings
	KM planning and improvement	Projects on time Projects on budget Projects meeting original performance goals
Customer satisfaction	All	Customer surveys, interviews, complaints, and unexpected events

membership needs to be broad and talented. Education programs and retreats to understand complex issues are useful. Overlapping committee membership with marketing and strategic planning and with the governing board planning committee is essential. The committee should be part of the HCO's "brain trust," along with board leadership, senior management, the medical executive committee, and the performance improvement council.

The committee should make liberal use of subcommittees and task forces, with a goal of identifying and resolving many issues close to their point of origin. The projects in the portfolio should be adequately staffed; full-time managers and implementation staffs are required to move the larger projects. Senior management's listening activity should identify and pursue both opportunities and issues with a goal of increasing the on-time, on-budget, and on-performance outcomes.

There are at least three critical points in the planning committee strategy, beginning with the relationship between the organization's strategic plan and its KM plan. The strategic plan (Chapter 15) is developed as a stakeholder consensus on the direction of improvement. It will identify the organization's most pressing needs. Senior management must align the KM plan with the strategic plan. The path to that is through extensive dialogue with customer units, helping them design their requests, and using subcommittees and task forces to resolve concerns.

The second point is to provide sufficient staff, including KM associates and time contributed by customer units, to ensure that the projects are implemented on time, on budget, and on performance. That requires effective management both inside and outside KM. Inside, KM must meet its goals with customer-responsive services and staff project teams. Outside, the KM projects are mirrored by PITs' efforts to change work processes and generate the planned benefits. All of these steps—capital for the strategic and KM plans, planning project implementation teams, subcommittees and task forces removing roadblocks—take time and money.

The third point is to make sure that funding is adequate for implementation. Many HCOs struggle to find it. The question is the perennial "How can I drain the swamp when I'm surrounded by alligators?" The record of excellent HCOs shows that it has a two-part answer. Part one is the deliberate search for easy gains or "low-hanging fruit." The documented experience has shown that most HCOs have readily available improvements that pay off simultaneously in reduced wasted staff time, better quality, and lower costs. The first step in this dynamic is reducing clinical error. It's done by using the service excellence model and applying both empowerment and continuous improvement. If the initial projects are well selected and well implemented, they will generate cash flow. The role of senior management is to keep the cash coming.

The second step is to assess the inherent cost of KM budgets with great care, including the total cost of ownership. Taken into consideration should be implementing redundant systems, budgeting for upgrades, and providing for ongoing training. However, these costs should be offset by overall efficiencies in the delivery of care, which likely means cost savings, but not necessarily revenue generation, although there may be pockets of increased revenue.

The second part is that while resource consumption is important, the central management questions for KM are not "How much are we spending?" but "What are we getting for the money?" and "How much should we spend?" It is possible to operate KM at an insufficient scale and not recognize it. The customers of KM may be satisfied with service. The cost may be below reported benchmarks. The critical test, which must be explored by the board finance committee, senior management, and the KM planning committee, is not whether current performance is acceptable but whether an additional investment would gain important returns. One way to approach this is through a periodic audit by an outside expert, who can compare service as well as cost and identify the technological opportunities. In addition, the audit team can evaluate all the KM activities in light of other HCOs' achievements, such as the Baldrige Award applications[43] and the HIMSS Value Suite, which captures vignettes of value from use of KM using the STEPS (satisfaction, treatment/clinical, electronic information/data, prevention/patient education, savings) methodology.[44]

Promoting the Use of Knowledge

In addition to sustaining a strong forward motion through the KM planning committee, the information retrieval function and some aspects of the data reliability function are likely to need ongoing management support. The data communication functions of KM now work at or near 6 sigma levels (three failures per million operations). An HCO with recurring data communications difficulties should seek a thorough review by a skilled consultant organization. Similarly, the security function should be audited periodically by an independent consultant and should offer protection equivalent to similar organizations.

The definitions of many clinical quality measures have moved to national or international levels. Data collection is built into much special-purpose software. Specification and adjustment have also been automated. As a result, counts and benchmarks for these measures are highly reliable. Reports of quality measures require continuing managerial attention. Only significant variation should be pursued. When the variation is not statistically significant, studying it will be time wasted. Worse, some individuals or processes may be identified incorrectly as contributors. This is particularly likely and particularly dangerous when measures are applied to individual physician performance. Physicians' practices are filters; one doctor can accumulate a disproportionate fraction of difficult cases, testing the limits of statistical adjustment. Physician practices are small, resulting in large standard errors. A single patient can cause substantial distortion.

The solution is threefold:

1. *Incorporate residual variation (i.e., sigma) in the reported data.* This helps associates learn the underlying principles and their implications. It is increasingly easy to do using statistical process control software.
2. *Pursue as OFIs only those cases that are different from the goal by 3 sigma (one per thousand) or that have a nonstatistical justification.* If a smaller error is ignored and there is a special cause that can be corrected, the opportunity will arise again in the next period. The delay is cheaper than the cost of error.
3. *Provide local statistical consultation to managers and PITs.* The consultant needs only basic competence in statistics. Complex questions will be answered via the web or consultation with topical experts. The purpose of local consultation is to guard against pursuing the impossible and to make sure that all associates are protected against incorrect criticism.

Using Outside Contractors and Vendors

KM, like many units of HCOs, can be provided by employees of the organization, by outside contractors, or by almost any combination of the two. The fact that measures are available for all important KM performance dimensions makes a flexible approach to the ownership possible. A well-managed organization seeks the best profile on the KM unit scorecards, whether it means internal ownership or contracting. Every HCO relies heavily on commercial vendors for both hardware and software. Larger HCOs tend to employ the CIO and retain the contracting functions for specialized services. Smaller ones tend to contract for comprehensive service.[45] KM is a highly technical area, where the expertise of an outside vendor may be of great value. It pays to understand the opportunities and hazards of outside contracting and to evaluate the opportunities specifically, in terms of the documented record. At least one organization surveys and ranks major KM vendors.[46]

Several kinds of assistance from outside contractors are available for information systems (IS):

1. *Integrated software support.* Commercial companies develop *enterprise systems*— integrated comprehensive software that serves well-managed HCO activities such as a clinical support service or a logistic function (e.g., supply management). The companies that provide the software also maintain it, incorporating changes imposed by outside agencies and technological advances. These vendors sometimes offer customization services as well.
2. *Finance.* Leases and mortgages on hardware are generally available from a variety of outside sources. Software is usually available for purchase or lease from the software vendor. However, transaction costs are associated with dealing with several different companies and using general institutional debt for information systems. An outside contractor can consolidate the financing and offer a comprehensive system on a single lease.

3. *Consultation and planning.* Assistance in analyzing current capabilities, benchmarking, developing an IS plan, and selecting hardware and software is available from consultants. Larger organizations frequently rely on independent consultants to assist them in identifying all information opportunities and selecting a coordinated package.

4. *Facilities management.* A few companies that specialize in HCO needs operate on-site data processing services under contract. These companies also arrange for financing for the facilities and can be hired for consultation and planning.

5. *Joint developmental ventures.* For those HCOs in a position to develop new or improved applications, collaboration with an established vendor is highly desirable. The vendor brings experience, extra personnel, capital, and a marketing capability if the development succeeds.

In a complex, rapidly moving technical field, the use of a consultant is often prudent. Consultants can assist materially with the IS plan. Few HCOs have the expertise to forecast developments in hardware, software, and applications. Both management consulting firms and IS specialists offer consulting services. There are advantages to each type of company, but the key criteria should be a record of successful engagements and a willingness to match competition or benchmark values on actual performance.

Facilities management of KM—contracting or outsourcing the entire operation—has appealed to both large and small organizations. As with other departments, internal KM should be compared to outsourcing alternatives in terms of specific performance measures. The desired arrangement is based on the best value for the organization as a whole. In the short run, that value is measured by the operating measures in Exhibit 10.7. The contractor should accept those measures and the annual goal-setting process. In the long run, value must be reflected in the HCO's strategic scorecard. The contracting firm is expected to name an on-site leadership team with technical skills and knowledge comparable or superior to those the organization could employ. The on-site managers are supported by the broader experience and specialized knowledge of the contractor's other employees. In concept, the model provides a much richer resource than most HCOs could provide on their own. Lower-level employees may work for either the contractor or the HCO.

A role remains for internal leadership. The KM planning committee remains in place. It has a major role in selecting and working with contractors. It negotiates the annual performance goals. Contractors have no incentive to limit the hospital's costs and usually will profit from an excessive program for improvement. Thus, even with a facilities management contract, the KM planning committee and hospital governance have the responsibility to require justification, select improvements, and pace the evolution of the information system.

Healthcare systems generally centralize much of KM. They standardize definitions to provide comparative and benchmarking data. They require complete standardization of accounting and internal auditing, which virtually mandates standard software. They can frequently negotiate volume discounts on hardware and software. Training, local planning, and some user support for clinical and other systems must remain decentralized, although teaching aids can be standardized and modern communication allows expert backup that was formerly obtainable only from consultants. The performance measures are critical, as they are in selecting outside vendors. Each hospital in the system is entitled to service and price as good as or better than it could achieve on its own. But each hospital is obligated to produce and implement a plan of KM improvement.

Additional Resources

Glandon, G. L., D. H. Smaltz, and D. J. Slovensky. 2013. *Information Systems for Healthcare Management*, 8th ed. Chicago: Health Administration Press.

Green, M. A., and M. J. Bowie. 2010. *Essentials of Health Information Management: Principles and Practices*, 2nd ed. Clifton Park, NY: Delmar.

McWay, D. C. 2009. *Legal and Ethical Aspects of Health Information Management*, 3rd ed. Clifton Park, NY: Delmar.

Senge, P. M. 1995. *The Fifth Discipline: The Art and Practice of the Learning Organization*. New York: Doubleday.

Wager, K. A., F. W. Lee, and J. P. Glaser. 2013. *Health Care Information Systems: A Practical Approach for Health Care Management*, 3rd ed. San Francisco: Jossey-Bass.

Notes

1. Stefanelli, M. 2002. "Knowledge Management to Support Performance-Based Medicine." *Methods of Information in Medicine* 41 (1): 36–43.

2. U.S. National Center for Biotechnology Information, National Library of Medicine. 2014. "PubMed.gov." [Online information; retrieved 6/30/14.] www.ncbi.nlm.nih.gov/pubmed.

3. Henry Ford Health System. 2009. Malcolm Baldrige National Quality Award Application, p. 19.

4. U.S. Department of Health and Human Services. 2014. "About ONC." [Online information; retrieved 7/12/14.] www.healthit.gov/newsroom/about-onc.

5. *Ibid.*

6. U.S. Department of Health and Human Services. 2014. "Health IT Regulations." [Online information; retrieved 7/12/14.] www.healthit.gov/policy-researchers-implementers/meaningful-use-regulations.

7. Sarasohn-Kahn, J. 2014. "Here's Looking at You: How Personal Health Information Is Being Tracked and Used." California Healthcare Foundation. [Online information; retrieved 7/21/14.] www.chcf.org/publications/2014/07/heres-looking-personal-health-info/.

8. Hernandez, S. R. 2014. "What's Private and What's Not?" California Healthcare Foundation. [Online information; retrieved 7/21/14.] www.chcf.org/about/extras/big-data-privacy.

9. Sharp HealthCare. 2007. Malcolm Baldrige National Quality Award Application, p. 17.

10. World Health Organization. 2014. "International Classification of Diseases (ICD)." [Online information; retrieved 6/25/14.] www.who.int/classifications/icd/en/.

11. *Ibid.*

12. American Hospital Association. 2013. *Hospital Statistics 2014 Edition.* Chicago: Health Forum.

13. Joint Commission. 2004. "The Joint Commission and CMS Align to Make Common Performance Measures Identical." *Joint Commission Perspectives* 24 (11): 1.

14. Rode, D. 2001. "Understanding HIPAA Transactions and Code Sets." *Journal of AHIMA* 72 (1): 26–32.

15. Roach, M. C. 2001. "HIPAA Compliance Questions for Business Partner Agreements." *Journal of AHIMA* 72 (2): 45–51.

16. National Quality Forum. 2014. "About Us." [Online information; retrieved 7/12/14.] www.qualityforum.org/story/About_Us.aspx.

17. U.S. Department of Health and Human Services. 2014. "Quality Measures." [Online information; retrieved 7/12/14.] www.qualitymeasures.ahrq.gov/.

18. Electronic Healthcare Network Accreditation Commission. 2014. "Glossary of Terms." [Online information; retrieved 7/21/14.] www.ehnac.org/wp-content/uploads/2014/01/EHNAC-Glossary-of-Terms-20140121.pdf.

19. Ries, M. 2009. "Tele-ICU: A New Paradigm in Critical Care." *International Anesthesiology Clinics* 47 (1): 153–70.

20. Kobb, R., N. R. Chumbler, D. M. Brennan, and T. Rabinowitz. 2008. "Home Telehealth: Mainstreaming What We Do Well." *Telemedicine Journal & E-Health* 14 (9): 977–81.

21. Brown, S. M. 2010. "Information Technologies and Risk Management." In *Risk Management Handbook for Health Care Organizations*, 6th ed., edited by R. Carroll. San Francisco: Jossey-Bass.

22. U.S. Food and Drug Administration. 2014. "Cybersecurity." [Online information; retrieved 7/21/14.] www.fda.gov/medicaldevices/productsandmedicalprocedures/connectedhealth/ucm373213.htm.

23. Centers for Medicare & Medicaid Services. 2013. "Medical Privacy of Protected Health Information." [Online information; retrieved 6/30/14.] www.cms.gov/Outreach-and-Education/Medicare-Learning-Network-MLN/MLNProducts/downloads/SE0726FactSheet.pdf.

24. Gostin, L. O. 2001. "National Health Information Privacy: Regulations Under the Health Insurance Portability and Accountability Act." *Journal of the American Medical Association* 285 (3): 3015–21.

25. Glitz, R., and C. Stanton. 2010. "The Health Insurance Portability and Accountability Act (HIPAA) of 1996." In *Risk Management Handbook for Health Care Organizations*, 6th ed., edited by R. Carroll. San Francisco: Jossey-Bass.

26. See R. P. Solomon, "Information Technologies and Risk Management"; P. J. Para, "Evolving Risk in Cyberspace and Telemedicine"; and K. S. Davis, J. C. McConnell, and E. D. Shaw, "Data Management." 2010. In *Risk Management Handbook for Health Care Organizations*, 6th ed., edited by R. Carroll. San Francisco: Jossey-Bass.

27. Health Information and Management Systems Society. 2014. "Mobile Health IT." [Online information; retrieved 7/21/14.] www.himss.org/mobilehealthit/roadmap.

28. Brigl, B., E. Ammenwerth, C. Dujat, S. Graber, A. Grosse, A. Haber, C. Jostes, and A. Winter. 2005. "Preparing Strategic Information Management Plans for

Hospitals: A Practical Guideline SIM Plans for Hospitals: A Guideline." *International Journal of Medical Informatics* 74 (1): 51–65.

29. Anderson, J. G. 2003. "A Framework for Considering Business Models." *Studies in Health Technology & Informatics* 92: 3–11.

30. Glaser, J. 2004. "Back to Basics Managing IT Projects." *Healthcare Financial Management* 58 (7): 34–38.

31. Ross, J. W., and P. Weil. 2002. "Six IT Decisions Your IT People Shouldn't Make." *Harvard Business Review* 80 (11): 84–91.

32. Lenz, R., and K. A. Kuhn. 2004. "Towards a Continuous Evolution and Adaptation of Information Systems in Healthcare." *International Journal of Medical Informatics* 73 (1): 75–89.

33. Griffin, J. 1997. "The Modern CIO: Forging a New Role in the Managed Care Era." *Journal of Healthcare Resource Management* 15 (4): 16–17, 20–21.

34. Leviss, J., R. Kremsdorf, and M. F. Mohaideen. 2006. "The CMIO: A New Leader for Health Systems." *Journal of the American Medical Informatics Association* 13 (5): 573–78.

35. Runy, L. A. 2008. "The Changing Role of the CMIO." *Hospitals & Health Networks* 82 (2): 37–42.

36. Moore, R. A., and E. S. Berner. 2004. "Assessing Graduate Programs for Healthcare Information Management/Technology (HIM/T) Executives." *International Journal of Medical Informatics* 73 (2): 195–203.

37. Brettle, A. 2003. "Information Skills Training: A Systematic Review of the Literature." *Health Information & Libraries Journal* 20 (Suppl. 1): 3–9.

38. Health Information and Management Systems Society. 2014. Home page. [Online information; retrieved 7/1/14.] www.himss.org.

39. Glandon, G. L., D. H. Smaltz, and D. J. Slovensky. 2013. *Information Systems for Healthcare Management*, 8th ed. Chicago: Health Administration Press.

40. Sjoberg, C., and T. Timpka. 1998. "Participatory Design of Information Systems in Health Care." *Journal of the American Medical Informatics Association* 5 (2): 177–83.

41. Glandon, Smaltz, and Slovensky (2013, 230–32).

42. Bates, D. W., S. Saria, L. Ohno-Machado, A. Shah, and G. Escobar. 2014. "Big Data in Health Care: Using Analytics to Identify and Manage High-Risk and High-Cost Patients." *Health Affairs* 33 (7): 1123–31.

43. U.S. Department of Commerce. 2014. Malcolm Baldrige Award Recipients. [Online information; retrieved 7/10/14.] http://patapsco.nist.gov/Award_Recipients/index.cfm.

44. Health Information and Management Systems Society. 2014. "Value Suite." [Online information; retrieved 7/21/14.] www.himss.org/valuesuite.

45. Menachemi, N., D. Burke, M. Diana, and R. Brooks. 2005. "Characteristics of Hospitals That Outsource Information System Functions." *Journal of Healthcare Information Management* 19 (1): 63–69.

46. KLAS. 2014. Home page. [Online information; retrieved 7/1/14.] www.klasresearch.com.

11 HUMAN RESOURCES

1. *Treating the human resource as an investment:*
   - Manage the human resource through careful planning and recruitment, and with ongoing support.
   - Reward the value added by skilled associates.
   - Use the transformational culture to build retention.
   - Identify and respond to associates' development needs.

2. *Measuring and improving associate loyalty:*
   - Ensure safety and comfort in the workplace.
   - Identify and address opportunities for improvement (OFIs) from surveys and collective assessments.
   - Listen and respond to OFIs from individual comments.

3. *Promoting service excellence:*
   - Train workers to exceed expectations in meeting customers' needs.
   - Train managers in responding to workers' needs.
   - Provide rewards for exceptional effort in customer service.

4. *Building a competent workforce and an attractive workplace environment:*
   - Train associates for teamwork.
   - Maintain a healthy work environment.
   - Implement a value of respect.
   - Develop rewards and incentives for excellent performance.

5. *Building workforce diversity:*
   - Encourage individual leadership development plans.
   - Identify and assist high-potential associates for advancement.
   - Leverage workforce differences with cultural sensitivity.
   - Maintain succession plans for key positions.

Questions for Discussion

These questions are about applying the chapter content. It's often helpful to discuss them with classmates or mentors, gaining different perspectives on the issues.

1. You are talking with the superintendent of schools in your HCO's community, who is a potential governing board member. Explain to her the HCO's human resource strategy, assuming that the HCO implements the *WMHO*/Baldrige approach.

2. Why is workforce diversity important in HCOs? Why are some ethnic groups, women, and members of the lesbian, gay, bisexual, and transgender community underrepresented in higher-paying positions? What steps can be taken to improve diversity?

3. The local news calls, having found the HCO's IRS Form 990. The reporter notes that the CEO and several employed physicians are listed with generous compensation. She'd like an explanation of the HCO's policy. What's the best answer? What are the key takeaways you want the reporter to put in her story?

4. Suppose you found yourself in management of an organization that was in trouble on all the strategic scorecard measures in Exhibit 1.11. Where would you start recovery—with operations, finance, workforce loyalty, or customer loyalty? What might a successful recovery strategy look like?

5. The chapter argues not that the human resource be treated fairly but that the HCO promote among individual associates the perception that they are treated fairly. Is that really an important distinction? Why? This chapter notes that perceived fairness requires that senior leadership "go beyond the letter of the law." What happens if the senior leaders do not meet that standard?

Purpose

The purpose of human resources (HR) is

> **to sustain and increase the contribution of the associates to the HCO's mission by designing and implementing policies and programs to improve the skills, effectiveness, engagement, and commitment of associates.**

In fulfilling its purpose, HR becomes a central force that shapes and sustains the culture of empowerment and transformation, a major contributor to improvement goals, and a critical component of strategy development.

An HCO's associates often include several hundred or thousand people, working in one of dozens of job classifications, many of which are licensed or certified clinical specialties. Most are employed, but others work under long- and short-term service contracts. All physicians are affiliated through a privilege contract (Chapter 6), and some are employed. A significant number of associates are volunteers.

Excellent HCOs rely on the service excellence model shown in Exhibit 2.2. The service excellence emphasis on investment—that is, developing, rewarding, and retaining the human resource as an asset rather than viewing it simply as a cost—is a radical departure from the tradition of bureaucratic organizations. The investments add at least 10 percent to payroll costs. They must be recovered by improved efficiency or increased patient volumes. High-performing HCOs like North Mississippi Health Services (NMHS) and Henry Ford Health System (HFHS) implement the model aggressively.[1] They view their associates as their most valuable resource and are willing to invest in them whenever evidence shows the investment will improve capability, loyalty, and engagement. These characteristics are measured directly by satisfaction and engagement surveys, turnover, and absenteeism rates, and indirectly by quality of care, patient satisfaction, cost of care, and workplace safety measures.

NMHS describes its HR strategy as shown in Exhibit 11.1, a comprehensive and complex effort to create, recruit, retain, and develop the human resource. When HR is successful, caregiving and other work teams are committed to the mission. They know their jobs and they know each other. The team can respond quickly to patient or customer need. Delays, injuries, and accidents to patients or associates are infrequent. Empowered associates identify and correct conditions interfering with mission achievement. Teams find ways to improve efficiency of care that cover the cost of initiatives in Exhibit 11.1.

Functions

The functions of HR shown in Exhibit 11.2 are essential to implement the service excellence strategy. HR supports the transformational culture by training

EXHIBIT 11.1
North
Mississippi
Health Services'
Human
Resources
Strategy

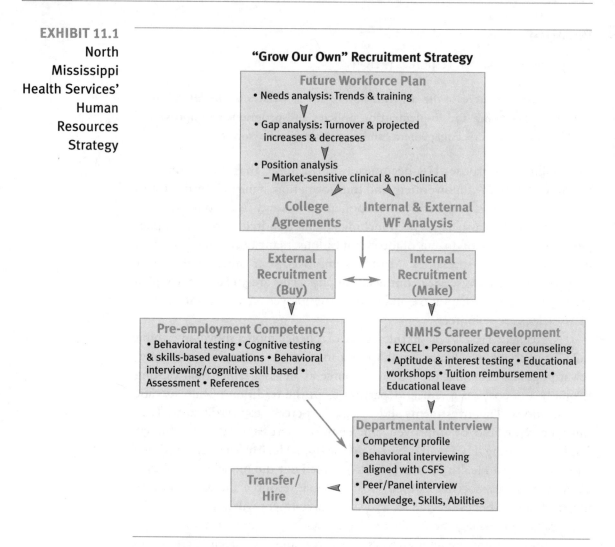

Source: North Mississippi Health Services Baldrige National Quality Award Application. 2012. [Online information; retrieved 1/28/14.] http://patapsco.nist.gov/Award_Recipients/PDF_Files/2012_North_MS_ Application_Summary.pdf.

virtually all associates in work processes, evaluating each associate's abilities and supporting their development, training all managers in transformational management, and advising on all human resource issues. In addition, it carries out the traditional HR functions of recruitment, compensation, benefits management, and collective bargaining, adapted to the transformational model.

Workforce Planning

Workforce planning allows the organization adequate time to respond to changes in the exchange environment with replacement, increases, or decreases in the numbers of associates. The workforce plan is a subsection of the organization's strategic plan (discussed in Chapter 15). It develops forecasts of the number of persons required in each skill by year for three to five years in the future. It also projects additions and attrition and even specifies the planned

EXHIBIT 11.2 Functions of Human Resources

Function	Description	Example
Workforce planning	Development of employment needs by job category	Forecast of RNs required and available by year
	Strategic responses in recruitment, downsizing, training, compensation	Strategy for recruitment, retention, and workforce adjustment
Workforce development	Recruitment, selection, and orientation	Advertising, career promotion, assistance to schools and colleges
		Credentials review, interviewing
	Associate safety	Accident reduction programs, OSHA reports
	Harassment-free environment	Review mission/vision/values, key workplace policies
	Diversity	Special programs for women and minorities
	Skills training	Specific skill training and continuous improvement courses
	Leadership development and succession planning	Programs to prepare first-line managers
		Identification and support of candidates for upper management
	Service recovery	Training in identifying service failures and responding
	Cultural competence	Training in cultural issues affecting care
Workforce maintenance	Employee services	Health promotion, child care, social activities offered to associates
	Workforce reduction	
	Grievance management	Counseling, grievance, and collective bargaining management
	Regulatory compliance	Validation and reporting of employment regulations
Empowerment, transformation, and service excellence	Management education	Programs of human relations skills, continuous improvement skills, meeting management
	Service recovery	Programs in service standards
		Training for service recovery
Compensation and benefits management	Position control	Central review of number of positions and employees
	Wage and salary administration	Market surveys of compensation, benefits
		Issuance of paychecks, transfer of payroll deductions
	Incentive compensation	Distribution of incentives earned
	Benefits administration	Disbursements and usage data
	Records management	Protection and analysis of employment data
Collective bargaining	Response to organizing drives, negotiation, and contract administration	Management of union collective bargaining contracts
Continuous improvement	Ongoing review of performance of the associate force	Identification of potential shortage situations, recruitment or retention OFIs
		Continued improvement of workforce satisfaction, retention, safety
	Ongoing review of HR activities	Human resources department operational scorecard improvements
	Identification of OFIs and establishment of improvement goals	

OFI: opportunity for improvement; OSHA: Occupational Safety & Health Administration; RN: registered nurse retirement of key individuals. It includes a succession plan for managerial positions. The medical staff plan (see Chapter 6) is a component. More specific plans are made for the coming year. NMHS "continually assesses its workforce needs" through

1. the annual budget process that projects volumes by work unit and senior leadership assignment;
2. hospital leaders use external staffing benchmarks and best practice reviews to determine staffing needs and evaluate staffing to volumes;
3. outpatient areas, such as clinics or home health, project staffing based on historical appointment data combined with projected demographic and/or population changes;
4. a new computerized scheduling system . . . maximizes staffing effectiveness, allowing leadership to monitor staffing to volumes in real time.[2]

A task force that includes representatives from human resources, planning, finance, nursing, and medicine guides workforce planning. HR works closely with the employing departments to translate the plan to workforce adjustments and plans for individuals, including hires, promotions, training, separations, and compensation changes. HR establishes guidelines for the use of temporary labor such as overtime, part-time, and contract labor. The plan is coordinated with new programs and capital requests. The revised plan is coordinated with the facilities plan because the number and location of employees determine the requirements for many plant and guest services. The final package must be integrated into the long-range financial plan. Finally, it must be approved by the governing board. The approved plan establishes each unit's goals for the coming year.

Workforce Development

High-performing HCOs commit to continued development for every associate. Building and maintaining the best possible workforce require recruitment, selection, training, and managing diversity. Most of these functions are provided in close collaboration with the associates' work units.

Recruitment, Selection, and Orientation

Retention of proven associates is generally preferable to recruitment because the cost of recruiting new personnel is surprisingly high—usually 20 to 30 percent of the annual compensation[3]—and the risk of an unsatisfactory outcome is lower for both the organization and the associate. However, expansions, changes in services, and associate life cycles result in continuing recruitment needs at all skill levels. Even under the best retention program, about 10 percent of the workforce will depart and be replaced each year.

A uniform protocol for recruitment and selection establishes policies for the following activities:

1. *Position approval.* Recruitment is for a specific vacancy identified through position control (described below).
2. *Job description.* Each position must be described in enough detail to identify education and training, licensure, and experience requirements to determine compensation and to permit equitable evaluation of applicants. Descriptions are developed by the operating managers and approved and recorded by human resources.
3. *Classification and compensation.* Wage, incentive, and benefit levels must be assigned to each recruited position. These must be kept consistent with the external market, similar job descriptions, collective bargaining contracts, and regulations. HR maintains the classifications. Each class has an associated pay scale, benefit entitlement, and incentive program.
4. *Applicant pool promotion.* HR develops and administers the policies following Equal Employment Opportunity Commission[4] and other compliance requirements and the design, placement, and frequency of media advertising, including use of the organization's website. Both HFHS and NMHS devote substantial effort to promoting healthcare careers in their communities. They partner with local schools and colleges to support formal training and encourage interest. They offer scholarships and other benefits to their employees who want to advance.
5. *Initial screening.* "Self-screening," exposing applicants to the mission, vision, and values of the organization and the detailed job description, is used to inform applicants about expectations before they apply. HR screening normally includes verifying professional certifications, verifying data on the application, contacting references, and checking criminal records and listings in the National Practitioner Data Bank.[5] Applicants may also undergo background checks for credit and driving records and a brief physical examination, which may include drug testing. Structured interviews are increasingly popular and are believed to be effective.
6. *Final selection.* Applicants who pass the initial screening are subjected to more intensive review, usually involving the immediate supervisor of the position and future teammates. HR monitors compliance with state and federal equal opportunity and affirmative action regulations and with the job description and requirements.
7. *Orientation.* New associates should learn the organization's mission and values, its policies to encourage their contribution, and its associate support services. They need assistance in a variety of areas, ranging from maps that show how to navigate their workplace to counseling on selecting their benefit options. HR offers a basic orientation program. The new associates' supervisor arranges a unit- and job-specific orientation and assigns more experienced colleagues to be preceptors or coaches.

8. *Probationary review.* Employees begin work with a probationary period, which concludes with a review of performance and usually an offer to join the organization on a long-term basis. Often, increased benefits and other incentives are included in the long-term offer. Line supervisors conduct the probationary review, with advice from HR.

For the medical staff leaders and higher supervisory levels, search committees are frequently formed to establish the job description and requirements, encourage qualified applicants, carry out screening and selection, and assist in convincing desirable candidates to accept employment. HR acts as staff for the search committee and ensures that the intent of organization policies has been met. Internal promotion is often desirable for these positions.

Associate Safety

In 2011, hospitals had 6.8 work-related injuries and illnesses for every 100 full-time equivalents; the healthcare industry overall had 2.7, and all private industries had 2.3. Illness and injury from hospital work can be kept at low levels by constant attention to safety. Back injuries, needle sticks, and associate infections are preventable. Hazards such as repeated exposure to low levels of radioactivity or small quantities of anesthesia gases can be reduced. The Occupational Safety and Health Act identifies standards for safety in the workplace, supports inspections, and levies fines for noncompliance.[6]

Much of the direct control of hazards is the responsibility of the clinical engineering and facilities maintenance departments. Infection prevention is an important collaborative effort of housekeeping, plant engineering, nursing, and medicine to protect the patient and the associate. Employee protection in well-run organizations stems from procedures developed for patient safety. Oversight responsibility for the environment of care is required by The Joint Commission and is useful in coordinating efforts and monitoring overall achievement. HR is usually assigned the following functions:

- Monitoring and analyzing safety and complaint measures, benchmarks, federal and state regulations, and professional literature for organization-wide opportunities for improvement (OFIs)
- Maintaining or coordinating the completion of material safety data sheets—profiles of hazardous substances with information on safe handling that must be filed with the Occupational Safety & Health Administration and systematically distributed to associates who are exposed to the substance
- Providing or assisting with training in and promotion of safe procedures and practices
- Negotiating contracts for workers' compensation insurance or managing settlements where the organization self-insures

Healthy Work Environment

A healthy work environment is an essential requirement for recruiting and retaining associates. HR is responsible for meeting the requirements and submitting statistics for the Occupational Safety and Health Act, which mandates workers' compensation for injury, establishes safe practices, and collects worker safety statistics.[7] It is also responsible for "clearly and regularly" communicating and "effectively" enforcing policies forbidding sexual harassment.[8] The regulations in these areas recognize and reward careful efforts to prevent problems. Excellent HCOs strive to exceed legal requirements, making physical and psychological safety a given.

Harassment is both illegal and a serious infraction of the value of respect. In addition to unacceptable activities by individuals, a hostile environment can be a violation of civil rights law. It is one in which the employee has specifically complained about practices that "unreasonably interfere with an individual's work performance" or create "an intimidating, hostile, or offensive working environment" and the employer has taken no steps to correct the practices.[9] Leading institutions go beyond the law with healthy work environment initiatives. These have enhanced associate satisfaction and retention, patient safety, and the organizations' financial viability.[10]

Diversity

The more successful HCOs make a deliberate and vigorous effort to represent the racial, ethnic, gender, lesbian, gay, bisexual, and transgender (LGBT) makeup of their community in their medical staff, management group, and workforce.[11] They adapt job requirements to family needs and work to promote women in management.[12] While this may be driven in part by a belief in social justice, it is also supported by sound marketing theories. Many people seek healthcare from caregivers who resemble them in gender, language, sexual identity, or culture. Increasing attention to the needs of female workers has clearly influenced the structure of employment benefits and the rules of the workplace.[13] Human resources monitors workforce diversity, guards against discriminatory activity, and designs programs that assist all associates to reach their full potential.

Leadership diversity is believed to promote associate engagement. It may eliminate health disparities.[14] Despite its advantages, limited evidence suggests that diversity implementation is not widespread.[15] Surveys show that women and minorities are still underrepresented in management.[16]

Training

Training is a major component of HR activity, and an important aspect of associates' work life. It averages about ten days per year for full-time employees.

The array of offerings in a large HCO includes the following:

- *Orientation.* This is a review of the organization's mission, history, vision, values, major assets, and marketing claims as well as policies and benefits of employment.
- *Technical skills.* Modern protocols and work processes require precise completion of highly technical activities. Although appropriate professional education provides a foundation, it cannot ensure proficiency and current competence. HR operates an ongoing educational activity for all associates. Content is developed by the profession or activity involved. HR assists with learning tools and facilities.
- *Continuous improvement and performance measurement.* This is basic education in continuous improvement and safety practices, including the reason for, meaning of, and application of concepts; how to use several basic tools; and how improvement teams work. Advanced training includes project management skills and more sophisticated analytic tools.
- *Guest relations programs.* These involve role-playing, scenario planning, and group discussion techniques that demonstrate ways to carry out service standards and that reinforce responses that show caring behaviors to patients and visitors.
- *Work policy change rollouts.* These review the objectives and implications of major changes in compensation, benefits, and work rules.
- *Retirement and financial planning.* This is offered to workers for assistance with understanding retirement benefits and planning for retirement transitions.
- *Outplacement assistance.* This is for persons who are being involuntarily terminated through reductions in workforce.
- *Benefits management.* This is guidance on options and procedures for using benefits, including efforts to minimize misuse.[17]
- *Major organizational change rollouts.* These explain permanent or temporary actions, such as new facilities and programs that would be of interest to associates.
- *Formal continuing education.* Opportunities to advance professionally through study in accredited outside programs are supported by flexible hours and scholarships. Both continuing education and degree programs are supported.
- *Healthy lifestyle management.* Health education and disease prevention classes are provided in order to support a healthy workforce.

HFHS claims:

Our commitment to building a learning and development infrastructure for our entire workforce supports Learning and Continuous Improvement as a core value. The HFHS University, established in 2004, enables us to deploy a high-quality, consistent, and convenient education and training platform across

HFHS. A web-based learning management system provides employees with easy classroom or online course registration for required and elective courses from work or home. Each employee has a personal learning site that tracks assigned courses, course completion, transcripts, and certificates. Employees completed 217,598 courses in 2008. Average training per leader was 57.2 hours in 2008.[18]

Leadership Development and Succession Planning

Leadership development begins with identification of promotable associates, who are offered extra learning opportunities through special assignments, advanced training, expanded mentoring or coaching, committee responsibilities, and activities outside the organization, often called *talent management*. Their potential is made clear to them, and their favored position is soon grasped by their peers. In addition, leaders are recruited from outside the HCO.

HFHS describes best practice in developing leaders:

> The HFHS Leadership Competency Model . . . defines the leadership attributes that all HFHS leaders are expected to demonstrate. Self-assessments, 360-degree assessments, personality assessments . . . and supervisor evaluations during the performance management process support evaluation against the competency model. Leaders use results in collaboration with their supervisors to create personal development plans to address gaps in leadership competencies and behaviors. Actions may include course work and development opportunities available through the HFHS University leadership development curriculum and/or external opportunities that align with and support expected leadership competencies. Many leaders, including our physicians, improve their personal leadership through diverse opportunities beyond HFHS, such as professional education, community service, and leadership positions in professional organizations and societies.[19]

Employees discuss career progression with their supervisors during the performance management process. HFHS supports these discussions by providing defined career paths for various job functions; daily, online, system-wide job postings of all available positions; and the Careers for Life Center, which offers career counseling, professional development programs, remedial courses and workshops, and a library of career planning resources.[20]

HFHS states:

> Results [of engagement surveys] are segmented by business unit, department, and key workforce demographics. Results are compared against internal segments and against a national database of medians and top quartile results for health care organizations. All leaders attend four hours of training prior to

receiving their assessment results and develop impact plans with their individual work groups, targeting two Q12® items for improvement and entering improvement plans into the online [commercial] engagement tool. Progress is monitored throughout the year at regularly scheduled meetings and through pulse surveys.[21]

At more senior levels, the program becomes more intense. Succession planning identifies potential replacements for all senior executive team members, their direct reports, and other key leadership positions. Steps include the following:

- Each leader completes a competency needs assessment for their position using the HFHS Leadership Competency Model.
- Each leader identifies three to five potential successors in "ready now," short term," and "long term" categories against the needs assessment.
- The list of high-potential candidates is reviewed and confirmed by next-level leadership.
- Each manager uses the "Development Guide and Roadmap" to help them assess strengths and opportunities for growth, interpret 360-degree assessments, and create specific team member development plans.
- All leaders are required to have a development plan to promote engagement. For employees identified as high potential, additional steps help create a development plan aligned with the position for which they have been identified.
- Senior leaders share succession plans as a team, identifying opportunities to spread talent across units.[22]

Service Recovery

Service recovery is a program that empowers workers to recover from patient service mistakes.[23] It must be taught to associates and first-line supervisors so that they are comfortable using it and they use it correctly. The primary purpose is to retain customer loyalty in situations in which the organization has failed. Its secondary purpose is to create a record of unexpected events that can be used to identify and address OFIs. When an associate feels that a customer has been treated in a substantially substandard manner, he or she corrects the problem as fully as possible and is authorized to compensate the customer appropriately as well. Patients and families may be given flowers, free meals, free parking, and even waiver of hospital charges, as indicated by the seriousness of the shortfall. All such transactions are reported in depth; these records identify process weaknesses and generate OFIs.

Service recovery is believed to improve customer satisfaction and reduce subsequent claims against the hospital. It has been proven cost-effective in other industries.[24] It is an extension of a long-standing procedure of completing written records of unexpected events. Because many of the events are clinical, service recovery is a foundation for a more elaborate program of potential malpractice claims management, described in Chapter 5.[25] The direct cost of the program can be managed with expenditure limits and required documentation. Its contribution is difficult to measure but almost certainly exceeds its cost. The program's success obviously depends on the organization's performance level. A hospital must have sound processes in place and a reasonable record of performance to make service recovery feasible.

Cultural and Linguistic Competence

Cultural competence is a set of complementary behaviors, practices, and policies that enables a system, an agency, or individuals to work and effectively serve pluralistic, multi-ethnic, and linguistically diverse communities.[26] The Joint Commission standards address food preferences, translation services, equal-standard-of-care provision, patient assessment and education (literacy and language appropriate), appropriateness of environment, and ongoing staff education.[27] Language barriers, religious beliefs, unconventional views of illness and alternative remedies (from birth to death), and diseases or conditions that may emanate from the patient's country of origin reduce patient satisfaction but also impair outcomes.[28] Cultural competence needs are met by training and the availability of coaches, ethics committees, and counselors. Linguistic services include bilingual/bicultural staff, trained medical interpreters, and qualified translators.

Cultural competence
A set of complementary behaviors, practices, and policies that enables a system, an agency, or individuals to work and effectively serve pluralistic, multiethnic, and linguistically diverse communities.

Training for all associates in contact with patients and for the specialist coaches, counselors, and interpreters is an HR responsibility. Without a deliberate support program, sensitivity to the cultural and linguistic perspectives of patients and their families is often inconsistent and ineffective.[29] Leading HCOs collect patient population data and use it to plan for and evaluate effectiveness of cultural and language services.[30,31]

Workforce Maintenance

The retention strategy of excellent HCOs is supported by a battery of employee services, management of workforce reductions, counseling and mediating grievances, and compliance with various federal and state regulations.

Employee Services

HR provides a number of personal services to associates. Workplace wellness and employee assistance programs have been shown to reduce absenteeism and health insurance costs. Childcare also reduces absenteeism.

Specific offerings are often tailored to the employees' needs. Charges are sometimes imposed to defray the costs, but some subsidization is usual. Commonly found programs include the following:

- *Workplace wellness*—health-risk screening, smoking cessation, nutritional advice, and exercise programs
- *Employee assistance*—counseling and therapy sessions to assist with substance abuse, stress management, and mental health–related issues
- *Infant and child care*
- *Social events*—major corporate events and recognition of employee contributions
- *Recreational sports*—sponsored teams and events
- *Credit unions*
- *Voluntary payroll deduction*—for various purposes such as retirement, tax benefits, and charitable donations to organizations such as United Way

Workforce Reduction

Changes in population, technology, competition, payment for care, and the economy can force any HCO to make substantial involuntary reductions in its workforce. Because job security is an important recruitment-and-retention incentive, such reductions must be handled well.[32,33] Good practice pursues the following rules:

- Workforce planning is used to foresee reductions as far in advance as possible, allowing natural turnover and retraining to account for much of the reduction.
- Temporary and part-time workers are reduced first.
- Personnel in at-risk jobs are offered priority for retraining programs and positions in needed areas.
- Early retirement programs are used to encourage more senior (and often more highly compensated) employees to leave voluntarily.
- Terminations are based on seniority or well-understood rules, judiciously applied.

Using this approach has allowed many HCOs to limit involuntary terminations to a level that does not seriously impair the attractiveness of the organization to others.

Grievance Administration

Well-managed HCOs provide an authority independent of the normal accountability for employees who believe, for whatever reason, that a complaint or question has not been fully and fairly answered. The intent is to resolve these concerns fairly and quickly. Human resources departments often offer ombudsman-type programs that provide an unbiased counselor for concerns of any kind. Personnel in these units are equipped to handle a variety of problems, from health-related issues, which are referred to employee assistance programs or occupational health services, to complaints about supervision or work conditions to sexual harassment and discrimination. The office's success depends on its ability to meet worker needs before they develop into confrontations or more serious dissatisfaction.

A few of the matters become formal grievances. The traditional collective bargaining contract includes a formal grievance process that often becomes adversarial in nature. The elements of transformational management—sound, clearly communicated policies, thorough education, servant leadership, and systems that emphasize rewards over sanctions—minimize adversarial situations. Effective management training produces supervisors who respond promptly to associates' questions and problems and who have substantially fewer grievances.

These processes are appropriate in both union and nonunion environments. They should make the formal review process typically found in union contracts, leading to resolution by an outside arbitrator, unnecessary in the vast majority of cases. Grievances that go to formal review encourage an adversarial environment. "Solving the problem" is implicit in servant leadership. It improves both the work and worker engagement.

Regulatory Compliance

Federal regulations regarding equal opportunity require that no discrimination occurs on the basis of sex, age, race, creed, national origin, sexual orientation, or disabilities that do not incapacitate the individual for the specific job. Laws that cover affirmative action require special recruitment efforts and priority for equally qualified women, African Americans, and Hispanics. (Religious organizations may give priority to associates of their faith under certain circumstances.) The regulations include wage and hour laws, the Family and Medical Leave Act of 1993, Title VII of the Civil Rights Act of 1964, and the Americans with Disabilities Act of 1990. HCOs are required to document compliance with these rules and may be subject to civil suits by applicants who are dissatisfied. HR monitors and documents compliance. Many associates are contract workers rather than employees. They work in the HCO for companies that provide services, such as food service and supply management. HR is responsible for verifying that the employing company has followed procedures consistent with the HCO's values and the law.

Compensation and Benefits Management

Employee compensation includes direct wages and salaries, shift differentials and premiums, bonuses, retirement funds, and a substantial number of specific benefits supported by payroll deduction or supplement. Federal law defines employment status and requires withholding of Social Security and income taxes from the employee and contributions by the employer. Other employment benefits are automatically purchased on behalf of the employee via the payroll mechanism. Compensation constitutes more than half the expenditures of most HCOs. From the organization's perspective, such a large sum of money must be protected against both fraud and waste. From the employee's perspective, accuracy regarding amount, timing, and benefit coverage should be perfect.

The growing complexity of compensation has been supported by highly sophisticated computer software, with each advance in computer capability soon translated to expanded flexibility of the compensation package. The latest developments in payroll have been increased use of bonuses and incentive compensation as well as "cafeteria" benefits, which allow more employee choice. Well-run organizations now use payroll programs that process both pay and benefit data for three purposes: payment, monitoring and reporting, and cost accounting. This software permits HR to manage compensation issues in the human resources department through position control, wage and salary administration, benefit administration, and retirement fund administration.

Position Control

The HCO must protect itself against accidental or fraudulent violation of employment procedures and standards and must ensure that only duly employed persons or retirees receive compensation. This is done through a central review of the number of positions created, called **position control**.

Position control
A system of payroll control that identifies specific positions created and filled.

Creation of a position generally requires multiple approvals, often including the chief operating officer. HR monitors the positions created to ensure compliance with recruitment, promotion, and compensation procedures and to ensure that each individual employed is assigned to a unique position.

Position control protects only against paying the wrong person, hiring in violation of established policies, and issuing fraudulent checks. It does not protect against overspending the labor budget. The number of hours worked outside position-control accountability is significant.

Wage and Salary Administration

Most HCOs operate at least two payrolls and a retirement plan disbursement system. One payroll covers personnel hired on an hourly basis, requiring reporting of actual compensable hours for each pay period—usually two weeks. The other covers salaried, usually supervisory, personnel paid a fixed amount per period—often monthly. Contract workers are often compensated through nonpayroll systems. Tracking these payments is important to measure the full cost of the workforce.

Wage and salary administration covers all of these disbursements for personnel costs and includes the following activities:

- *Compensable hours and compensation due.* The activity of verifying hours and compensation is applicable only to hourly personnel. The operating unit is accountable for the accuracy of hours reported and for keeping hours within budget agreements. HR verifies authorization, applies the appropriate pay rate, and applies policies establishing differentials. Computerized systems also identify other elements, such as the worker's location or activity, to support cost-finding activities. The data become an important resource for further analysis.

- *Compensation scales.* Each position is classified and assigned a compensation grade. Human resources conducts or purchases periodic salary and wage surveys to establish competitive pay scales for representative grades. At supervisory and professional levels, these surveys cover national and regional markets. For most hourly grades, the local market is surveyed.
- *Seniority, merit, and cost-of-living adjustments.* Compensation is sometimes adjusted for seniority, merit, or cost of living. Seniority and cost-of-living raises are not directly related either to the market for employment or to the success of the organization. Merit raises—increases in the base pay reflecting the individual employee's skill improvements—are difficult to administer objectively and tend to become automatic. Leading organizations are moving to replace all three adjustments with improved compensation scaling and performance-oriented incentive payments.

Fair compensation should meet three general criteria:

1. *Compensation should equal long-run economic opportunities for similar positions elsewhere.* The test of compensation is the market. Compensation consistently below market rates creates difficulty in recruiting and retaining professionals. Compensation consistently above market rates impairs the competitive position of the organization.
2. *Compensation should reflect actual contribution to the HCO's strategic goals.* This is usually implemented through incentive programs that recognize achievement of operational and strategic goals.
3. *Compensation should encourage professional growth and fulfillment consistent with organizational needs.* Incentives to learn and grow are part of a good compensation program.

Incentive Compensation

The market demand for competitive performance has made tangible reward for individual achievement desirable, and improved information systems have made it possible.[34] An organization built on rewards and the search for continued improvement is strengthened by a system of compensation that supplements personal satisfaction and professional recognition. HCOs have advanced significantly toward this goal.

Certain constraints must be recognized in designing an incentive compensation system:

- The resources available will depend more on the organization's overall performance than on any individual's contribution. They may be severely limited through factors outside the organization's control. The incentives must recognize this reality, emphasizing overall performance (the strategic scorecard) over unit performance (the operational scorecard).

- Equity and objectivity are expected in the distribution of the rewards.
- The individual's contribution is difficult to measure.
- Group rewards attenuate the incentives to individuals. The larger the group, the more the attenuation.
- The incentive program must avoid becoming a routine or expected part of compensation. These constraints suggest a *gain-sharing incentive system* based on both strategic and unit performance, with negotiated unit goals, and applied to the individual's work team. Gain-sharing approaches suggest that primary worker groups can effectively set expectations consistent with the needs of the larger organization and that the effort to do so leads to measurable improvement in achievement. Under a gain-sharing compensation system, annual longevity salary increases disappear as incentive pay increases, and incentives provide a substantial portion of compensation, particularly for senior management.

Benefits Administration

Many of the social programs of Western nations are related directly or indirectly to employment, through programs of payroll taxes, deductions, and entitlements. These programs are fixed in place by a combination of market forces, direct legal obligation, and tax-related incentives. HCOs and other employers in the United States support extensive programs of nonwage benefits, which add as much as 30 percent beyond salaries and wages to the costs of employment and are generally exempt from income and Social Security taxes. The exact participation of each employee differs, with major differences depending on full-time or part-time status, grade, seniority, and employee selection. In general, five major classes of employee benefits and employer obligations exist beyond wage compensation:

1. *Payroll taxes and deductions.* The employer is legally obligated to contribute premium taxes to Social Security for pension and Medicare benefits and to collect a portion of the employee's pay for Social Security and withholding on various income taxes. Certain funds, such as uninsured healthcare expenses and child-care expenses, can be exempt from income taxes by the use of pretax accounts. In unionized companies, dues are usually deducted from hourly workers' pay. While the deductions represent only a small handling cost to the employer, they are an important convenience to the employee.

2. *Mandatory insurance.* Employers are obligated to provide workers' compensation for injuries received at work, including both full healthcare and compensation for lost wages. They are also obligated to provide unemployment insurance, covering a portion of wages for several months following involuntary

termination. Under the Affordable Care Act, all but the smallest HCOs are obligated to provide health insurance.

3. *Vacations, holidays, and sick leaves.* Employers commonly pay full-time and permanent employees for legal holidays, additional holidays, vacations, and sick leaves. Some also compensate certain other non-worked time such as educational leaves, jury duty, and military reserves duty. They grant unpaid leaves for family needs, in accordance with the Family and Medical Leave Act,[35] and for other purposes as they see fit. As a result, only about 85 percent of the 2,080 hours per year that nominally constitute full-time employment is actually worked by hourly workers. The nonworked time becomes an extra cost to the organization when the employee must be replaced by part-time workers or by overtime premiums. It is also an important factor in the cost of full-time versus part-time employees. Part-time positions often share in employment benefits only on a drastically reduced basis.

4. *Voluntary insurance programs.* Defined contribution retirement programs are offered by most large HCOs. The specified contribution and agreed-on deduction are deposited into a tax-advantaged account. Life insurance and travel and accident insurance are also common. Various tax advantages are available for these protections. The programs are subject to state laws, the federal Employee Retirement Income Security Act, and income tax laws.

5. *Other perquisites.* A wide variety of other benefits of employment can be offered, particularly for higher professional and supervisory grades. Generally, perquisites are shaped by a combination of tax and job-performance considerations. Educational programs, professional society dues, and journal subscriptions are used. The Internal Revenue Service (IRS) requires Form 990 reporting of community benefit and executive compensation/perquisites for tax-exempt organizations (nonprofits). Benefits such as cars, club memberships, and expense accounts have come under increased scrutiny by the IRS. Public reporting has reduced nonwage benefits for executives.[36] Added retirement benefits—actually income deferred for tax purposes—and termination settlements are used to defray the risks of leadership positions. All of the perquisites must meet tests of reasonableness to avoid inurement concerns.

In managing employment benefits, HR strives to maximize the service excellence objective of mission achievement. Four courses of action are characteristic of well-run departments, three relating to program design and one to program administration:

1. *Program design for competitive impact.* The value of a given benefit is in the eye of the employee, and demographics affect perceived value. A married mother might prefer child care to health insurance because her husband's employer already provides health insurance. A single person whose children are grown

might prefer retirement benefits to life insurance. Employee surveys help predict the most attractive design of the benefit package. Recent trends have emphasized cafeteria-style benefit plans, where each employee can select preset combinations.

2. *Program design for cost-effectiveness.* Several benefits have an insurance characteristic such that actual cost is determined by exposure to claims. Health insurance, accident insurance, and sick benefits are particularly susceptible to cost reduction by benefit design. Health insurance, by far the largest of these costs, is minimized by the use of defined contribution approaches, including copayments, premium sharing, and selected provider arrangements. It may also be reduced by health promotion activities.[37] Accident insurance premiums are reduced by limiting benefits to larger, more catastrophic events. Duplicate coverage—where the employee and the spouse who is employed elsewhere are both covered by insurance—can be eliminated to reduce cost. Costs of sick benefits can be reduced by eliminating coverage for short illnesses and by requiring certification from a physician early in the episode of coverage.

3. *Program design for tax implications.* Income tax advantages are a major factor in program design. Many advantages, such as the exemption of health insurance premiums, are deliberate legislative policy. Details are subject to constant adjustment through both legislation and administrative interpretations. As a result, it is necessary to review the benefit program periodically for changing tax implications, in terms of both current offerings and the desirability of additions or substitutions.

4. *Program administration.* Almost all of the benefits can be administered in ways that minimize their costs. Strict interpretation of benefits can be received well by employees if it is fair, courteously administered, and accompanied by documentation in the benefit literature initially given employees. Preventing insured claims is important. Absenteeism and on-the-job injuries are reduced by effective supervision, and health promotion, counseling, and employee risk management assist toward this end. Unemployment liability is reduced by better planning and use of attrition for workforce reduction. HR affects all these activities through employee services, supervisory training, workforce planning, and occupational safety programs.

Records Management

HR maintains a large and sensitive information base about the workforce. This record is computerized, with the content organized around eight core files of information, as shown in Exhibit 11.3. These files contain individual records, including specific competency assessments and development plans. They support the workforce measures and many of HR's operational measures.

Human resources files, like patient records, must be protected against unauthorized access and misuse. Persons with access to the files must be trained in proper use. More serious questions arise after these basic concerns

File	Uses
Position control	
List of approved full- and part-time positions by location, classification	Provides a basic check on number and kinds of people employed
Personnel record	
Personal data, training, development plan, employment record, hearings record, benefits use	Provides tax and employment data aggregated for descriptions
Workforce plan	
Record of future positions and expected personnel	Shows changes needed in workforce
Succession plan	
Specific replacement candidates for managerial and other critical posts	Plans internal promotion possibilities for all key positions
Payroll	
Current work hours or status, wage, or salary level	Generates paychecks Provides labor-cost accounting
Employee satisfaction	
Results of surveys by location, class	Assesses employee satisfaction
Training schedules and participation	
Record of training programs and attendance	Generates training output statistics and individual records
Benefits selection and utilization	
Record of employee selection and use of services	Benefits management and cost control

EXHIBIT 11.3
Core Files of
HR Records
Management

have been met. Reduction of dissatisfaction, turnover, absenteeism, grievances, accidents, and illness is a goal of HR. It is clearly proper, even desirable, to study variations in measures such as supervisory effectiveness that can be improved by systems redesign, counseling, and education. Analyses based on worker characteristics (e.g., age, sex, race) or performance (e.g., illness, grievances) are often ethically questionable and can be illegal. Some facts, such as drug-test data, are potentially destructive and libelous if false. Some companies have attempted to deny employment opportunities in situations that present a high risk of occupational injury. For example, female nurses in their childbearing years have been denied employment in operating rooms because of the known pregnancy risks related to exposure to some anesthetics. When questions involving inferences about such matters arise, a review by the HCO's ethics committee or institutional review board is wise.

A sound policy must balance the advantages of investigation against its dangers. The following guidelines help:

- *Information access must be limited to a necessary minimum group.* Those with access are taught the importance of confidentiality and the organization's expectation that individuals' rights will be protected.
- *Formal approval must be sought for studies of individual characteristics that affect personnel performance.* Often a specific committee, including associates of the organization's ethics committee, is designated to review study proposals. Criteria for approval include protection of individual rights, scientific reliability, and evidence of potential benefit.
- *Actions should make associate restrictions or sanctions a last resort.* Considerable effort should be made to find nonrestrictive solutions. In the operating room example, avoiding potentially harmful gases or implementing special safety practices should be considered before employment is restricted.
- *When used, sanctions or restrictions must offer the individual the greatest possible freedom of choice.* The right of the individual to take an informed risk should be respected, and it may reduce the organization's ultimate liability. Material safety data sheets (Chapter 12) are designed to promote intelligent choices. Such a sheet would be required in the operating room example. Its purpose is to promote safety and informed choice. A nurse may accept employment, weighing the risks in light of her lifestyle.

Collective Bargaining

HCOs are subject to state and federal legislation that governs the right of workers to organize a union for their collective representation on economic and other work-related matters. Federal legislation generally supports the existence of unions; state laws vary. Collective bargaining is a declining element in the United States, to the point that, in 2013, only 7.2 percent of all health industry employees were union members.[38] Unionization differs significantly by state, with the northeastern states and California most unionized. Unionization is far more common in urban areas. In hospitals, unskilled workers and members of the building trades are the most likely to be organized. Nurses are next most likely; other clinical professionals are rarely organized. Periodic efforts to organize attending physicians and resident physicians have gained little headway.[39]

The National Labor Relations Board (NLRB) regulates unions and organization efforts. It requires unions to organize within specific job classes: physicians, registered nurses, all professional personnel other than doctors and nurses, technical personnel (including practical nurses and internally trained assistants and technicians), skilled maintenance employees, business office clerical employees, guards, and all other employees. Any organizing vote must gain support of a majority of all the associates of a given class.[40] An NLRB ruling in 1999 redefined medical residents as employees (rather than students) and permitted them to organize as a separate group.[41] The NLRB maintains that physicians in private practice are independent contractors and thus are not eligible to organize. Well-managed HCOs respond to organizing drives by hiring legal counsel to guide them in fulfilling their NLRB rights and obligations.

Unions are likely to continue to be important in specific institutions and job classes but are unlikely to expand dramatically. Well-run HCOs seek to discourage unionization and establish nonadversarial, collaborative relationships with existing unions. Such a strategy is actualized through transformational management, which explicitly recognizes employee needs without requiring union representation. Well-run organizations use experienced bargainers, have expert legal counsel, and promote union participation in ongoing performance improvement teams (PITs) and planning activities. They will accept a strike on issues that substantially disrupt the exchange environment for patients or associates, but as a strategy they avoid strikes whenever possible. Considerable supervisory education is necessary to implement this policy. Supervisors should know the contract and abide by it, but whenever possible their actions should be governed by the goals of transformational management. Any distinction between unionized and nonunionized groups should be minimized.

Continuous Improvement

HR supports continuous improvement in its own unit and throughout the organization. Its customers are both associates and employing units. The department also prepares its own OFIs and goals and implements its own improvements. HR will measure its own performance using multidimensional measures. Most of the functions can be benchmarked on cost and quality against competitors and nonhealthcare service organizations. Exhibit 11.4 shows typical OFIs and likely outcomes for HR improvement.

People

Human Resources Professionals

Human resources management emerged as a profession after World War II, in response to the complexities created by union contracts, wage and hour laws, and benefits management. HCOs were sheltered from these developments for several years, but as the need arose, HCOs moved to establish an identifiable human resources system and to hire specially trained leadership for it. Human resources professionals have a distinctive curriculum of formal education and a recognizable pattern of professional experience, and they may be voluntarily credentialed as a professional in human resources (PHR).[42] Healthcare practitioners have an association—the American Society for Healthcare Human Resources Administration, an affiliate of the American Hospital Association.[43] Well-run organizations now recruit professionals with experience in the healthcare or service industry to fill their human resources

EXHIBIT 11.4
Typical
Improvements
for Human
Resources

Indicator	Opportunity	Example
Potential RN shortage	Expand RN recruitment program	Install expanded part-time RN program, emphasizing retraining, child care, flexible hours
High health insurance costs	Promote more cost-effective program	Revise health insurance benefits Install managed care Promote healthy lifestyles
Low associate incentive payments	Redesign incentive pay program	Expand eligibility for incentives, improve measurement of contribution
Low employee satisfaction	Identify common causes and address individually	Improve employee amenities Offer special training for supervisors with low employee satisfaction
Inadequate operational performance improvement	Support line review of root causes	Conduct focus groups on motivation Seek evidence of worker dissatisfaction Review incentive programs
Labor costs over goal	Support orderly employment reduction	Curtail hiring in surplus categories Design and offer early retirement program Start cross-training and retraining programs

RN: registered nurse

director or vice president positions. Professional training and experience contribute to mastery of the several areas in which laws, precedents, or specialized skills define appropriate actions.

Organization of the Human Resources Department

HR is organized by function, to take advantage of specialized skills and processes. Exhibit 11.5 shows a typical accountability hierarchy for a large HCO with labor union contracts. Small organizations often use consulting organizations for support. (Collective bargaining is less common in small institutions.)

In multistate healthcare systems, HR tends to be decentralized by work site. While some activities, such as records management, can be centralized, most require frequent contact with employees and supervisors, demanding a local presence. Some policies are driven by state laws, which vary. A central office can monitor planning, support more elaborate educational programs, operate a uniform information system, and promote consistency of many policies. Decentralized representatives available in each site concentrate on implementation of these programs. Similarly, human resources services can be

EXHIBIT 11.5 Organization of a Large Human Resources Department

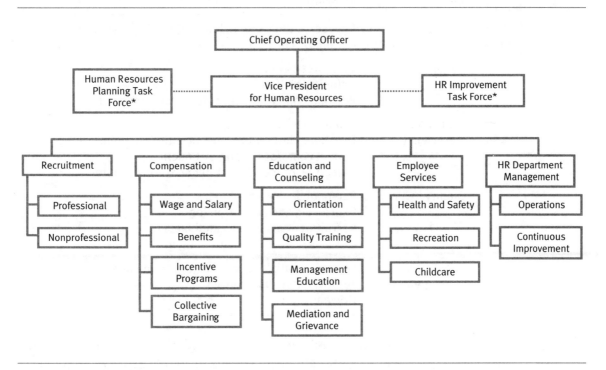

*Dotted lines show advisory relationships. The two task forces draw broadly from within and outside the human resources department.

contracted from outside vendors. The use of multidimensional performance measures makes contracting useful, and contracts can be arranged for specific functions or the entire human resources unit. Outsourcing all or part of human resources services is probably a viable solution for small organizations.

Measures

HR requires two measurement systems. One measures the workforce itself; supports planning; and identifies OFIs for recruitment, training, or compensation. The other measures the unit's own performance, using the standard operational measures template. Exhibit 11.6 lists many of the commonly used measures for describing and assessing the workforce.

Measures of the human resource are an important part of the annual environmental assessment. The values for most demand, cost, efficiency, quality, and satisfaction measures can be compared with benchmarks, with competitors, and with the organization's own history. OFIs can be identified and pursued. They are often in specific units of the HCO or job classes. For example, satisfaction or efficiency may be lower in one or two service lines, allowing a focused PIT to identify improvements. The workforce itself changes only slowly. Improvement goals are possible, but they sometimes take several years to achieve.

EXHIBIT 11.6
Measures of
the Human
Resource

Dimension	Measure
Workforce characteristics	Age, sex, ethnic origin, language skills, profession or job, training, certifications, other
Demand	New hires per year Unfilled positions Positions filled with short-term contract labor
Costs and efficiency	Labor costs/unit of output Overtime, differential, and incentive payments Benefit costs/associate, by benefit Human resources department costs/associate
Quality	Personal development plans Skill levels and cross-training Recruitment of chosen candidates Analysis of voluntary terminations
Satisfaction and engagement	Employee satisfaction or engagement surveys Turnover and absenteeism Grievances

An additional set of measures is important in assessing the department itself, as shown in Exhibit 11.7. More than 250 metrics exist for various details of department operation, and consulting companies provide benchmarks and consultation services.[44] The quality of HR services includes the measures of the workforce as shown in Exhibit 11.6. Specific goals can be set and achieved by HR. Many require collaboration with operating units, but the improvements should be reflected in their measures as well.

The use of both workforce and effectiveness metrics helps identify goals for both the strategic focus on investing in the human resource and the departmental operation.

Managerial Issues

HR has grown rapidly in recent years because leading HCOs have discovered the critical contribution it can make to sustain the human resource as an investment. Several issues—adequate funding, consistent senior leadership, and perceived fairness—can make or break the HR program.

Adequate Funding

Modern HR is an expensive support activity. In budget discussions, the question is often raised about the appropriateness of the expenditures. It can be tempting to protect profit margins by cutting HR costs. The model used by high-performing HCOs is "Spend enough on HR to build a loyal, engaged associate group." While benchmarks on HR operational measures are useful, the right cost of HR is the minimum necessary to optimize the human

EXHIBIT 11.7
Measures
of Human
Resource
Management

Dimension	Concept	Representative Measures
Demand	Requests for human resources department service	Requests for training and counseling services Requests for recruitment Number of employees*
Cost	Resources consumed in department operation	Department costs Physical resources used by department Benefits costs, by benefit
Human resources	The workforce in the department	Satisfaction, turnover, absenteeism, grievances within the department
Output/ efficiency	Cost/unit of service	New hires per year Hours of training provided per employee Cost per hire, employee, training hour, etc.
Quality	Quality of department services	Goals from measures of the workforce Time to fill open positions Results of training Audit of services Service-error rates
Customer satisfaction	Services as viewed by employees and supervisors	Surveys of other units' satisfaction with human resources Employee satisfaction with benefits, training programs, etc.

*Employees automatically receive many services from human resources and thus are a good indicator of overall demand for service.

resource. The evidence shows that when HR strategy is included in organizational strategic planning, the overall HCO performance is improved in the following ways: finding talent in advance for key job openings, stressing organizational culture and values in the selection process, and basing individual or team compensation on goal-oriented results.[45]

Consistent Senior Leadership

As discussed in Chapter 2, the organization's culture is supported through leadership actions and reinforced through consistent messages to associates and other key stakeholders. Senior leadership controls this consistency with two major themes:

1. *Making the mission, vision, and values real.* Service excellence organizations use their mission, vision, and values constantly. The mission, vision, and values are always public, widely disseminated, and referenced in debate. Management must promote them, respect them, and live by them.

2. *"Walking the talk" with the associates.* The messages to the associates are
   - We are truly and deeply committed to our mission (otherwise, we would not be offering incentive pay for mission achievement, providing all this training, and supporting service recovery).
   - We value not only your effort but also your opinion (otherwise, we would not spend so much time doing surveys and inviting you to meetings).
   - We want to help you grow and be promoted (otherwise, we would not talk about a personal and professional development plan).
   - We support your engagement in meaningful work in a healthy work environment (otherwise, we would not invest in your satisfaction and a culture of empowerment).

As with any communications campaign, these messages must be repeated thousands of times, with high consistency, to be credible. Senior leadership must make a visible presence throughout the organization, and it must respond in ways that convince associates that they have been heard. That means simple problems are fixed, complicated problems are explained, progress toward solutions is publicized, and roadblocks to progress are removed. The test of success is the associates' belief that management has been fair and aggressive in attacking the improvement agenda. It is measured by surveys, face-to-face meetings, incidents, and retention statistics.

Perceived Fairness

An associate's rewards—compensation, learning opportunities, recognition, and work conditions—are perceived to be fair when the associate believes a similar effort elsewhere would receive similar returns. The HR processes that set compensation, evaluate individual performance, distribute incentives, resolve conflicts, and open learning and promotion opportunities must all pass intense scrutiny. Evaluations must be unbiased. Pay must be systematically matched to competitive opportunities. Bonuses and promotions must be distributed on the basis of individual contribution, and learning opportunities must be distributed on the basis of organizational need. The test is stronger than the absence of a hostile environment; it must be the presence of a healthy, comfortable, and supportive work environment. HR and senior leadership must see that fair processes are in place, enforced, and respected. That, of course, means that leaders must go beyond the letter of the law themselves.

Additional Resources

Davidson, M. N. 2011. *The End of Diversity as We Know It: Why Diversity Efforts Fail and How Leveraging Difference Can Succeed*. Oakland, CA: Berrett-Koehler.

Fried, B., and M. D. Fottler. 2015. *Human Resources in Healthcare: Managing for Success*, 4th ed. Chicago: Health Administration Press.

Ulrich, D., J. Younger, W. Brockbank, and M. Ulrich. 2012. *HR from the Outside In: Six Competencies for the Future of Human Resources*. New York: McGraw-Hill.

Notes

1. North Mississippi Health Services (NMHS). 2012. Application for the Malcolm Baldrige National Quality Award. [Online information; retrieved 6/17/14.] http://patapsco.nist.gov/Award_Recipients/index.cfm; Henry Ford Health System (HFHS). 2009. Application for the Malcolm Baldrige National Quality Award. [Online information; retrieved 6/17/14.] http://patapsco.nist.gov/Award_Recipients/index.cfm.

2. NMHS (2012, 21).

3. Kocakulah, M. C., and D. Harris. 2002. "Measuring Human Capital Cost Through Benchmarking in Health Care Environment." *Journal of Health Care Finance* 29 (2): 27–37.

4. U.S. Department of Labor. 2014. "Equal Opportunity Employment." [Online information; retrieved 6/21/14.] www.dol.gov/dol/topic/discrimination/.

5. National Practitioner Data Bank. 2014. "How to Get Started." [Online information; retrieved 5/27/14.] www.npdb.hrsa.gov/hcorg/howToGetStarted.jsp.

6. Occupational Safety & Health Administration. 2013. "Worker Safety in Hospitals." [Online information; retrieved 5/27/14.] www.osha.gov/dsg/hospitals/index.html.

7. Occupational Safety & Health Administration. 2014. Home page. [Online information; retrieved 4/23/14.] www.osha.gov.

8. U.S. Equal Employment Opportunity Commission. 1990. "Policy Guidance on Current Issues of Sexual Harassment." Notice N-915-050. [Online information; retrieved 5/27/14.] www.eeoc.gov/policy/docs/currentissues.html.

9. *Ibid*.

10. American Association of Critical-Care Nurses. 2014. "Healthy Work Environments Initiative." [Online information; retrieved 5/28/14.] www.aacn.org/WD/HWE/Content/hwehome.content?menu=hwe.

11. Joint Commission. 2014. "Advancing Effective Communication, Cultural Competence, and Patient- and Family-Centered Care for the Lesbian, Gay, Bisexual, and Transgender (LGBT) Community: A Field Guide." [Online information; retrieved 5/28/14.] www.jointcommission.org/lgbt/; Dreachslin, J. L. 2007. "The Role of Leadership in Creating a Diversity-Sensitive Organization." *Journal of Healthcare Management* 52 (3): 151–55.

12. Myers, V. L., and J. L. Dreachslin. 2007. "Recruitment and Retention of a Diverse Workforce: Challenges and Opportunities." *Journal of Healthcare Management* 52 (5): 290–98.

13. McCracken, D. M. 2000. "Winning the Talent War for Women. Sometimes It Takes a Revolution." *Harvard Business Review* 78 (6): 159–67.

14. Dotson, E., and A. Nuru-Jeter. 2012. "Setting the Stage for a Business Case for Leadership Diversity in Healthcare: History, Research, and Leverage." *Journal of Healthcare Management* 57 (1): 35–46.

15. Davidson, M. N. 2011. *The End of Diversity as We Know It: Why Diversity Efforts Fail and How Leveraging Difference Can Succeed*. Oakland, CA: Berrett-Koehler.

16. Foundation of the American College of Healthcare Executives. "A Race/Ethnic Comparison of Career Attainments in Healthcare Management: 2008." [Online information; retrieved 5/27/14.] www.ache.org/PUBS/research/Report_Tables.pdf; Foundation of the American College of Healthcare Executives; "A Comparison of the Career Attainments of Men and Women Healthcare Executives: 2012." [Online information; retrieved 5/27/14.] www.ache.org/pubs/research/2012-Gender-ExecSummary.pdf.

17. Clement, D. G., M. A. Curran, and S. L. Jahn. 2015. "Employee Benefits." In *Human Resources in Healthcare: Managing for Success*, 4th ed., edited by B. J. Fried and M. D. Fottler. Chicago: Health Administration Press.

18. HFHS (2009, 23).

19. *Ibid.*

20. *Ibid.*, p. 24.

21. *Ibid.*, p. 25.

22. *Ibid.*, p. 24.

23. Leebov, W. 2012. *Resolving Complaints for Professionals in Health Care.* CreateSpace Independent Publishing Platform.

24. Bendall-Lyon, D., and T. L. Powers. 2001. "The Role of Complaint Management in the Service Recovery Process." *Joint Commission Journal on Quality Improvement* 27 (5): 278–86.

25. Boothman, R. C., A. C. Blackwell, D. A. Campbell Jr., E. Commiskey, and S. Anderson. 2009. "A Better Approach to Medical Malpractice Claims? The University of Michigan Experience." *Journal of Health and Life Sciences Law* 2 (2): 125–59.

26. Evans Sr., R. M. 2014. "Workforce Diversity." In *Human Resources in Healthcare: Managing for Success*, 4th ed., edited by B. J. Fried and M. D. Fottler. Chicago: Health Administration Press.

27. Joint Commission. 2010. *Cultural and Linguistic Care in Area Hospitals: Final Report.* Oakbrook Terrace, IL: Joint Commission; U.S. Department of Health and Human Services, Office of Minority Health. 2013. *National Standards for Culturally and Linguistically Appropriate Services in Health and Health Care.* [Online information; retrieved 5/27/14.] www.thinkculturalhealth.hhs.gov/Content/clas.asp.

28. Cohen, J., B. Gabriel, and C. Terrell. 2002. "The Case for Diversity in the Health Care Workforce." *Health Affairs* 21 (5): 90–102.

29. Tschurtz, B. A., R. G. Koss, N. J. Kupka, and S. C. Williams. 2011. "Language Services in Hospitals: Discordance in Availability and Staff Use." *Journal of Healthcare Management* 56 (6): 403–18.

30. Dreachslin, J. L., and V. L. Myers. 2007. "A Systems Approach to Culturally and Linguistically Competent Care." *Journal of Healthcare Management* 52 (4): 220–26.

31. Lewis, M. G. 2007. "A Cultural Diversity Assessment and the Path to Magnet Status." *Journal of Healthcare Management* 52 (1): 64–70.

32. Woodward, C. A., H. S. Shannon. C. Cunningham, J. McIntosh, B. Lendrum, D. Rosenbloom, and J. Brown. 1999. "The Impact of Re-engineering and Other Cost Reduction Strategies on the Staff of a Large Teaching Hospital: A Longitudinal Study." *Medical Care* 37 (6): 556–69.

33. Burke, R. J., and E. R. Greenglass. 2001. "Hospital Restructuring and Nursing Staff Well-Being: The Role of Personal Resources." *Journal of Health & Human Services Administration* 24 (1): 3–26.

34. Milkovich, G., J. Newman, and B. Gerhart. 2013. *Compensation*, 11th ed. New York: McGraw-Hill/Irwin.

35. U.S. Department of Labor. 2014. "Family and Medical Leave Act." [Online information; retrieved 5/27/14.] www.dol.gov/whd/fmla/.

36. GuideStar. 2014. Home page. [Online information; retrieved 5/27/014.] www2.guidestar.org/Home.aspx.

37. Aldana, S. G. 2001. "Financial Impact of Health Promotion Programs: A Comprehensive Review of the Literature." *American Journal of Health Promotion* 15 (5): 296–320.

38. U.S. Bureau of Labor Statistics. "Economic News Release." [Online information; retrieved 5/27/14.] www.bls.gov/news.release/union2.t03.htm.

39. For background on this topic, see Hoff, T. J. 2000. "Physician Unionization in the United States: Fad or Phenomenon?" *Journal of Health & Human Services Administration* 23 (1): 5–23.

40. Gullett, C. R., and M. J. Kroll. 1990. "Rule Making and the National Labor Relations Board: Implications for the Health Care Industry." *Health Care Management Review* 15 (2): 61–65.

41. Hein, J. G., Jr. 2000. "Employment: NLRB Empowers Residents to Unionize." *Journal of Law, Medicine & Ethics* 28 (3): 307–309.

42. HR Certification Institute. 2014. Home page. [Online information; retrieved 5/27/14.] www.hrci.org/.

43. American Society for Healthcare Human Resources Administration. 2014. Home page. [Online information; retrieved 5/27/014.] www.ashhra.org.

44. PricewaterhouseCoopers. 2014. "Saratoga: Human Capital Measurement." [Online information; retrieved 5/27/14.] www.pwc.com/extweb/service.nsf/docid/de40ffb0d40981d385256f17005397cd.

45. Platonova, E. A., and S. R. Hernandez. 2013. "Innovative Human Resource Practices in U.S. Hospitals: An Empirical Study." *Journal of Healthcare Management* 58 (4): 290–303.

12 ENVIRONMENT OF CARE

Critical Issues in the Environment of Care

1. *Designing space for improved patient outcomes:*
   - Architecture and equipment that emphasize safe design and materials.
   - Deliberate attention to a visually welcoming atmosphere.
   - Investment in preventive maintenance.

2. *Planning the best use of space:*
   - Space allocation assigned to one central office.
   - Formal, open process for review of requests for expansion.
   - Periodic review of space use to determine continuing need.

3. *Using benchmarks and goals to support security, sanitation, maintenance, and materials management services:*
   - Zero harm as an achievable goal for safety.
   - Delighting customers and internal customers.
   - Training, support, and rewards for service employees and supervisors.

4. *Using contract services to improve performance:*
   - Contracting with outside suppliers to ensure near-benchmark performance.
   - Specification of service requirements in cost, quality, and satisfaction dimensions.
   - Benchmarking and comparison of service.

5. *Developing evacuation and emergency plans capable of handling natural disasters, large-scale accidents, and the possibility of terrorism:*
   - Internal plans for response.
   - Drills and testing.
   - Coordination with other community agencies.

Questions for Discussion

These questions are about applying the chapter content. It's often helpful to discuss them with classmates or mentors, gaining different perspectives on the issues.

1. To accommodate a rapidly growing and aging community, it is necessary to expand capacity for long-term care by constructing a new wing. How would you determine the primary

health concerns for this population, and how would you develop the plan and design to meet their medical needs and improve their satisfaction?

2. Your organization will contract with an orthopedic implant supplier. What steps would you take in selecting vendors, writing contract specifications, and administering a contract?

3. Patient satisfaction surveys criticize overall appearances and attitudes of employees. How would you design an improvement program for your HCO? What lessons in hospitality might be transferable from the hotel industry?

4. Your community HCO is in a large coastal city and in hurricane territory. What issues should your disaster plan address, and how does the HCO develop an effective response?

5. You have an offer from a vendor to outsource your entire supplies function. How would you evaluate that offer?

Purpose

The purpose of managing the environment of care is to

provide safety for all persons in the HCO;

provide the physical environment required for the mission, including all buildings, equipment, and supplies;

plan for contingencies and implement risk mitigation strategies;

and

maintain reliable guest services at satisfactory levels of economy, attractiveness, and convenience.

Functions

Environment-of-care functions can be grouped into six major categories, as shown in Exhibit 12.1. It is noteworthy that the functions include the management of all the plant, equipment and supplies, and many nonclinical services for guests and associates. The functions range from lawn mowing and snow removal to security, signage, and meals to the life-support environments of surgery and intensive care. Everything must be done well—from sweeping the entranceway to maintaining intensive care unit equipment—with the number one goal to ensure safety for all persons.

Facilities Design, Planning, and Space Allocation

The HCO's physical facility—often an array of buildings of various ages and several locations—is a resource that must be planned to accommodate future technology and market changes, designed or redesigned to fit user needs, acquired, and uniquely allocated to meet the needs of specific activities in the context of environmental responsibility. The planning and design function is centralized to ensure consistency across the HCO.

Planning Facility Requirements

Healthcare facilities are built for their users; thus, plans begin with identifying specific needs and architectural specifications. Plans continue through the management of construction contracts and the lifecycle of maintenance, renovation, and eventual replacement.

As shown in Exhibit 12.2, the **facilities master plan** begins with an estimate of the space needs of each service or activity proposed in the services plan. Space needs must be described by location, special

Facilities master plan

A document that begins with an estimate of the space needs of each service or activity proposed in the services plan.

EXHIBIT 12.1 Functions of Environment of Care

Function	Activities	Examples
Facilities design, planning, and space allocation	Using design to improve performance	Patient-, associate-, and environment-friendly designs
	Planning, building, acquiring, and divesting facilities	Facilities management plan
		Construction and renovation management
		Facilities leasing and purchase
		Space allocation
	Promoting environmental sustainability	LEED certification
		Recycling
Facilities maintenance and guest services	Housekeeping	Cleanliness
	Groundskeeping	Landscaping and decorating
	Transportation	Snow removal
		Parking
	Support for associates, patients, and visitors	Food service
		Signage and wayfinding
	Preventive maintenance	Preventive maintenance schedules
Environment-of-care safety and regulatory compliance	Safety	Accident and harm prevention and risk management; elimination of hazards
	Security	24/7 facility security and risk mitigation
	Hazardous materials and waste	Chemical and radiation hazard management
	Fire safety	Fire prevention and management
	Medical equipment	Maintaining and repairing medical equipment
		Compliance with Safe Medical Device Act
	Utilities	Utility backup and failure prevention
Materials management	Purchasing, receiving, storing, and distributing supplies	Clinical supplies
		Foodstuffs
		Drugs
		Office supplies
		Medical gases
		Value analysis and selection of supplies
Emergency management and disaster preparedness	Emergency preparedness	Preparing for large-volume disasters—internal and external
		Weather-related disasters
	Life safety and fire protection	Response to internal fire or safety problem
Performance improvement	Customer-focused identification of OFIs	Ensuring that internal and external customer needs are met
	Contracting with service vendors	Developing a long-range vision
	Coordinating multiyear plans	Maintaining competitive services

LEED: Leadership in Energy & Environmental Design; OFI: opportunity for improvement

EXHIBIT 12.2
Facilities
Planning
Process

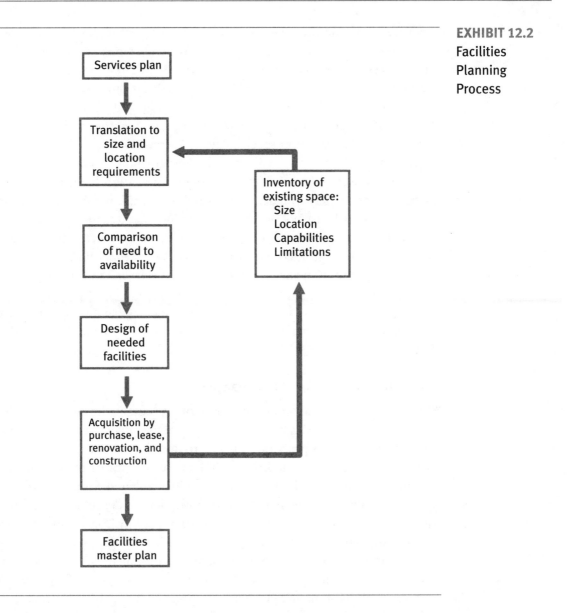

requirements, and size. Need is compared to available space, and deficits are met at the lowest cost. *Conversion*—the simple reassignment of space from one activity to another—is the least expensive, but so many healthcare needs require specific locations and requirements that renovation, acquisition, or construction are frequently necessary. The final facilities master plan shows the future location of all services and documents the renovation, acquisition, or construction necessary in terms of specific actions, timetables, and costs.

Sizing of Facilities

Facilities are sized based on forecasts of demand. Methods for the actual calculation will get quite complex. Often several methods of forecasting are used to improve confidence in the forecast. For example, surgeries will be categorized by type of room and square footage required. Each type of room will have several sources of demand that are forecast separately. Duration of operations will be studied carefully. Trade-offs will be required; a room designed for a certain specialty might be highly inefficient for other demands. Trade-offs must also be evaluated between the efficiency of high load factors and the increased associate satisfaction from specialization. A simulation model might be constructed to evaluate trade-offs between alternative designs and load factors.

In general, plans minimize costs by using high load, or occupancy, factors. Part of performance improvement is minimizing the allowance. For example, it is usually possible to schedule maintenance in times of low demand. Unattractive times can be filled by using incentives—discounts, faster service to customers, or extra pay to associates. Facilities where emergency demand is often encountered, such as obstetrics and coronary care, will require standby capacity, which may reduce expected occupancy, sometimes as low as 50 percent. These allowances cannot be changed by internal performance improvement, but they can be changed by centralizing to larger facilities.

Using Design to Improve Performance

Poor HCO design is an important cause of preventable hospital errors, infections, and work-related stress and injuries. For example, poor ventilation with two or more patients per room can lead to nosocomial infections, while inadequate or inappropriate lighting is linked to suboptimal patient outcomes and medication errors. Better, safer, and evidence-based design environments promote healing and satisfy healthcare staff.[1] Several design elements are recognized to be important: private rooms, sound control, air quality, ecological impact, signage, and information stations. New design must address wireless communication, delivery robots, and appearance. Bronson Methodist Hospital's facility in Kalamazoo, Michigan, introduced many improvements, including art, light, nature elements (such as a central garden courtyard), and information technology (such as touch-screen kiosks).[2] Bon Secours St. Francis Medical Center, a hospital in Richmond, Virginia, uses natural elements such as fountains, meditative gardens, and a chapel that opens to walking paths[3] not only for patients, families, and associates but for the surrounding community, ascribing to the urban planning principles of New Urbanism.[4]

Money spent on design innovations and upgrades can be recovered through operational savings and increased revenue. In a study of 19 replacement hospitals, 75 percent experienced overall average increases of 15 percent in admissions, 33 percent in outpatient visits, and 2.5 percent in operating margins in the first year.[5] Investing in better hospitals requires that leadership recognize the need for and plan strategically to promote an environment to minimize stress. Good design is an evolution, rather than an adoption of radical changes.[6] Improved design is clearly an important component of a successful continuous improvement program. Hospitals and health systems have begun to follow performance-based building practices, such as applying for LEED (Leadership in Energy & Environmental Design) certification, to maximize ecological **sustainability**,[7,8] as well as decreasing waste, reducing their environmental footprint, and promoting public environmental health.[9]

> *Sustainability*
> The quality of not being harmful to the environment or depleting natural resources, thereby supporting long-term ecological balance.

Renovation, Construction, and Acquisition

Implementing the facilities master plan requires a comprehensive program of real estate and building management that indicates the way the requirements will be met. The unfilled needs, including renovations, must be expanded into specifications and drawings for both space and fixed equipment and translated to reality. Real estate must sometimes be acquired, contracts let, progress maintained, and results inspected and approved before the facility can be occupied. In large projects, several years elapse between approval of the facilities plan and opening day. Plans have specific, carefully developed time schedules.

Real estate is acquired through purchase or lease. It is possible to lease all or part of a facility, including a single lease for a building and equipment designed and constructed specifically for the HCO. Major equipment can also be leased. Real estate transactions generally require governing board approval, and the finance department is always involved (see Chapter 13).

Major construction and renovation usually call for extensive outside contracting. The traditional approach is to retain an architect, a construction management firm, and a general contractor. Construction financed directly by public funds, such as that of public hospitals, usually must be contracted via formal competitive bids. Private organizations frequently prefer more flexible arrangements, negotiating contracts with selected vendors. Recent innovations have simplified the contracts by combining various elements; turnkey construction involves a single contract to deliver the finished facility. Advantages of speed and flexibility are cited, and costs likely can be reduced if the HCO is well prepared and supervises the process carefully. Small renovation projects are often handled by internal staff. As an interim step, the organization can provide design and construction management, preparing the plans and contracting with specific subcontractors.

Regardless of the size or complexity of the project, any project to change the use of space should be carefully planned in advance and closely managed as it evolves. A sound program includes the following:

1. Review of the space and equipment needs forecast
2. Identification of special needs

3. Trial of alternative layouts, designs, and equipment configurations
4. Development of a written plan and specifications
5. Review of code requirements and plans for compliance
6. Approval of plan and specifications by the operating unit
7. Development of a timetable identifying critical elements of the construction
8. Contracting or formal designation of work crew and its accountability
9. Ongoing review of work against specifications and timetable
10. Final review, acceptance, and approval of occupancy

Involvement of end users, especially caregiving associates and physicians, in planning and specifying the space requirements from idea conception to completion maximizes space functionality and stakeholder satisfaction and minimizes costly change orders.

Space Allocation

The criterion for allocating existing space is conceptually simple. Each space should be used or disposed of in the way that optimizes achievement of the organizational mission. In reality, this criterion is difficult to apply. Activities tend to expand to fill the available space. As a result, there are always complaints of shortages of space and an agenda of possible reallocations or expansions. When activities shrink, the space is often difficult to recover and reuse. Space is highly valuable and unique: The third floor is not identical to the first. Space also confers prestige and symbolic rewards. Space next to the doctors' lounge, for example, is more prestigious than space adjacent to the employment office. As a result, space allocation decisions tend to be strenuously contested.

Each unit that seeks substantial additional space or renovation must prepare a formal request and gain approval from the space office before submitting a new program or capital proposal. The following guidelines assist in space management:

- Space management is assigned to a single office that permits occupancy and controls access to space. The office participates in new programs and capital budget review activities (see chapters 8 and 13), where most changes originate, and designs appropriate ad hoc review for other requests.
- A key function of the space management office is the preparation of the facilities master plan. Internal consulting and marketing staff assist in the preparation. The draft plan is derived from the services plan, and the final version becomes part of the planning package. The facilities master plan includes forecasts of specific commitments for existing and approved space; plans for acquisition of land, buildings, and equipment; plans for renovation and refurbishing requirements for existing space; and plans for new construction.
- The facilities master plan is incorporated into the long-range financial plan and annual review and approval processes.

- The plant services department implements acquisition, construction, and renovation. Details of interior design are reviewed and approved by units that will use the space. Financing is managed by the finance department.

Facilities Maintenance and Guest Services

A safe and attractive environment of care helps determine the impressions and attitudes that people form about an organization. It is a central component of the HCO's culture and important in promotional activity, not only to patients but also to associates. An excellent environment-of-care system is safe, reliable, convenient, attractive, and economical. It includes facilities, supplies, equipment, security, waste disposal, food service, and maintenance services. Exhibit 12.3 shows several HCO environments, nonhealthcare organizations with which they are commonly compared, and their special needs. All of these environments must provide safety, comfort, sanitation, and, except for the smallest, food service. All of them have needs unique to healthcare. At the

Activity	Facility	Nonhealth Counterpart	Special Needs
Primary care	Small office	Small retail store	X-ray machine Drugs and clinical supplies Clinical waste removal
Outpatient specialty care	Medical office building	Shopping mall	Special electrical and radiologic requirements Drugs and clinical supplies Clinical waste removal Disaster preparation
Long-term care	Nursing home	Motel	Extra fire safety and disability assistance Drugs and clinical supplies Clinical waste removal Pathogenic organisms Special air handling 24-hour security
Acute and intensive care	Hospital	Hotel	Extra fire safety and disability assistance Drugs and clinical supplies 24-hour security Disaster and terrorism preparation Dangerous chemicals High-voltage radiology Radioactive products Clinical waste removal Pathogenic organisms Special air handling Emergency utilities preparation

EXHIBIT 12.3
Facilities Maintenance Requirements

extreme, the acute care hospital provides complete environmental support not only for patients but also for staff and visitors. It must have extra supplies of power and water to allow it to operate through disruptions of those services. It requires narrower tolerances on temperature, humidity, air quality, cleanliness, and wastes. It has high volumes of human traffic and, as a result, has high risks of personal and property safety, including a risk of direct terrorist attacks. Several hazards, including fire, chemical spillage, radiation, infection, and criminal violence, can be life threatening to employees, visitors, and patients. The well-run organization uses carefully designed, conscientiously maintained programs to make these services transparent, reliable, and risk free.

Facilities Maintenance

Facility maintenance includes decorating; maintaining lighting, water, heating, and air-conditioning; supplying power; and cleaning and repairing all buildings and grounds. The components are shown in Exhibit 12.4. These activities are required for any facility, even a single family home. They are more complex in HCOs because the facilities are large and multistory and have large traffic volumes, and some must operate 24/7/365. Special needs arise from many clinical activities. Facilities maintenance must respond to local conditions, including weather, and be performed in compliance with a variety of federal regulations established by the Occupational Safety and Health Administration (OSHA) and the Environmental Protection Agency (EPA).

Preventive maintenance

The care and servicing by personnel for the purpose of maintaining equipment and facilities in satisfactory operating condition by providing for systematic inspection, detection, and correction of incipient failures either before they occur or before they develop into major defects.

The objective of **preventive maintenance** is to keep the facility and its equipment like new so that patients, visitors, and staff perceive the environment

EXHIBIT 12.4
Facilities and Preventive Maintenance Services

Housekeeping
Interior design
Routine cleaning
  General patient areas
  High-risk patient areas
  Nonpatient areas
  Special problem areas
Odor control
Sound control

Utilities management
Electrical power
Heating, ventilation, and air-conditioning
Lighting
Communications support
Gases supply

Groundskeeping
Landscaping
Grounds maintenance
Recycling

Hazardous waste management
Safeguarding hazardous materials
Material safety data sheets
Clinical waste removal

Maintenance and repair services
Building and utility maintenance
Equipment maintenance

positively or neutrally. The goal is achieved by fixing or replacing equipment before it is broken. Well-managed plant systems schedule preventive maintenance for all the mechanical services and specific building areas. They regularly inspect general-use equipment (such as elevators and air-handling units) and plant conditions (such as floor and wall coverings, plumbing, roofs, and structural integrity). They perform repairs and routine maintenance as needed, and their logs are used to assess replacement needs. A significant fraction of mechanics' time is devoted to preventive maintenance, and adherence to the schedule is one measure of the quality of the department's work.

Outside vendors are used to maintain many specialized equipment items. Well-run organizations tend to place the responsibility for managing the contract on the unit that uses the equipment, if only one unit is involved. The plant department is responsible for equipment in general use, such as elevators, heating, and air-conditioning. Actual contracting for all equipment maintenance is centralized through materials management, which must consult with the responsible units.

Housekeeping and groundskeeping must maintain campuses (of millions of square feet) efficiently and at standards to ensure visual attractiveness and to control microbial and other hazards. Some services, such as snow removal and exterior lighting, must be available around the clock. In well-run HCOs these activities are conducted to explicit standards of quality and are monitored by inspectors using formal survey methods. These activities also interact with important programs for environmental safety. Continuous improvement, training, and carefully specified equipment and supplies are used to attain high levels of cleanliness and safety.

Cleaning and landscape services are frequently subcontracted. The most common contracts are for management-level services. The outside firm supplies procedures, training, and supervision; the workers are hourly employees. Large organizations with access to central services for training and developing methods may be able to justify their own management.

Decorating and landscaping are performed with an understanding of public taste and the cost of specific materials. Colors, fabrics, and designs are selected for comfort, durability, and conformity with the applicable life-safety code (rating for fire retardancy and prevention). The best decor creates an attractive ambiance but consists of materials that do not show wear and are durable, fire rated, and easy to clean. Careful initial design leads to higher capital costs, lower operating costs, and greater user satisfaction. Evidence-based design environments have been shown to contribute to improved patient outcomes.[10]

Guest Services

Large numbers of patients, visitors, and staff become the guests of HCOs and require a variety of services. People expect to come to a facility; park; find what they want; get certain amenities such as waiting areas, lounges, or the cafeteria; and leave without even recognizing that they have received service. They expect, and are fully entitled to, strenuous efforts by the HCO to maintain a safe environment. Those who access the organization by telephone or electronic communication expect a similarly complete, prompt, and unobtrusive response. The organization's attractiveness is diminished if the services listed in Exhibit 12.5 are either inadequate or intrusive.

Coordinated management of guest services stresses the importance of a satisfactory overall impression. Guest services occur in multiple locations and encounters. For example, receptionists and security personnel need training in handling recurring situations consistently; current knowledge of the location of each inpatient, event, or activity; and a central source for advice on unexpected events. Training in service management, recognition of potentially serious situations, and HCO geography are necessary to do the job well.

Food Service

The preparation of food for patients, staff, and guests has become a service similar to the food services of hotels, airlines, and resorts. Food service should provide inexpensive, nutritious, appealing, and tasty meals that encourage good eating habits. HCOs typically offer a choice of entrees, appetizers, and desserts to each patient. "On demand" food service is popular. Patient meals must also be provided to a variety of clinical specifications. Soft, low-sodium, and sodium-free diets account for up to half of all patient meals. Patients are often susceptible to food bacteria, so food service must be conducted to exceptional standards of safety in preparation and distribution.

In addition to patient meals, about an equal number of meals are provided to associates and guests, usually in cafeterias. Visitors and employees expect greater variety, a range of prices, and service at odd hours. A snack

EXHIBIT 12.5 Guest Services: Workforce, Patient, and Visitor Support	*Security Services* Guards Employee identification Traffic control Facility inspection and monitoring *Parking Services* *Food Service* Cafeteria and vending service Patient food service Routine patient service Therapeutic diets	*Communication and Transportation Services* Telephone and television Messenger Tube transport systems Reception and guidance Signage Parking Internet access Public website design and maintenance Intranet design and maintenance Telephone reception

bar, a coffee shop, and a variety of vending machines with food and drinks are among common offerings. Food service also supports home care and meals-on-wheels distribution.

Food service is frequently contracted. Contract food suppliers meet the quality and cost constraints through centralized menu planning, well-developed training programs for workers and managers, and careful attention to work methods.

Food service is supplemented by therapeutic dietetics, a clinical support service. Clinical dietitians focus on nutritional therapy in acute and post-acute settings. They provide nutritional education and consultation and the preparation of special diets to meet medical needs.

Environment-of-Care Safety and Regulatory Compliance

The environment of care is highly regulated by licensure, accreditation, and statutory requirements. For accredited organizations in all settings, the six environment-of-care functional areas described in this section require management plans to reduce risks and threats to safety. Furthermore, each of these management plans must include: risk assessment; staff development; emergency response and procedures; inspection, testing, and maintenance; information collection and evaluation; performance monitoring; and annual evaluation.[11]

Safety and Risk Management

Safety should be a universal concern in HCOs. Risks arising from both patient care and the environment are overseen by a risk management committee with representatives from senior management, legal counsel, clinical services, and support services. The committee is charged to develop and protect a culture of safety, monitor the risk management process, and evaluate safety threats and opportunities for improvement (OFIs). Its duties are often split between clinical and environmental subcommittees. An environmental safety officer is charged with implementing safety improvements. Improvements can include process revision, equipment and facilities redesign, and expanded training for associates.

All adverse events and safety concerns are routinely reported and reviewed by a risk manager or teams accountable to the patient safety committee. These "adverse event" reports (often called by other names) provide alerts for individual corrective action or recovery and statistics on the frequency and seriousness of events that can identify correctable processes. Variation in reporting is a known problem. Training, recognition, and examples are used to create a blame-free culture, where associates feel comfortable in identifying errors and other safety issues. As associates attain greater psychological safety, the number of reports often increases. While complex and rigorous, patient quality and safety programs that identify the source of adverse events and take corrective action achieve substantially improved patient outcomes and business metrics.[12]

Security

Security services are necessary to protect associates, visitors, patients, and property. There are recognized hazards of theft, property destruction, and personal injury to associates and visitors. Both associates and visitors can commit violent acts.[13] The hazard is particularly high in urban areas[14] and at night. High-quality security services are preventive. They control access, monitor traffic flow, and provide and verify employee identification. They work with risk management and facilities planning to create an environment that is reassuring to guests and discouraging to persons with destructive intentions. Digital cameras and emergency call systems amplify the scope of surveillance. Special attention must be given to high-risk areas, such as the emergency department and parking areas. Uniformed guards serve as a visible symbol of authority, to respond to questions and concerns, and to provide emergency assistance in those infrequent events that exceed the capability of reception personnel.

Security is frequently a contract service. It must be coordinated with local police and fire service. Municipal units sometimes provide the contract service, particularly in government hospitals. Not-for-profit HCOs usually do not pay local taxes in support of local fire and police service. As a result, agreements on the integration of taxpayer services with HCO associates are necessary.

Hazardous Materials and Waste

Environmental needs and the hazards of biological and clinical wastes complicate HCO's waste management. Waste disposal must meet increasingly stringent EPA standards and state and local laws that protect the safety of landfills, water supplies, and air. Many cities require segregation of nonclinical wastes to permit recycling. Federal and state laws govern burning and shipment of wastes. Federal laws govern handling and disposal of medical waste[15] and other hazardous materials, such as chemical, biological, radiological, and nuclear that may be used in terrorist attacks.[16] Emergency response plans must include requirements for personal protective equipment and clear assignment of tasks, locations, and training to prevent healthcare workers from exposures.

Within the HCO, wastes must be handled correctly and efficiently. Clinical wastes are known to transmit contagious diseases, such as hepatitis and HIV. Additionally, procedures should outline the steps to be taken for decontaminating patients who seek emergency medical care after being exposed to hazardous materials. Specially designed systems for decontamination and waste management must be carefully planned. Personnel who are most likely to come into contact with hazardous materials or waste contamination (e.g., emergency department, housekeeping, and nursing staffs) must be trained. Drills must be conducted for unusual threats.

Following are five basic approaches to managing hazardous materials:

1. *Restricting exposure at the source.* Good design and good procedures for use reduce bacteriological and chemical contamination. Air- and water-handling systems can be made almost completely safe. Special handling is necessary for contaminated wastes. Human vectors in the spread of infection are harder to control, and they include both caregivers and plant personnel. Hand hygiene, or hand washing, is basic to infection prevention; it takes repeated training and reinforcement to achieve improved patient outcomes.[17] Development of comprehensive control systems and monitoring of actual infection rates are clinical functions usually assigned to an infection control committee, which includes persons from facilities maintenance, housekeeping, and central supply services.

2. *Cleaning and removal.* The housekeeping department is usually responsible for cleaning and removing hazardous substances. Techniques are adjusted to the level of risk. Special cleaning materials and associate protective gear are necessary for handling spills of hazardous material.

3. *Attention to exposed patients, visitors, and associates.* Trauma or infection from contaminants can occur either during patient treatment or in cleaning and disposing of equipment. Needle sticks are a common safety hazard for clinical associates. The OSHA standard to protect workers from exposure to bloodborne pathogens requires employers to maintain an exposure control plan, ensure the use of personal protective equipment, provide initial and ongoing training, maintain records, report exposures to the required bodies,[18] and initiate post-exposure prophylaxis, if indicated.[19] Well-designed clinical waste–removal systems protect associates and guests. Any associate or guest believed to be injured or exposed should receive care following protocols recommended by the Centers for Disease Control and Prevention. Workers' compensation insurance covers treatment costs and loss of income for any employee injury.

4. *Epidemiologic analysis of failures.* Studies of the incidence of specific illnesses and injuries can identify process improvements and, in the case of communicable diseases, detect impending epidemics. The work requires special training in epidemiology.

5. *Strategic management of waste disposal.* HCOs have sewage and solid wastes to dispose of. The basic strategy is to select supplies that minimize waste, to recycle whenever possible, and to meet special handling needs. Used needles and blades represent a particular problem and are handled through a dedicated collection system from point of use to ultimate destruction.

HCOs usually contract for hazardous materials and waste removal. The contractor team is deeply integrated into the HCO to coordinate these activities. They work side by side with employees on the job and on numerous process improvement teams (PITs).

Fire Safety

A life-safety program protects persons and property from fire hazards. The life-safety management plan must include provisions for staff education on life-safety issues, a plan for emergency procedures, and periodic plan review. In addition, the plan must address facility-wide and area-specific fire response, evacuation routes, and specific roles and responsibilities of personnel at and away from a fire's point of origin and in preparing for building evacuation. Additional written policies must address recognized hazards and construction projects.[20] State licensure, Joint Commission accreditation,[21] and Medicare certification requirements enforce compliance.

The National Fire Protection Association Life Safety Code requires routine inspection and maintenance of facilities and often dictates specifications of new construction. Although facilities must comply with code in effect when they are opened, when a renovation is made to an area, all violations of current code must be corrected. The degree of departure from current code is an important factor in renovation and remodeling plans. An old building may contain many violations and be costly to renovate.

Although these provisions are frequently viewed as onerous, fire safety is one area where U.S. HCOs approach zero defect. Reported fires and fire injuries are extremely rare.

Medical Equipment

HCOs require a wide variety of specialized medical equipment that must be maintained near optimum operating condition and repaired or replaced as necessary. Apparatus-like ventilators, magnetic resonance imaging machines, ultrasound equipment, multichannel chemical analyzers, electronic monitoring equipment, heart and lung pumps, and surgical lasers and robots have become commonplace. The acquisition, maintenance, and replacement of this equipment require specially trained personnel (usually called biomedical or clinical engineers), who can be either employees or contractors. Their understanding of purposes, mechanics, hazards, and requirements allows them to increase the reliability of the machinery and reduce operating costs.

The role of clinical engineering includes the following activities:

- Assisting the user department or group to develop specifications, review competing sources, and select medical equipment
- Verifying that power, weight, size, and safety requirements are met
- Contracting for preventive and routine maintenance, or arranging training for internal maintenance personnel

- Periodically inspecting equipment for safety and effectiveness
- Developing plans for replacement when necessary

Utilities

Most HCOs need highly reliable supplies of all utilities. Utilities for most outpatient offices are no different from those for other commercial buildings, but inpatient hospitals operate sophisticated utility systems that provide air, steam, and water at several temperatures and pressures and filter some air to reduce bacterial contamination.[22] The enhanced performance requires extra safeguards against failure.

Electrical systems are particularly complex. Feeds from two or more substations, approaching the hospital from different directions, are desirable. In addition, the hospital must have on-site generating capability to sustain emergency surgery, ventilator, safety lighting, and communication operations. Critical areas must be able to switch to the emergency supply automatically.

Several utilities are unique to hospitals. Most hospitals pipe oxygen and suction to all patient care areas. Many also pipe nitrous oxide to surgical areas. Many hospitals use pneumatic tubes to transport small items such as paper records, drugs, and specimens. A few use robot cart systems to transport large supplies.

Materials Management

HCOs typically spend 25 to 30 percent of their budget on supplies. Most supply costs are represented in the following inventory groups, which are either large volumes of inexpensive items (such as foodstuffs) or relatively small volumes of expensive items (such as implants):

- Surgical supplies and implants
- Pharmaceuticals, intravenous solutions, and medical gases
- Foodstuffs
- Linens
- Dressings, kits, and supplies for patient care

Materials management concentrates supply purchases under a single unit that is responsible for meeting standards of quality and service at a minimum total cost. The materials management function includes the supply chain activities shown in Exhibit 12.6.

Materials managers work with users, including clinical users like the pharmacy and therapeutics committee, to identify the most economical supplies consistent with patient needs. Many of the costliest supplies are physician-preference items. Their use is standardized through the protocol-setting process. Buyers then negotiate prices, manage inventories, and maintain accounting records of use.

EXHIBIT 12.6
Functions
of Materials
Management

Material selection and control
Specifications for cost-effective
    supplies
Standardization of items
Reduction in the number of items

Purchasing
Standardized purchasing procedures
Competitive bid
Annual or periodic contracts
Group purchasing contracts

Receipt, storage, and protection
Reduction of inventory size
Control of shipment size and frequency
Reduction of handling
Reduction of damage or theft
Economical warehousing

Processing
Elimination of processing by purchase
    or contract
Improved processing methods
Reduced reprocessing or turnaround
    time

Distribution
Elimination or automation of ordering
Improved delivery methods
Reduced end-user inventories
Reduced wastage and unauthorized
    usage

*Revenue enhancement and cost
    accounting*
Uniform records of supplies usage
Integration of clinical ordering and
    patient billing systems

Improvement of materials management lies in systems that achieve the lowest overall costs, rather than those that simply purchase at the least expensive price.[23,24] End-user involvement—often on *value analysis committees*—to specify supplies is a critical component. Working with PITs and end users, materials management personnel strive to standardize items, reduce the number of different items purchased, establish criteria for appropriate quality, and eliminate unnecessary purchases. They examine alternative processes and identify improved methods and new supply specifications. For example, disposables may be compared to reusable alternatives.

Most important, the large volumes of standardized materials can be controlled more carefully for quality, and the high quantity can be leveraged to negotiate lower prices. The purchasing process itself uses long-term contracting and competitive bidding to reduce prices. Most well-managed organizations now use **group purchasing**—cooperatives that use the collective buying power of several organizations to leverage prices downward. Some large vendors offer comprehensive materials management, providing a complete service at competitive costs.

Group purchasing
Alliances that use the collective buying power of
several organizations to leverage prices downward.

Vendors can reduce the cost of the materials-handling system. Automation of inventories, ordering, and billing reduces handling costs. Most major vendors supply just-in-time service, effectively bearing the cost of inventory management as part of their activities. Vendors guarantee specific quality levels and are certified to comply with standards of the International Standards

Organization. Compliance eliminates the need for routine sampling of received goods. Centralized storage protects against theft and damage. Careful accounting and division of duties guard against theft and embezzlement. Some bulk supplies are delivered by robots to reduce costs. Finally, electronic records of supply usage provide data for cost analysis.

Emergency Preparedness and Disaster Management

HCOs must have a planned and systematic response to emergencies and disasters. The programs shown in Exhibit 12.7 are deliberate efforts to ensure operations continue under exceptionally stressful circumstances (e.g., natural and manmade disasters) or to systematically improve outcomes of emergency management. The Joint Commission standards include these (and more) general standards for life-safety protection and emergency management.[25]

Emergency management includes four phases: mitigation, preparedness, response, and recovery.

Emergency preparation for unplanned and unexpected mass-casualty events—such as natural disasters, pandemics, large-scale accidents, civil disturbance, or terrorist attacks—is an important and expected function of community HCOs. *Disaster* is defined as any event that suddenly increases demand substantially beyond the HCO's normal capacity. Advance warning, medical needs, and the number and severity of injuries differ greatly depending on the disaster. Terrorist attacks have drawn the nation's attention, but the most common disasters are storms and large-scale accidents such as fires and mass-transport crashes.[26]

When disaster strikes, people turn instinctively to the hospital. Victims are brought by rescue vehicles, in private cars, or by other means. Even a large

Program	Examples
Emergency preparedness	Disaster plan Disaster training and routine drills Disaster utilities and communications management Leadership involvement Collaboration with community response partners Annual review and approval by senior leadership Evaluation of all disaster occurrences and drills to identify OFIs
Life safety and fire protection	Evacuation plans and routes Routine inspection and testing of fire suppression equipment Preparation for radioactive or chemical contamination Life-safety training and drills

EXHIBIT 12.7
Emergency Management Requirements

OFI: opportunity for improvement

emergency service can face 20 times its normal peak load with little warning. Word of disaster spreads quickly through local radio, television, phone conversations, and social media (e.g., Twitter, Facebook). The hospital may be inundated with visitors, families, and well-meaning volunteers in addition to the sick and injured. Communication with other community agencies is essential, and normal channels are often overwhelmed or inoperable.

The clinical response to mass casualties begins with **triage**, a method for sorting patients according to the urgency of their need for care. Although specific events vary, generally only a small fraction of victims require hospitalization. A great many more require ambulatory treatment. Temporary stabilization is often important. The Centers for Disease Control and Prevention maintains a website of clinical information for both professionals and the public. It provides advice on treatment responses and mass-casualty management.[27]

Triage
A method of sorting patients according to the urgency of their need for care.

An effective HCO response requires a detailed plan; normal operations must be suspended to the extent possible so that personnel, space, equipment, and supplies can be reallocated to the "surge."[28] The design of the plan is a major project that requires the coordinated efforts of virtually all HCO leadership.[29] The elements of the response include

- rapid assembly of clinical and other personnel;
- inclusion of HCO leaders;
- reassignment of tasks, space, and equipment;
- establishment of supplementary telephone and radio communication;
- triage of arriving injured;
- temporary shelter for the homeless;
- continued care of patients already in the hospital;
- housing and food for hospital associates; and
- provision of information to the media, volunteers, and families.

The American Hospital Association (AHA) maintains a disaster preparedness website[30] and prepared an analysis of needs in the first 48 hours following an attack. The AHA identified additional areas that must be addressed to respond to terrorist activity:

- Communication and notification
- Disease surveillance, disease reporting, and laboratory identification
- Personal protective equipment
- Dedicated decontamination facilities
- Medical/surgical and pharmaceutical supplies
- Mental health resources

Others have noted that extended disasters, such as September 11, 2001, and Hurricane Katrina, severely stress associates, and provision for relief and rehabilitation for associates is important.[31]

Training for disaster is difficult, and results are uncertain.[32] The plan must be tested as realistically as possible, and the test often uncovers substantial weaknesses. Once tested, the plan must be rehearsed periodically and include drills with mock casualties and postdrill evaluation.[33,34]

The hospital's response must be coordinated with other community resources. Police, fire, and public health organizations are immediately involved, and schools, churches, and businesses can be converted for emergency needs. Coordination requires careful collaboration on roles, alternative plans, public messages, communications, and central leadership.[35] A military-type command structure is necessary to reduce confusion and address rapidly changing situations. Government public safety personnel generally assume this role, under emergency powers.

The disaster response requires broad involvement from all associates. The need to convert spaces, enhance communication, expand supply distribution, and arrange utilities gives the facilities management department a central role.

Performance Improvement

Performance improvement for environment-of-care services must deal with three realities:

1. The services must view themselves as competing for customer approval. Satisfaction of customer requirements, including both price and quality, must be the consuming objective.
2. Many environment services are delivered by long-term contract with outside vendors, often called *strategic partners*. The contracts must meet terms that include continuous improvement. No vendor or employed service team can consider itself independent of benchmarks and competing suppliers. HCOs can solicit offers from competing companies and compare outside competition to their internal capability. The selected provider should be able to document near-benchmark performance on the operational scorecard, and the contract should explicitly reference continued benchmarking, annual goals, and improvement.
3. As a result of strategic partnerships and of the capital requirements for environmental services, improvement planning must adopt a multiyear horizon.

Environment-of-care services must seek "world class" benchmarks and best practices. A housekeeping service, for example, should compare its performance to hotels. Food service must draw its benchmarks from commercial restaurants. At the same time, environment-of-care services must meet the specific needs of sick patients and integrate their services with the other systems of the HCO. Improvement opportunities often include process revisions, cross-training, revised scheduling, and special needs that must be coordinated with other units.

Major change in environmental services, such as replacing a vendor, requires long time windows and multiyear forecasting. For example, consider an organization that has operated its own inventory for many years. Its existing storage and distribution equipment is still useful but is aging and already less efficient than current models. As long as the equipment is still serviceable, contract inventory management may not be price competitive, but when the organization faces a major investment to replace that equipment, contract services are suddenly more attractive. Similarly, an opportunity to use the existing space for more productive activities will make contract service more attractive. These needs must be anticipated months or years in advance to gain maximum advantage.

People

Managers and Professional Personnel

Environment of care has a few widely recognized educational programs. Contract management firms that have extensive on-the-job training programs may be the best source for management talent. A bachelor's degree in engineering is generally considered necessary for facility operation managers, particularly if construction responsibilities are included. Some large organizations also employ architects, a profession with both formal education and licensure.

The American Society for Healthcare Engineering is a professional association that offers publications and educational opportunities.[36] There are licensure requirements for professional engineers and architects in a consulting practice, but they do not apply to employment situations. The AHA offers five certificates in facilities services: certified healthcare environmental services professional, certified healthcare facility manager, certified materials and resource professional, certified professional in healthcare risk management, and certified healthcare constructor.[37] These certifications stress experience and practical training, and they are open to high school graduates.[38] Clinical engineers have baccalaureate degrees in engineering and a sequence of professional recognition.[39] Maintenance services on clinical equipment are provided by biomedical equipment technicians. Materials managers should acquire purchasing and supply chain management knowledge, including general business education and relevant experience. Much of the needed knowledge can also be acquired through a well-supervised work experience, which need not be in healthcare. A professional association—Association for Healthcare Resource & Materials Management—provides educational materials and services to supply chain professionals.[40] Security managers frequently have active police experience and at least a bachelor's degree in their field. Food service managers have a bachelor's degree and extensive experience in bulk food preparation.

Several professions are involved in environmental safety. Infection prevention is within the purview of an infection prevention practitioner—a nurse or another clinician with special education and training in infectious diseases and epidemiology or certification by the Association for Professionals in Infection Control and Epidemiology—and generally an infectious disease physician consultant. Organizations with high-voltage radiation therapy services usually employ a radiation physicist who can also assist with radiation safety standards and compliance with the Nuclear Regulatory Commission. Large organizations employ toxicologists to assist with control of chemical contamination. There is an engineering specialty known as safety engineering. Consultative services are available in many of these areas. The Centers for Disease Control and Prevention and local public health departments may also have useful resources.

Outside Contractors

All plant services except facilities planning can be provided by contract with outside vendors. The plant functions and their components differ little from hospital to hospital, allowing contractors to develop significant advantages in specialized knowledge. Facilities construction, facility operation, maintenance and guest services, and clinical engineering are often provided by outside vendors. Some supply companies provide complete management of the supply function. Two forms of contracting arrangements are used. In one, all the associates of the service work for the contractor. In the other, probably more common, form, management personnel work for the contractor while hourly workers are the HCO's employees. The contractor supplies processes, training, performance measures, and supervision in both models.

The contract should specify the performance measures to be used in the operational scorecard. The HCO should negotiate annual improvement goals with the contractors as it does with internal suppliers. It should monitor performance against the goals and independently audit and benchmark as many of the measures as possible. The contract should be periodically reopened, allowing change of vendor if necessary. The vendor competes against similar vendors and against the possibility of internal operations and wins the competition because it does as good a job overall as any alternative.

Training Needs

As environmental control methods and equipment become more sophisticated, workers require orientation, process training, and continuing education on an ongoing basis. In addition to job content, purpose, and method, employee training for several environment-of-care areas must include guest relations. As participation on improvement teams increases, associates must be trained in performance improvement fundamentals. Much technical training is assigned to contractors, but elements such as orientation and supervision must be integrated with the HCO's training.

Supervisors need mastery of the work methods and explicit training in supervision. In many settings, the folklore of the transactional boss who gives orders and has special privileges must be replaced with an understanding of the supportive transformational leader who is obligated to find answers to employee questions. Formal training, including case studies and role-playing, establishes the desired model. Constant reinforcement is necessary to keep it in place. Supervisors also need advanced training in performance improvement, budgeting, and regulatory compliance.

Associate training programs must be carried out at a high school level, and in many communities they must be available in several languages. The emphasis is on action, practice, graphics, and only lastly words. All training programs present important opportunities to build the employee's pride in craftsmanship and loyalty to the organization.

Incentives and Rewards

The most important incentives are nonmonetary. Pride of achievement is probably the most important. It is supported by prompt reporting of formal measures, well-designed methods, appropriate training, and responsive supervision. Recognition of achievement includes both encouragement from the supervisor and celebration of team achievements. The amount of recognition should be tailored to the level of achievement: Supervisors should recognize any positive response; coworkers should recognize above-average results; and the organization at large should recognize extraordinary achievement.

Explicit monetary incentives are most powerful as supplements to nonmonetary incentives. Even a small payment serves to show the seriousness of management intent. The gain-sharing approach, with negotiated goals and ongoing measures of progress, is effective. When contractors manage the service and employees work for the HCO, the incentive must be comparable to opportunities in similar HCO job classes.

Organization

Exhibit 12.8 shows a general organizational model for plant systems in a large HCO. Any element in Exhibit 12.8 can be contracted to an outside firm. Facility planning and space allocation are the most likely to be retained internally. A contract manager employed by the institution must be designated at the level of the contract. For example, if food service is contracted, the guest services manager is designated as contract manager. Contract managers are often supported by committees made up of various users. The committees form a platform for addressing OFIs arising in the services.

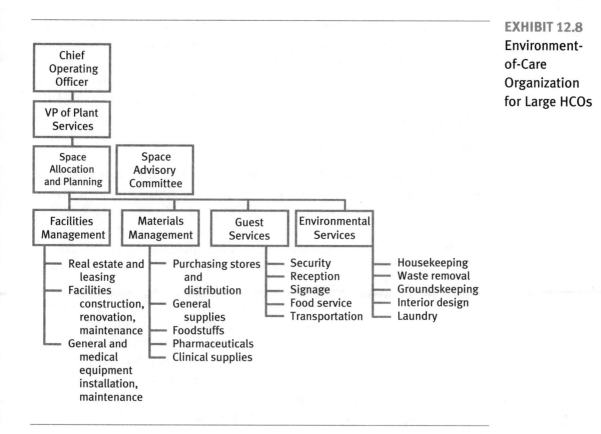

EXHIBIT 12.8
Environment-of-Care
Organization
for Large HCOs

Measures

All environmental services must first be reliable and safe, then satisfactory to associates and guests, and finally efficient. Measures for the six dimensions of the operational scorecard are well developed and can usually be benchmarked from other HCOs or comparable services in other industries. Human resources measures are similar to those in clinical and other support systems. Customer satisfaction measures recognize that all the other units of the organization are internal customers. Many services also have external customers: patients, families, and other guests.

Demand is usually forecast by analysis of historical data on the incidence and duration of demand for each identified physical resource. Peak loads are frequently important. Analysis of cyclical fluctuation and other variation in demand is frequently required to set sound resource expectations.

Many activities of the plant system require short-term forecasts, with horizons ranging from hours to months. For example, operating room activity may require that plant services be able to raise or lower room temperature in advance of surgical start times. Efficiency in supply and service processes, such as housekeeping, heating, and food service, depends on careful adjustment to variation in demand. Inventory usage forecasts can be used to minimize out-of-stock items and emergency trips, and to maintain optimum inventory levels and ordering cycles. The preparation of these forecasts is normally the obligation of the appropriate environment-of-care unit, with guidance from finance and planning. Experienced managers can often make useful subjective refinements to statistically prepared forecasts.

Resource Consumption and Effectiveness

Environment-of-care services and products are used by all units of any HCO. Some products and services are sold to patients or customers, but most are consumed by HCO units. Managing the efficiency and effectiveness of these services requires careful accounting, as shown in Exhibit 12.9. Establishing a **transfer price** based on the unit cost allows an in-house "sale" that emulates a market purchase and substantially clarifies accountability. Modern cost accounting (Chapter 13) has allowed accurate estimates of unit cost for most of the goods and services provided by environmental care. The alternative to transfer pricing is cost allocation, which simply assigns a portion of costs based on some approximation, such as allocating housekeeping costs on square footage of space.

Transfer price

Imputed price for an item of goods or service transferred between two units of the same organization, such as housekeeping services provided to nursing units. The transfer price is based on cost of individual units.

Transfer pricing has three important advantages:

1. The unit cost of producing the service can be benchmarked, improving the producing unit's goal setting.

EXHIBIT 12.9 Implications of Cost Accounting on Environmental Services	*Costing Method*	*Impact on Producing Activity*	*Impact on Consuming Activity*
	Transfer pricing	Total cost per unit of service (TC/U) is calculated using activity-based costing TC/U can be benchmarked TC/U can be compared to that of the competition	"Buys" service and controls units consumed Units/patient or customer can be benchmarked, established by protocol, or established by evaluating customer needs and satisfaction
	Cost allocation	Total direct cost (TDC) for producing activity TDC can rarely be benchmarked	Receives an allocated "indirect cost" charge for service Indirect cost cannot be benchmarked Consumer has no incentive to control use

2. The unit cost can be compared to competing alternatives, such as purchasing instead of making the service or centralizing producers for efficiency.

3. The consuming unit can benchmark the volume of service used and establish OFIs to optimize the quantity of service. (Note that the "optimum" service is the one that best fulfills the user's mission, but it is not necessarily the least expensive.)

Quality

Exhibit 12.10 shows important measures of quality of environment-of-care services. Compliance of a product or service with technical specification can be measured. Many processes can be inspected by unbiased experts, who score

Type	Approaches	Examples
Outcomes	Technical standards	Many environmental services have explicit technical standards developed by organizations such as the National Institute of Science and Technology or the American Society for Quality
	Incident counts	Guest and associate accidents Delay and failure rates Service interruption rates
	Surveys	Guest and associate satisfaction
	User complaints	Service complaints
Process	Raw materials	Technical standards Compliance to purchase specification Failures and returns
	Service/product inspections	Food preparation Cleanliness Job completion
	Contract compliance	Return rates On-time supplies delivery
	Supply failures	Back-ordered items
	Inventory wastage	Losses of supplies
	Automated monitoring	Atmospheric control Power and utility failure
Structure	Facility	Life-safety compliance
	Equipment	Elevator inspections
	Worker qualifications	Stationary engineer coverage

EXHIBIT 12.10
Measures of Quality for Environment-of-Care Services

the result. Many services have automated records of failure or delay. Others can be estimated from user or inspector surveys.

Inspections are critical to laundry service, food service, supplies, maintenance, and housekeeping. Subjective judgment is usually required, but it is reliable when inspectors are trained and follow clear standards for cleanliness, temperature, taste, appearance, and so on. The frequency of inspection is adjusted to the level of performance, and performance is improved by training and methods rather than by negative feedback. Work reports—brief notes that identify specific events or issues—reveal correctable problem areas in plant maintenance and materials management.

Benchmarks and scientific standards for these values are widely available. Numerous consultants offer information on labor standards for laundries, kitchens, and the like and on cost standards for energy use, construction, renovation, and security. The AHA publishes a manual of materials management supply-cost benchmarks.[41] Constraints on costs are derived from two sources—the competitive prices of outside vendors and the internal needs developed from the budget guidelines. The former are preferable wherever they can be obtained.

Managerial Issues

The focal points for senior leadership attention to the environment of care include facilities planning and space allocation, the selection and management of outsourcing contracts, and the integration of facilities operations with other activities. The first two of these often generate expensive and difficult decisions. The third is an important source of failures in efficiency, safety, and associate satisfaction.

Facilities Planning and Space Allocation

Facilities planning and space allocation present unique management problems. Space has important symbolic and cultural implications (like "the corner office") as well as major practical implications. It is immutable and unique. Each square foot is exactly that, but because of location, it is different from every other square foot. The decisions have profound implications for individual stakeholders. Conflict is normal and must be systematically managed. Management and governance focus all decisions on the mission.

Facilities planners use the best available objective data to forecast future needs, make their work as transparent as possible, draw all affected parties into the discussion at an early stage, establish and live by the rules for making the decisions, and allow appeals. The strategy for preventing and resolving conflict is to make sure that facts, rather than influence, determine the outcome and to aim for financial success necessary to remain competitive.

Selection and Management of Outsourcing Contracts

The questions of what to outsource, with whom to outsource, and how to ensure the effectiveness of outsourced services are all challenging. Managers have a duty to see that objective measures and benchmarks are in place for the entire environment of care. With these measures in place, the opportunities for improvement are clear to all. Questions such as "Should we outsource?" or "Should we change suppliers?" convert to "What improvements must we make to reach benchmark, and how do we achieve them?" In this format, the current supplier is usually given a chance to improve, and it usually does. Supplier change is not necessary because the current supplier changes to do the job better.

Service managers make it clear that the benchmarks are realistic goals and provide the support to learn and change so that progress can be made. They establish a culture in which ignoring the opportunity is unacceptable. If the service is contracted, the contract manager reinforces the culture, recognizing that service alternatives do exist but that retaining the current supplier is often the best choice.

Integration of Facilities Operations with Other Activities

Vendors and their associates cannot be viewed as outsiders. "Strategic partner" means "part of our team." Many issues arise from the coordination between clinical services and plant services. New food service systems must coordinate with nursing, patient transportation must adapt to new facility layouts and service needs, and new patient care protocols require new supplies and new delivery methods. PITs must incorporate all the involved services, regardless of contract status.

PIT participation is valuable in three senses. First, the exchange of information leads to a better result, particularly with a skilled vendor that has experience at many HCOs. Second, participants gain insight into the underlying customer needs. They come away from the process understanding why the improvement was necessary and more committed to making it work. Third, participation is a reward. PIT assignments empower associates and provide an opportunity to reward effort.

Additional Resources

Guenther, G., and R. Vittori. 2013. *Sustainable Healthcare Architecture*, 2nd ed. New York: Wiley.

Joint Commission. 2014. *2014 Environment of Care Essentials for Health Care*. Oakbrook Terrace, IL: Joint Commission Resources.

_____. 2012. *Emergency Management in Health Care: An All-Hazards Approach*, 2nd ed. Oakbrook Terrace, IL: Joint Commission Resources.

_____. 2010. *Environment of Care Management Plans*, 3rd ed. Oakbrook Terrace, IL: Joint Commission Resources.

———. 2009. *Planning, Design, and Construction of Health Care Facilities*, 2nd ed. Oakbrook Terrace, IL: Joint Commission Resources.

Kros, J. F., and E. Brown. 2013. *Health Care Operations and Supply Chain Management: Strategy, Operations, Planning, and Control*. San Francisco: Jossey-Bass.

Ledlow, G. R., A. P. Corry, and M. A. Cwiek. 2007. *Optimize Your Healthcare Supply Chain Performance: A Strategic Approach*. Chicago: Health Administration Press.

Puckett, R. P. 2012. *Foodservice Manual for Health Care Institutions*, 4th ed. AHA Press.

Rich, C. R., J. K. Singleton, and S. S. Wadhwa. 2013. *Sustainability for Healthcare Management*. New York: London: Routledge.

Shore, D. A. 2014. *Launching and Leading Change Initiatives in Health Care Organizations: Managing Successful Projects*. San Francisco: Jossey-Bass Public Health.

Verderber, S. 2010. *Innovations in Hospital Architecture*. New York: Routledge.

Notes

1. Ulrich, R. S., L. L. Berry, X. Quan, and J. T. Parish. 2010. "A Conceptual Framework for the Domain of Evidence-Based Design." *Health Environments Research and Design Journal* 4 (1): 95–114.

2. Bronson Methodist Hospital. 2005. Malcolm Baldrige National Quality Award Application. [Online information; retrieved 6/1/14.] www.baldrige.nist.gov/Contacts_Profiles.htm.

3. Hewitt, D. H. 2010. "Models from Past Mold the Future in Evidence-Based Health Care Design." *Health Progress* 91 (2): 9–13.

4. Bernard, P. J. 2010. "New Urbanism Drives Hospital Site Plan." *Health Progress* 91 (2): 21–25.

5. Hosking, J. E., and R. J. Jarvis. 2003. "Developing a Replacement Facility Strategy: Lessons from the Healthcare Sector." *Journal of Facilities Management* 2 (2): 214–28.

6. Hosking, J. E. 2004. "What Really Drives Better Outcomes?" *Frontiers of Health Services Management* 21 (1): 35–39.

7. Green Guide for Health Care. 2014. Home page. [Online information; retrieved 6/1/14.] www.gghc.org/.

8. Zimring, C. M., G. L. Augenbroe, E. B. Malone, and B. L. Sadler. 2008. "Implementing Healthcare Excellence: The Vital Role of the CEO in Evidence-Based Design." Healthcare Leadership White Paper Series, No. 3. Atlanta, GA: Center for Health Design, Georgia Institute of Technology.

9. Rich, C. R., J. K. Singleton, and S. S. Wadhwa. 2013. *Sustainability for Healthcare Management*, 21–36. New York: Routledge.

10. Ulrich et al. (2010).

11. Joint Commission. 2013. "Environment of Care Management Plans: Making Sure Your Plans Get the Job Done." *Joint Commission Perspectives* 33 (6): 6–7.

12. Barnas, K. 2011. "ThedaCare's Business Performance System: Sustaining Continuous Daily Improvement Through Hospital Management in a Lean Environment." *Joint Commission Journal on Quality and Patient Safety* 37 (9): 387–99.

13. Smith, M. H. 2002. "Vigilance Ensures a Safer Work Environment." *Nursing Management* 33 (11): 18–19.

14. Smith, M. H. 2002. "Condition Critical: Study Shows Many Hospitals Located in High-Crime Areas." *Health Facilities Management Magazine*. [Online article; retrieved 3/15/06.] www.hfmmagazine.com/hfmmagazine/index.jsp.

15. Environmental Protection Agency. 2014. "Medical Waste." [Online information; retrieved 6/1/14.] www.epa.gov/osw/nonhaz/industrial/medical.

16. Occupational Safety & Health Administration. 2006. "OSHA/NIOSH Interim Guidance: Chemical, Biological, Radiological, and Nuclear—Personal Protective Equipment Selection Matrix for Emergency Responders." [Online information; retrieved 6/1/14.] www.osha.gov/SLTC/emergencypreparedness/cbrnmatrix/index.html#Introduction.

17. Song, X., D. C. Stockwell, T. Floyd, B. L. Short, and N. Singh. 2013. "Improving Hand Hygiene Compliance in Health Care Workers: Strategies and Impact on Patient Outcomes." *American Journal of Infection Control* 41 (10): 101–105.

18. Occupational Safety & Health Administration. "Bloodborne Pathogens Standard." 29 CFR 1910.1030. [Online information; retrieved 6/15/14.] www.osha.gov/pls/oshaweb/owadisp.show_document?p_table=STANDARDS&p_id=10051.

19. Kuhar, D. T., D. K. Henderson, K. A. Struble, W. Heneine, V. Thomas, L. W. Cheever, A. Gomaa, and A. L. Panlilio; U.S. Public Health Service Working Group. 2013. "Updated U.S. Public Health Service Guidelines for the Management of Occupational Exposures to HIV and Recommendations for Postexposure Prophylaxis." *Infection Control and Hospital Epidemiology* 34 (9): 875–92.

20. National Fire Protection Association. 2012. *Fire Code Handbook, 2012 Edition.* [Online information; retrieved 6/1/14.] www.nfpa.org/catalog.

21. Joint Commission. 2014. "Environment of Care." In *Comprehensive Accreditation Manual for Hospitals.* Oakbrook Terrace, IL: Joint Commission Resources.

22. Sehulster, L., and R. Y. Chinn. 2003. "Guidelines for Environmental Infection Control in Health-Care Facilities. Recommendations of CDC and the Healthcare Infection Control Practices Advisory Committee (HICPAC)." *Morbidity and Mortality Weekly Report, Recommendations and Reports* 52 (RR-10): 1–42.

23. Long, G. 2005. "Pursuing Supply Chain Gains." *Healthcare Financial Management* 59 (9): 118–22.

24. Beth, S., D. N. Burt, W. Copacino, C. Gopal, H. L. Lee, R. P. Lynch, and S. Morris. 2003. "Supply Chain Challenges: Building Relationships." *Harvard Business Review* 81 (7): 64–73, 117.

25. American Society for Healthcare Engineering. 2014. "The Joint Commission." [Online information; retrieved 6/1/14.] www.ashe.org/advocacy/organizations/TJC/#.U5u0YrFcb08.

26. McGlown, K. J. 2004. *Terrorism and Disaster Management: Preparing Healthcare Leaders for the New Reality.* Chicago: Health Administration Press.

27. Centers for Disease Control and Prevention. "Mass Casualty Event Preparedness and Response." [Online information; retrieved 6/1/14.] www.bt.cdc.gov/masscasualties.

28. Ginter, P. M., W. J. Duncan, and M. Abdolrasulnia. 2007. "Hospital Strategic Preparedness Planning: The New Imperative." *Prehospital & Disaster Medicine* 22 (6): 529–36.

29. Joint Commission. 2013. "New and Revised Requirements Address Emergency Management Oversight." *Joint Commission Perspectives* 33 (7): 14–15.

30. American Hospital Association. 2014. "Emergency Readiness." [Online information; retrieved 6/1/14.] www.aha.org/advocacy-issues/emergreadiness/index.shtml.

31. Reissman, D. B., and J. Howard. 2008. "Responder Safety and Health: Preparing for Future Disasters." *Mount Sinai Journal of Medicine* 75 (2): 135–41.

32. Williams, J., M. Nocera, and C. Casteel. 2008. "The Effectiveness of Disaster Training for Health Care Workers: A Systematic Review." *Annals of Emergency Medicine* 52 (3): 211–22.

33. Agency for Healthcare Research and Quality. "Tool for Evaluating Core Elements of Hospital Disaster Drills." [Online information; retrieved 6/1/14.] www.ahrq.gov/prep/drillelements.

34. Jenckes, M. W., C. L. Catlett, E. B. Hsu, K. Kohri, G. B. Green, K. A. Robinson, E. B. Bass, and S. E. Cosgrove. 2007. "Development of Evaluation Modules for Use in Hospital Disaster Drills." *American Journal of Disaster Medicine* 2 (2): 87–95.

35. Joint Commission. 2006. "Surge Hospitals: Providing Safe Care in Emergencies." [Online information; retrieved 6/15/14.] www.jointcommission.org/assets/1/18/surge_hospital.pdf.

36. American Society of Healthcare Engineers. 2014. Home page. [Online information; retrieved 6/1/14.] www.ashe.org.

37. American Hospital Association. 2014. "AHA Certification Center." [Online information; retrieved 6/15/14.] www.aha.org/certifcenter/index.shtml.

38. American Hospital Association. 2014. Home page. [Online information; retrieved 6/1/14.] www.aha.org.

39. American College of Clinical Engineering. 2014. Home page. [Online information; retrieved 6/1/14.] www.accenet.org.

40. Association for Healthcare Resource & Materials Management. 2014. Home page. [Online information; retrieved 6/1/14.] www.ahrmm.org.

41. Association for Healthcare Resource & Materials Management. 2005. *2005 Performance Indicators Study on Healthcare Supply Cost Management.* Chicago: AHA Publishing.

13 FINANCIAL MANAGEMENT

Critical Issues in Financial Management

1. *Supporting an evidence-based culture:*
   How accounting
   - Identifies and reports costs
   - Supports the annual goal-setting process
   - Provides analysis and forecasts for performance improvement teams (PITs)

2. *Providing adequate financial resources:*
   How finance
   - Identifies long-term financial needs
   - Manages debt and liquid assets to meet needs
   - Negotiates contracts with health insurers to maximize revenue
   - Develops ownership structures that facilitate strategic partnerships

3. *Promoting integrity:*
   How internal and external auditing
   - Ensure accuracy of numbers, even those involving complex calculations
   - Support a culture where honesty is expected
   - Protect the organization's assets

Questions for Discussion

These questions are about applying the chapter content. It's often helpful to discuss them with classmates or mentors, gaining different perspectives on the issues.

1. Why are performance measures so complicated? Concepts like *cost per case* or *percent postoperative infections* seem simple enough. Why must we use Financial Accounting Standards Board rules and National Healthcare Safety Network definitions, and maintain internal and external audits? What would happen if we didn't do these things? Would an HCO ever design its own measures that were different from the national ones?

2. Suppose you are on a PIT to evaluate an HCO's goal-setting processes. What criteria should the processes meet? How could the criteria be measured? How hard would it be to benchmark them? Beyond the measures, what else would you do to identify opportunities for improvement in the process?

3. A hard-working associate says to a senior manager, "Our unit just got the bill for human resources. It was huge! We had to pay for the mandatory training for our new supervisor, plus the annual HIPAA, harassment, and disaster management training. Why do we have to pay for this? How do we know we're getting a fair price?" How does the senior manager respond?

4. How much should the audit functions cost? The system described is expensive; many organizations complain that it is excessive. What exactly are the benefits the organization gains from those expenditures, and how are they measured? How will the organization judge whether the investment is wise?

5. How does the organization evaluate its capital and liquid asset management program? What questions would you ask, and what numbers would you ask for, if you were exploring this question with the chief financial officer and her financial management team?

Financial management of the HCO controls all the assets; posts and collects all the revenue; settles all the financial obligations; arranges all the funding; and makes major contributions to strategic planning, performance measurement, and cost control. It deals directly with all the units of the organization, from the governing board to the primary accountability centers. Its role in HCOs is not substantially different from its role in other industries, although some of the approaches are modified to accommodate not-for-profit structures, health insurance contracts, and the complexity of care delivery.

This chapter describes the contribution that finance makes to other systems (i.e., those tasks that it must do to make the whole succeed). Finance and accounting are subject to much study, regulation, and standardization. Comprehensive texts describe its overall operation. (Several are listed in the Additional Resources section at the end of the chapter.) Laws, regulations, contracts, and standard practices control what is done in countless specific situations. This chapter emphasizes the activities that distinguish the most successful HCOs—principally, budgeting, cost reporting and analysis, strategic financial planning and provision of capital, and expanded use of the audits.

Purpose

The purposes of the finance system are to support the enterprise by

recording and reporting transactions that change the value of the firm;

assisting operations in setting and achieving performance improvements;

performing a financial analysis of new business opportunities, new programs, and asset acquisitions to assist governance in strategic planning;

arranging capital and operating funds to implement governance decisions;

and

guarding assets and resources against theft, waste, or loss, and guarding the information against distortion.

These five purposes are accomplished through three general functions—(1) controllership, incorporating the first two; (2) financial management, incorporating the third and fourth; and (3) auditing, addressing the last. The finance activity is expected to maintain its own continuous improvement function and support the rest of the HCO in its improvement efforts. The activities that support these functions are shown in Exhibit 13.1.

EXHIBIT 13.1
Functions of the
Finance System

Function	Activity	Purpose
Controllership		
Transaction accounting	Capture data on all operational transactions	Record and control resources and sales
Financial accounting	Capture nonoperational transactions Create financial reports	Establish value of organization Report to owners and external stakeholders
Managerial accounting	Prepare cost and revenue data for monitoring and performance improvement Prepare special studies for planning and evaluation of improvements	Support all work teams with resource and output data Support PITs with forecasts and models
Goal setting and budgeting	Promulgate budget guidelines and budget packages Forecast major demand measures Compile operating, financial, and capital budgets	Support line management in setting performance goals Coordinate organization-wide activities Support strategic decisions
Financial Management		
Financial planning	Establish the long-range financial plan Conduct financial analysis of new business opportunities, new programs, and large asset acquisitions	Forecast the future viability of the organization Support analysis of alternative strategic opportunities Establish budget guidelines for profit, cost, and capital investment
Pricing clinical services	Develop pricing strategy and support specific price negotiations	Support maximum revenue to the institution and its physicians
Financial structures	Manage multiple corporate structures	Flexibility of financing and operating arrangements Containment of business risks
Securing and managing liquid assets	Manage debt, joint ventures, and stock and equity accounts	Minimize cost of capital Maximize return on assets
Managing multicorporate accounting	Manage working capital Maintain collections and payments	Minimize cost of working capital Settle the organization's accounts with patients, suppliers, and employees

EXHIBIT 13.1
Functions of the
Finance System
(continued)

Function	Activity	Purpose
Auditing		
Internal audits	Verify accounting transactions	Ensure accuracy of performance management reports Guard against loss and diversion of property
Compliance review	Review health insurance contracts, physician compensation, and pricing policies	Ensure compliance with law and regulation
External audits	Review accounting systems and decisions affecting financial reports	Attesting to accuracy of financial reports
Continuous Improvement of the Accounting and Finance Functions		
Stakeholder satisfaction	Monitor and benchmark satisfaction with accounting and financial performance	Ensure compliance with external requirements and satisfaction of customer and associate stakeholders
Improve performance	Identify, pursue, and implement OFIs	Implement more effective methods and results

OFI: opportunity for improvement; PIT: process improvement team

Controllership

Transaction Accounting

The transaction accounting function records and reports all transactions that affect the value of the firm and its subsidiaries. Transactions form the basis of all analysis and reporting. Most transactions are either *revenue transactions*—those that provide elements of care to patients or other services such as meals to families—or *expense transactions*—those that acquire resources such as personnel, supplies, and equipment. The physical transactions—such as patient days of care, hours worked, and drugs used—are generally captured by the knowledge management system described in Chapter 10. Accounting attaches a dollar value and assigns each transaction to a mission-related category. Once captured, valued, and assigned, the transactions support three different analyses—financial accounting, performance reporting, and managerial accounting studies. Transaction accounting keeps finance personnel involved in most areas of the organization.

Revenue transactions record virtually all the HCO's routine cash acquisition, except gifts, loans, and sales of assets. Computerization permits recording extensive detail: the patient, service, quantity, time, and unit or associate supplying the service. The record must meet Health Insurance Portability and Accountability Act confidentiality requirements.[1] When organized by individual patient, revenue transactions create the **patient ledger**—a detailed record of the individual services or supplies rendered to each patient. The ledger is a financial reflection of the electronic health record described in Chapter 10.

Patient ledger
Account of the charges rendered to an individual patient.

Expense transactions describe all commitments to pay cash. Data captured include the ordering or using person and unit, quantities, allocation, time, and prices of the resource purchased or disbursed. Cost ledgers are organized by type of resource (e.g., labor, supplies). The payroll system records hours worked by the employees, generates paychecks, and produces data on labor costs. The supply system provides count and cost data on supplies, issues checks for purchased goods and services, and maintains inventories.

General ledger
Technically, the record of all the firm's transactions; the term often refers to the fixed and collective assets, such as depreciation, that must be allocated to operational units.

Some expense transactions are internal rather than external exchanges; these are called **general ledger** transactions. General ledger entries assign capital costs through depreciation of long-term assets, adjust inventory values, and allocate expenses of central services. They tend to reflect resources that are shared by the organization as a whole rather than by individual accountability centers, and they tend to deal with resources that last considerably longer than one budget or financial cycle.

The value of most transactions is set by the market (i.e., the price of either a purchase or a sale), but because of general ledger transactions and the complexity of healthcare finance, external prices are not available for all transactions or all levels of aggregation. As a simple example, depreciation is an estimate of the loss in value of buildings and equipment based on an arbitrary assumption about the future life; the true change in value is unknown. It is priced according to widely accepted and audited rules so that the estimates are uniform and reliable, although not necessarily valid. More complicated issues arise from "bundled" revenue. Inpatient care is priced as a package based on diagnosis-related groups (DRGs). Several patient care teams treat most patients; the revenue for each team is not available. Although the pharmacy sells many prescriptions to outpatients for established market prices, it sells many to inpatients where payment is bundled and no pharmacy price is available. Exhibit 13.2 shows the availability of price information by level of aggregate. Estimates must be used when the transaction information is used in the shaded areas. They are prepared as a managerial accounting function.

Financial Accounting

Financial accounting fulfills a direct obligation to the organization's owners and creditors and to the public. It assembles the transactions to state as

Aggregate Level	Revenue Transactions	Expense Transactions			
		Labor	Supplies	Equipment	General Ledger
Item of care	Partial[1]	Partial	Yes[2]	No	No
Patient	Partial[2]	Partial	Yes	No	No
Responsibility center	Partial	Yes	Yes	Yes	No
Disease group	Partial	Partial[3]	Yes	No	No
Payer group	Yes	Partial[4]	Yes	No	No
Institution	Yes	Yes	Yes	Yes	Yes

EXHIBIT 13.2
Availability of External Price Information, by Type of Transaction and Level of Aggregate

Notes:
1. Certain expensive services, such as physician visits or operating room use, are priced at the transaction level in fee-for-service payment systems but not in case-based or capitation payment systems. An estimate of the direct labor cost is generally available when fee transactions exist.
2. The price paid by the patient or third-party intermediary is available under fee-for-service and case-based payment but not under capitation.
3. The cost of labor to serve patients is directly priced for the more expensive components, where the time expended is captured in the record. Some services (e.g., security) are provided on an aggregate, rather than an individual, basis. Bedside nursing, an expensive component of inpatient care, is accounted at the nursing unit level.
4. Disease-group and payer-group transactions are aggregated from individual patients and are subject to the same limitations, except that the totals paid by each payer are captured directly.

accurately as possible the position of the institution as a whole in terms of the value of its assets, the equity residual to its owners, and the change in value occurring in each accounting period.

Reporting Financial Information

Four reports have become standard for HCOs and most other nongovernmental enterprises:

1. Balance sheet
2. Income or profit-and-loss statement
3. Statement of sources and uses of funds
4. Statement of changes in fund balances

These summarize the financial activities and situation of the organization in a form now almost universal in the business world. The entries are defined by the Financial Accounting Standards Board (FASB).

Financial statements are usually issued monthly to the associates and annually to outside stakeholders. They are a critical report to the governing board, which is obligated to monitor performance and protect assets on behalf of the owners. They constitute the record of the board's discharge of its obligation to exercise fiscal prudence.

The annual statements are audited by the external auditor—a public accounting firm that attests that the statements follow the FASB rules, fairly represent the financial position of the organization, and are free of material distortion. Audited statements are the basis for most of the organization's financial communication with the outside world. Financial intermediaries often demand access to HCO finances as a condition of payment. Audited income statements and balance sheets must be reported to the federal government as a condition of participation in Medicare. Once filed, the reports are accessible to the public under the Freedom of Information Act. Several states now require public release of financial reports as well. HCOs that issue bonds on public markets are also required to reveal standard financial information, plus pro formas that forecast their performance in future years.

Not-for-profit HCOs have substantial obligations to report their financial activities through the Internal Revenue Service (IRS) Form 990. The form becomes public information. It is intended to monitor the public's return for the organization's privilege of tax exemption. It requires reporting of income, profit, executive compensation, and community benefit for parent corporations, major subsidiaries, and joint ventures. Community benefit is identified as charitable care, bad debts, Medicaid losses, community health activities, formal education, and research. The reporting schedule requires estimation of the actual cost of each benefit. The values reported on Form 990 are subject to a "reasonableness" test.[2] The IRS may eliminate an HCO's tax exemption in whole or in part on the basis of the values reported.

Well-managed HCOs deliberately publish their financial reports as part of their program of community relations. Subsidiaries of integrated systems, both for-profit and not-for-profit, are not automatically required to disclose their financial information, but many multihospital organizations make them public as basic community relations.

Revenue Accounting

Gross revenue
An entry to the patient ledger of the charge for a specific healthcare service; no longer a meaningful measure.

Net revenue
Income actually received, as opposed to that initially posted; equal to gross revenue minus adjustments for bad debts, charity, and discounts to third parties.

Bad debt
Cost for patients who were expected to pay for care but did not.

Individual charges are associated with each transaction to calculate **gross revenue**, but the charges have become meaningless under aggregate payment contracts. The actual amount paid—**net revenue**—has become the meaningful value. Patient ledger transactions are summed to generate net operating revenue generated from patient care reported in the income statement.

Under Form 990 requirements, net revenue also specifies charity care—care given to the needy without expectation of payment—and **bad debts**—costs for patients who were expected to pay but did not do so. Patient ledger data are also used in many case-based payment schemes to identify catastrophically expensive cases, called *outliers*, that qualify for special additional payments.

Nonoperational Transactions

Nonoperating revenue—income generated from non-patient-care activities, including gifts, investments in securities, and earnings from unrelated businesses—is also accounted on the income statement. It is an important contribution to overall profit for many HCOs. The funds flow statement and balance sheet include a number of nonoperational transactions. The sale of assets and the incurrence of debt (and the sale of equity in for-profit companies) generate cash for the firm. The purchase of capital goods, the retirement of debt (dividends and repurchase of stock in for-profit companies), and charges for restructurings consume cash. These are recorded with the cash transactions of operations in a statement of sources and uses of funds or funds flow. Subsidiary corporations can be used to handle major ongoing operations, such as donations, unrelated businesses, or joint ventures. Their summary results are included in the owning corporation's balance sheet.

> **Nonoperating revenue**
> Income generated from non-patient-care activities, including investments in securities and earnings from unrelated businesses.

Managerial Accounting

Managerial accounting restructures transaction data to support monitoring, planning, setting expectations, and improving performance. Opposite to financial accounting, it is oriented to produce information for internal organization uses, allowing management decisions about revision, continuation, and discontinuation of services and monitoring operational measures of cost, efficiency, and demand. It is organized around an internal chart of accounts that identifies every accountable unit. It records quantities and costs of resources consumed by the unit, such as labor and supplies (direct costs), and allocated to the unit, such as depreciation and shared central services (indirect costs or overhead). Traditional allocated costs were often crude approximations; activity-based costing improves the estimates and allows more resources to be treated as direct costs.

> **Managerial accounting**
> A process of restructuring transaction data to support monitoring, planning, setting expectations, and improving performance of accountability centers.

Managerial Accounting Reports

Managerial accounting reports identify the quantities and cost of resources consumed, the pricing mechanism (market priced, transfer priced, or allocated), and the assigned transfer and allocated costs. Unit management can classify these costs as fixed, variable, or semi-variable. These reports are now usually electronic. They are available in summary or in detail for each accountable unit and larger aggregates, and they provide drill-down to individual transactions.

Managerial reports are useful as an ongoing audit of management performance, as a source of detail when an unexpected event occurs, and as a data source for managerial analyses and construction of the following year's goals. The cost reports allow any level of management to say, "Our costs are equal to or better than goals" and to identify the opportunities for improvement (OFIs) for next year's goals.

Managerial Accounting Analyses

The data in the reports can be accumulated and aggregated to support analyses of variation and what-if projections that allow management to identify and evaluate alternatives. Common uses of managerial accounting analyses include the following:

- Preparing and analyzing transfer prices and cost-allocation estimates
- Analyzing and forecasting trends in demand, cost, output, and efficiency
- Developing new budget expectations, particularly for new or expanded services when the operating conditions have changed
- Understanding seasonal and day-of-week variation
- Comparing local production with outside purchase, often called make-or-buy decisions
- Comparing alternative protocols or work processes, particularly those substituting capital for labor
- Ranking cost-saving opportunities to identify promising areas in which to eliminate or reduce use
- Preparing forecasts for expanding or closing units

Managerial accounting analysis requires a cost-data archive (a system to retrieve relevant information), the ability to develop simulations and forecasts of future situations, and consultation on the limitations and applications of the data. Specific proposals often call for extrapolation to new work processes. Ideally, finance personnel work directly with accountability centers and internal consulting teams, helping them identify fruitful avenues of investigation, develop useful proposals, and translate operational changes to accounting and financial implications.

Activity-Based Costing

Historically, the precision and reliability of managerial accounting was limited by the difficulties of data collection and analysis. Large blocks of cost were allocated, rather than transfer priced, using formulas based on assumed proxies such as facility space, number of employees, total direct costs, or gross revenues.[3] Electronic databases permit a significantly more accurate process called activity-based costing (ABC).[4,5,6] ABC activities are work processes that can be defined as needed. They are often work processes under study by performance improvement teams (PITs).

ABC has three objectives:[7]

1. Show the resource elements of cost so that the producing unit or a PIT can compare to benchmark and evaluate changes in the activity.
2. Provide a transfer price for internal transactions. The transfer price can be compared to prices offered by external vendors. It also encourages the using unit to identify and control consumption.
3. Encourage the producing unit to think of the purchasing units as customers whose needs must be met.

ABC promotes control of services, the use of make-or-buy decisions, and improvement of processes that cross several accountability centers. Entire systems, including information services, finance, executive management, and human resources management, can be evaluated. Alternatives such as mergers, acquisitions, preferred partnerships, and alliances can be modeled. These large-scale reorganizations can change patterns of demand, introduce work processes that were previously impractical, and create other returns to scale. For example:

- A small clinic that fails to generate demand and has excessive fixed costs per case may become viable by a merger or partnership with an outside organization. (The market share served will increase, generating enough demand to cover the fixed costs.)
- The scope of clinical support services may be increased and transfer prices may be reduced by a merger. (The fixed costs will be spread over a larger base. Along with reduced costs, increased volume may improve quality.)
- The costs of governance and executive management may be reduced by merger. (Two senior management teams reduced to one, and the market share increased.)
- A major service, such as imaging, human resources management, financial management, or information services, can be purchased from a vendor. (The vendor has returns to scale and superior experience and is better positioned to keep up-to-date.)
- The capabilities of smaller units can expand while simultaneously lowering the cost of larger ones. Telemedicine programs for intensive care patients in small hospitals, which provide access to the advice of experienced intensivist physicians and allow centralized specialist monitoring of rural patients, are striking examples.[8]

Goal Setting and Budgeting

The controller's office supports the annual goal-setting process for the service lines and individual units. A section—the budget office—coordinates budget development and accounting reports, working closely with internal consulting and managing the extensive flows of information necessary to support the negotiations. The process takes several months, involves virtually everyone in the organization, and is the stimulus for continuous improvement and operational excellence. As shown in Exhibit 13.3, the environmental assessment and strategic analysis (chapters 4 and 15) lead to goals for the strategic scorecard. Each operating unit uses these and its own OFIs to identify improvements for the coming year. Goals are negotiated for all dimensions of the operational scorecards. Capital requests are separated from the operating goals and are subject to competitive review. The budget process establishes, and the budget documents, a quantitative

EXHIBIT 13.3
Integrating
Strategic and
Operational
Goal Setting

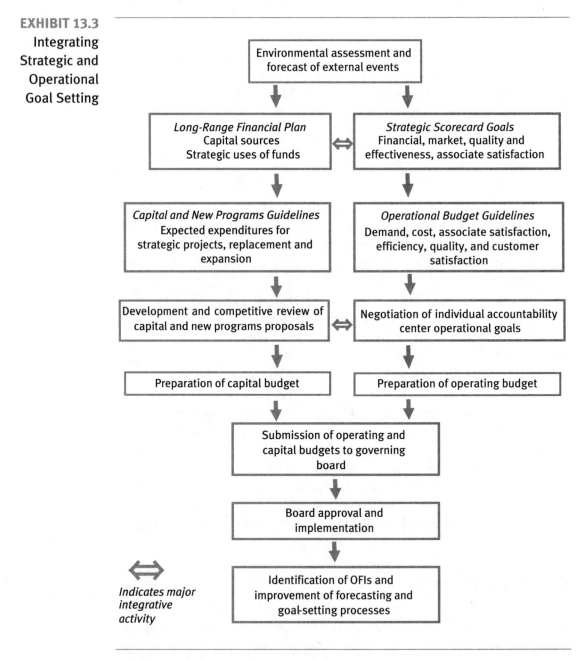

OFI: opportunity for improvement

consensus on expected operations, capital investment, and financing for the next fiscal year. Progress against the budget is monitored by operations managers and overseen by the budget office. The expectation is that all goals will be attained.

Budget Components

The budget describes expected financial transactions and other operational goals for each operating unit, by accounting period, for at least an entire year. Because it takes time to develop, the forecast must cover about 18 months into the future. Well-run institutions budget a second or even a third year in preliminary terms as part of their yearly budget cycle. Multiyear expectations encourage progress toward improvement goals.

The final budget has several components, as shown in Exhibit 13.4. The **operating budget** includes the following:

Operating budget
The aggregate of accountability-center expenditure budgets and the corporate revenue budget.

- *Accountability-unit budgets by reporting period and kind of resource.* Costs are negotiated with the other five dimensions of operational scorecards. The six dimensions comprise the unit goals for the coming year.
- *Aggregate expenditures budgets, or "roll-ups," that summarize larger sections of the organization that parallel the accountability hierarchy.* Similar aggregates are made of the goals for the other operational dimensions.

Budget	Contents	Use
Operating budget: Accountability centers	Accountability-center-level expectations for demand, costs, human resources, productivity, quality, and customer satisfaction	One- or two-year plan of accountability-center goals
Operating budget: Aggregate	Service line and other aggregate expectations for operational and financial measures	Monitor groups of accountability centers
New programs and capital budget	Approved capital expenditures by strategic category and funding sources	Manage investments in capital equipment and facilities
Financial budgets	Detailed pro forma of corporate income, expense, funds flow, and balance sheet	Verify capital management strategies and confirm the long-range financial plan
Cash budget	Projection of monthly cash flows	Manage working capital

EXHIBIT 13.4
Major Budgets and Their Relation to Strategic Goals

- *Revenue budgets that show expected income and profits for DRGs at organizational levels that parallel the payment aggregates.* Leading institutions report revenues only at aggregates that can be held accountable, now usually the service line.[9]

Financial budget
Expectation of future financial performance; composed of income and expense budget, budgeted financial statements, cash flow budget, and capital and new programs budget.

The **financial budgets** parallel the required financial reports. Three are more relevant to operations:

1. *The income and expense budget:* expected net income and expenses incurred by the organization as a whole by period
2. *The funds flow budget:* estimates of cash income and outgo by period, used by finance in cash and debt management
3. *The capital and new programs budget:* capital expenditures and new programs accepted by the governing board, with their implications for the operating and cash budgets by period and accountability center

The Budget Cycle

The budget development process follows an annual cycle, as shown in Exhibit 13.5. Completing the cycle takes about six months and demands substantial effort by every manager and executive as well as members of the governing board. During the remainder of the year, managers can focus on the analysis

EXHIBIT 13.5
Annual Goals and Budget Cycle

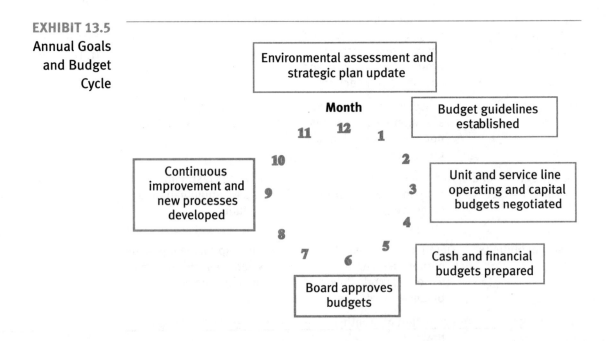

of operations and development of improved methods so that these are ready for implementation with the next cycle.

The operations budget process is managed by *packages*—specific bundles of information that are transferred from one unit or level to another—and timetables for package transfers.[10] The package concept allows the budget office to route information to the correct location, permitting many different teams in the HCO to work at once. Exhibit 13.6 shows the major steps, although the process is usually more complex than the graphic indicates. As a general rule, a specific information package is available for each accountability center or unit at each step, although later rounds of revision tend to focus on only a few unresolved areas.

The actual calculation is now computerized. Units have direct access to their own electronic files and can change resource requirements and some demand elements at will up to the package deadlines. At that time, they must submit the packages to central control, where aggregates are calculated and values are checked against historic records for errors or potential difficulties.

Negotiating the Operating Goals

The budget office initiates the process with forecasts of prices and unit activity; trends, benchmarks, and competitor data; and overall strategic goals.

- *Demand for major activity groups, such as primary care contacts, emergency visits, hospitalizations, births, and surgeries, are forecast using statistical analysis of market trends, combined with judgments of executive personnel.*[11] Forecasts for more detailed activities are derived from the major groups. They are developed first by the budget office and then refined for each unit by unit personnel.
- *Resource prices are forecast by type of resource from history and external references.* The purchasing unit usually prepares the price forecasts for supplies, human resources for personnel, and finance for transfer-priced resources. The unit forecasts the quantities of resources to be used. Budgeting software calculates cost.
- *Productivity forecasts are calculated mechanically as the ratio of forecast cost to forecast output.* Both physical and dollar values are important.
- *Quality, human resources, and customer satisfaction values are taken from historical data.* Trend analysis can be used if necessary. Benchmarks are obtained from a variety of sources.

The initial forecasts are *ceteris paribus*, continuation of past conditions. The unit managers and their supervisors respond with plans for the coming year. The forecasts, guidelines from the governing board, and benchmarks impose discipline on the process. Each unit and each measure should move toward benchmark, and the aggregate expectation must match the guidelines. The results of PITs are incorporated into the coming year's goals. The unmet benchmarks or values suggest the OFIs for study and their PITs during the coming year.

EXHIBIT 13.6
Major Steps
in Developing
Operations
Budgets

Month	Finance Activity	Operations Activity	Intent
1 Budget guidelines	Forecast strategic scorecard values for governing board	Distribute instructions, forms, and timetables	Provide targets and information for line managers' guidance
2–4 Operating goals and budget	Provide forecasts, historical, and comparative information to accountability centers and service lines Answer questions and requests for advice Tally proposed operating budgets, check against guidelines, suggest revisions	Negotiate operating goals using guidelines, competition, benchmarks, history, and values	Specify realistic operational expectations for coming year Improve competitive position and mission achievement
5 Cash and financial budget	Develop complete budget for board review Double-check financial implications		Prepare integrated package for board action
6 Board approval of budgets	Recommend final budget to board		Final review
7–11 Process improvement	Report on performance against budget Provide activity-based cost analysis and guidance on improvement opportunities Assist in evaluating new processes	Develop improved processes	Exploit opportunities to improve competitive position and mission achievement
12 Environmental assessment and strategic plan review	Present review of current performance, long-range forecasts, market analysis, and evaluation of current mission and vision	Review and understand competitive environment	Develop consensus on strategic OFIs, environmental conditions Reiterate relevant policy on quality, human resources, and operations

OFI: opportunity for improvement

Negotiating this result is often a substantial effort. It is important to keep the goals realistic. Achieving them allows unit teams to focus on future improvements, preparing for the following year's goals rather than fixing failures. Some organizations use two guidelines—one for minimally acceptable performance and a second stretch guideline for exceptional achievement. Incentives are established for exceptional effort. The unit's supervisors, including senior management, must assist the team in identifying and testing the goals and supporting PITs to develop better work processes. Senior management leads by pointing out benchmarks, making best practices available, encouraging innovation, and rewarding effective results. These actions are a central part of transformational management. They are radically different from the top-down, authoritarian approaches of earlier management systems.

Capital and New Programs Budget

Finance manages capital funds and is deeply involved in evaluating individual capital investment opportunities. Opportunities are evaluated in terms of contribution to mission. The evaluation process is described in detail in Chapter 14. It always includes the operating units involved and internal consulting. Projects can easily expand to include information and human resources management. The evaluation must be able to communicate across many elements of the HCO, including the governing board. It can be managed either by finance or by internal consulting. Finance's responsibilities include validating the forecasts for project costs, including capital and projected operating costs, and for benefits when they involve costs, efficiency, or revenues. Finance also manages the actual expenditures of capital as accepted projects are implemented.

Finance prepares the capital budget, which shows expected expenditures for new plant and equipment by accounting period and tracks the funds available to the enterprise. It manages the sources of capital funds, provides data for the long-range financial plan and the board's annual goal for investments, and prevents distortion of costs or benefits in proposals.

Guidelines for the Goal-Setting Process

The following are guidelines for a well-run goal-setting process:

1. *The budget and operating goals must constitute an integral whole.* At every level of the organization, the planned activities and goals must be consistent with each other. At higher levels, they must be consistent with the strategic plan, long-range financial plan, and annual environmental survey.

2. *Annual goals or guidelines from the governing board are a major force in gaining consistency and timely progress.* These are established at the outset of the process and include

- realistic forecasts of net revenue;
- a minimum acceptable return from operations;
- a target amount for capital expenditure; and
- corporate goals for customer satisfaction, quality, and associate satisfaction.

3. *The budget for capital expenses and new programs is separately developed and approved in a process that*
   - establishes quantitative forecasts of improvement in operational or strategic scorecards,
   - permits comparison of the value of programs,
   - allows the approval of new programs and even replacement capital to be adjusted quickly as conditions change, and
   - encourages deletion proposals for obsolete or uneconomical programs.

4. *Line managers are convinced of the realism of the goals, in terms of both organizational need and practical achievability.*[12] Senior managers are effective at negotiating goals and supporting lower managers in achieving them. Budget expectations are almost always achieved. Stretch goals may be used for higher risk or where extra effort is required. They are normally supported by increased incentives.

5. *Continuous improvement is the norm.* Goals move closer to benchmark or value over time. Improvements and benchmark performance are rewarded.

6. *The quality of data and the preparation of information by the budget office, as measured by time to completion, reliability, and ease of use, should improve from year to year, building on past work.*

7. *The budget process itself is subject to continuous improvement, becoming more rigorous over time.* An organization that is having difficulty establishing or meeting its budget must limit its attention to elementary concepts, concentrating on getting guidelines, forecasts, and improvement processes developed and accepted. A well-run organization with many years of budgeting experience will do extensive ABC and stretch scenarios. It also will extend the detail of its reporting, both by type of resource and by number of accountability centers. Similar growth in sophistication would occur in the capital and new programs budget.

Accountability centers and cross-functional team members should fully understand the market forces and planning processes that lead to the budget guidelines, participate in budget development, and be able to anticipate the general direction of the guidelines for at least two years into the future. When an effective dialogue takes place, quality and sophistication often improve as a result. Without effective dialogue, there is a constant danger of having the accountability centers adopt an adversarial or destructive approach to the budget.[13]

Monitoring Budget Achievement

Goals negotiated in the budgeting process are normally achieved. Operating units are expected to have used the continuous improvement process to develop, and if necessary test, new methods. Plans for necessary changes in equipment, supplies, and training will have been completed. (The achievement of stretch goals will be less certain, but the underlying preparation is still important.)

Any failure represents a serious management issue. It creates a direct problem (resources must be used to correct the specific failure) and an indirect one (those resources are drawn from the effort to identify and achieve next year's goals). In the rare cases where failure occurs, excellent HCOs respond with 90-day plans—specific reevaluations and corrective efforts to return to goal achievement. These plans are administered by the operating teams and their direct managers. The role of the budget office is to produce the reports that monitor progress, provide drill-down detail when needed, and alert senior management to potential failure. Assigning correction responsibility to the operations managers moves away from the blame culture and reinforces empowerment.

Financial Management Functions

The financial management function projects future financial needs, arranges to meet them, and manages the organization's assets and liabilities in ways that increase its profitability. Financial management in this sense is relatively recent, arising from the increased revenue base created by Medicare, Medicaid, and widespread private health insurance and from the opportunities for obtaining credit and equity. Before 1970, hospitals had two sources of funds—retained earnings and gifts. The growth of reliable income streams opened a broad spectrum of financing opportunities. The growth of multiple corporations, bonded indebtedness issued and reissued to minimize interest costs, and deliberate investment in joint ventures for profit are as telling a story of the healthcare industry as the development of heart transplants is. The five functions—financial planning, pricing, management of long-term capital, management of short-term assets and liabilities, and multicorporate accounting—are now essential to survival.

Financial Planning

Financial management is a forward-looking activity with a long time horizon. It begins with the generation of a long-range financial plan (LRFP), continues with the translation of plan values to annual guidelines, and results in establishing the institution's ability to acquire capital funds through debt or equity.

Developing the LRFP

The LRFP incorporates the expected future income and expense for every element of the strategic plan, specifying the amount and the time of its occurrence. It models the financial outcomes for various scenarios, reflecting

Pro forma
A forecast of financial statements establishing the future financial position of the organization for a given set of operating conditions or decisions.

possible future operating conditions. It is now commonly prepared with specialized software and counsel from a respected accounting firm. The software generates **pro forma** annual statements of income, asset and liability position, and cash flow for many years into the future, allowing senior management and the finance committee of the governing board to assess how well the HCO is prepared to fulfill its mission.

The structural changes in U.S. healthcare arising from the Affordable Care Act make a careful and sophisticated LRFP essential. It is clear that millions of Americans will move from uninsured to insured status. The structure of health insurance will shift to reward high-quality care and health maintenance, two core concepts of population health. Many Medicaid patients will receive care through accountable care organizations deliberately organized to keep them healthy. These changes will alter the array of service lines in most large HCOs. Primary care other than emergency will grow substantially. Chronic care and hospice services are likely to grow. Some surgical and acute inpatient services that have been growing rapidly are expected to stabilize, or even shrink. All of these trends can be identified by well-designed epidemiologic planning models integrated with LRFPs.

Activities such as bond repayments and major facility replacement require 30-year financial planning horizons. Although the accuracy of the estimates deteriorates in distant years, large financial requirements must be accommodated even though they are many years away. Most of the attention is focused on the first three to five years, when the irreversible decisions will be made. Topics of interest include the following:

- Cost of borrowing from various sources
- Cash flow required to support debt payments
- Efficiency improvements required to meet market constraints on revenue
- Financial prospects of specific service lines
- Identity and magnitude of various financial risks
- Overall prudence of the financial management

The LRFP process should include evaluation of the widest possible variety of alternative scenarios (what-ifs) that address future uncertainties, such as the following:

- The impact of inflation and the business cycle
- Changes in demand as a result of population shifts, technology, or competition
- Proposed federal and state legislation
- Trends in health insurance coverage and benefits
- Sources of donations, grants, and subsidized funding

- Alternative debt structures and timing
- Opportunities for joint ventures and equity capitalization

The HCO might respond by changing profit margin goals, revising debt structure, acquiring new equity investors, revising expansion strategies, acquiring or divesting units, or even merging or closing. The objective is to identify the optimum operating condition consistent with the mission and to evaluate that condition in terms of its acceptability. Unacceptable LRFP results can force a complete reevaluation of the strategic position, including the continued existence of the institution.

As indicated in Chapter 4, the financial plan is a critical reality check for the organization. The decision about the final plan—selecting the strategies that are best for the stakeholders as a whole—is made by the governing board. Financial management is responsible for generating information about the alternatives. Exhibit 13.7 shows the tests and the kinds of rethinking necessary to make the strategic plan fit financial realities. The financial ratios provide a way to benchmark financial performance. Bond-rating agencies use the ratios and other financial statement data to issue public ratings of the risk associated with long-term debt. Lower ratings (higher risks) bring higher interest costs on debt. A similar but less formal process operates with equity capital and, to some extent, with gifts. Thus, the institution's ability to acquire capital is directly dependent on its ability to construct a competitive LRFP.

The ideal LRFP generates operating costs substantially below expected revenues, creating a steady stream of profits. The organization can invest the funds in growth, community health, or service improvement and can amplify the investment with borrowed, donated, or invested capital. The ideal is not often achieved. High-performing HCOs use the plan to recognize danger

Test	External Source	Adjustment Required
Debt ratios	Bond market	Keep debt within bond-rating limits
Price	Buyers and intermediaries	Keep price competitive
Earnings	Bond and equity investment markets	Keep cash flow within bond-rating limits
Demand and market share	Competitor analysis	Keep demand forecast consistent with competitor and market conditions
Cost	Benchmarks, competition	Keep cost at or below (Expected revenue – Needed profit)

EXHIBIT 13.7
Tests and Adjustments in Financial Planning

signals in advance and make the necessary adjustments. Several principles guide their actions and are weighed as the plan is considered and adopted:

- *The necessary profit is the amount required to sustain the mission, replacing worn-out and outmoded facilities and equipment and expanding as community need grows.* Well-run not-for-profit HCOs have tended to seek returns in the range of 5 percent of total costs. Large for-profit organizations seek before-tax returns two to three times that high.
- *The criteria for investment decisions are biased toward liquidity and away from risk.* The bias toward liquidity means that most projects must justify themselves in terms of cash flow as well as community benefit. There are four basic causes of increased risk:
  1. Poor prior management has reduced financial capacity.
  2. Management systems lack the control required to meet stated goals.
  3. Individual proposals are inherently risky because they involve speculative goals outside conservative expectations.
  4. The rate of expansion exceeds what the organization can support.

     Well-run organizations guard against the first and second by building and sustaining effective management teams. They meet the third through the programmatic planning process, competitive review, and retention of skilled managers, and they meet the fourth by adhering to the capital investment limits suggested by the LRFP.
- *Portions of the available investment funds can be earmarked for strategic purposes, such as development of new markets, replacement of facilities, or implementing technology strategies like information systems.* Earmarking establishes a multiyear level for the category as a whole and forces evaluation of proposals within the category, rather than between category members and other categories.
- *Investment timing and capital management are frequently important.* Well-run organizations invest liquid assets wisely, avoid borrowing at peak interest rates, and refinance to take advantage of low rates.

Setting the Financial Budget Guidelines

The LRFP is used by the governing board to establish the annual strategic guidelines for revenue, profit, costs, and capital expenditures. The senior management team develops forecasts of market share, costs, and revenue and prepares a recommendation that translates the cash and profit requirements of the LRFP to the guidelines for the coming year or two. The finance committee of the governing board discusses the recommendation and alternatives and recommends the guidelines to the board as a whole. As noted, the board's action initiates the annual goal-setting process and is a more critical step than the final budget approval, which is often a formality because the negotiated goals meet the guidelines.

Pricing Clinical Services

The issues in pricing relate to three concerns: the unit of payment, the HCO mission, and the HCO's market strength. The traditional units of payment were fees for specific physician services and charges for hospital services and supplies. Insurance payment systems have moved to progressively broader aggregates in an effort to emphasize outcomes of care rather than inputs. Exhibit 13.8 shows the major options for pricing structures as sequential levels of risk taking and requirements for integration of the institution and its medical staff. All but Level 1 require increased collaboration. Caregiving associates must coordinate with each other, and the HCO must support and encourage that coordination.

An HCO with a community health mission, as opposed to an excellence-in-care mission, has a relatively straightforward pricing strategy. Its mission calls for maximizing health, reducing unnecessary use of services, and maintaining high efficiency for all services offered. Its strategic performance measures address the needs of community health as well as those of individual patients and associates. At least in theory and usually in reality, the community health mission minimizes the community's healthcare cost per capita, aligning the mission of the HCO with that of the insurers and insurance buyers. The HCO will accept all levels of Exhibit 13.8, with preference for the higher levels because they reward it and its caregivers for achieving the mission. Prices can then be evaluated based on the LRFP.

For HCOs that pursue an excellence-in-care mission, pricing is considerably more complex. The relationship between buyer and seller is adversarial and depends in part on the relative market power. The extent to which the seller has the ability to set the sales price measures monopoly-pricing power. The HCO is frequently in a monopoly situation with regard to uninsured purchasers, and the management of charges to these individuals is a matter of substantial board and societal concern.[14] Although many healthcare systems have acquired some monopoly power over private health insurance contracts,[15] major buyers—such as Medicare, Medicaid, and large commercial insurers—have the balance of market power. Medicare prices are set annually in the national political process.

The Medicare Payment Advisory Commission conducts research and holds hearings to develop market price recommendations. Medicaid payments are established by the states but are generally less than Medicare's. The terms are not negotiable for the individual HCO. For example, between 2000 and 2002, traditional Medicare moved most outpatient, rehabilitation, home, hospice, and mental health care from charges-based to episode-based payments. In 2009, the discussion was around reaching levels 4 and 5 in Exhibit 13.8— bundled payment for episodes of care offered jointly to the institution and its

EXHIBIT 13.8
Pricing
Structures for
Healthcare
Contracts

Structure	Example	Risk for Provider	Integration
1. Fee-for-service/charges	Cash payments, catastrophic and traditional health insurance	None beyond normal business risks	Traditional physician–HCO relationship
2. Negotiated fees and charges	PPO contracts, some traditional insurance contracts	Normal business risks, plus constraints imposed by contract limits	Traditional physician–HCO relationship
3. Fees for episodes of care negotiated separately between HCO and physicians	Medicare DRGs, APCs, some insurance contracts	HCO is at risk for the costs of and quantities of services ordered by physicians within the episode Physician has no additional risk	HCO must gain physician cooperation to meet its risk
4. Fees for episodes of care offered jointly to HCO and physicians	Single-price contracts for discrete episodes of care, such as cardiovascular surgery or chemotherapy	Both physician and HCO at risk for the cost of the episode	Requires physician–HCO collaboration on cost per episode
5. Fees subject to a group incentive	Contracts with penalties or bonuses for meeting utilization or quality targets, such as readmission penalties	Physician and HCO share limited risk for the cost, quality, and appropriateness of care	Requires physician–HCO collaboration on process improvements to meet specific targets
6. Capitation	Payment contracts independent of disease incidence or actual costs of treatment	Physician and HCO at unlimited risk for the cost of the episode and appropriateness of care	Requires physician–HCO collaboration on cost per episode, utilization, and disease incidence

APC: ambulatory patient classification; DRG: diagnosis-related group; PPO: preferred provider organization physicians, and incentives that reward the hospital and physician for more effective overall care, which minimizes readmissions of chronically ill patients.[16,17]

All HCOs must have a systematic pricing response that recognizes the reality of purchaser pricing power and the broad array of pricing structures. The impact of an offered price must be evaluated using the LRFP. All HCOs have high fixed costs, and as a result, profits are dependent on volume. To retain market share, they must meet most market demands in both price and service. As a practical matter, they cannot walk away from major insurers like Medicare. Pricing strategy cannot be set alone; it must be integrated with a strategy to manage the risks involved.[18]

The advanced levels in Exhibit 13.8 force more integration not only between each physician and the HCO but also among physicians. The pricing/risk management strategy must integrate a broad range of knowledge from practicing physicians, service line managers, clinical support services managers, and financial analysts. The time frame for strategy implementation must allow for individual learning and the development of effective teams.

The basic HCO response to the risk-sharing approaches in Exhibit 13.8 is an effective program of evidence-based medicine and evidence-based management, as described throughout this text. This holds cost per case to levels that are acceptable to insurers and generally ensures some profit under Medicare. Offers from private insurers will tend to move to the Medicare level. They must be evaluated against the financial needs reflected in the LRFP and the HCO's bargaining strength. Pricing and charging policies must also be established for uninsured patients. Pricing must include guidelines for charity care, arrangements for deferred payment, and management of delinquent accounts.

Securing and Managing Liquid Assets

Finance is responsible for managing all loans, bonds, and liquid assets. It evaluates alternative sources of funds and recommends the best solution to the governing board as part of the funds flow budget. It arranges borrowing; prepares supporting financial information; and manages repayment schedules, mandatory reserves, and other elements of debt obligation. It monitors the financial markets for opportunities to restructure financing. It manages liquid assets (cash and readily saleable investments). It manages endowments of not-for-profit HCOs.

Debt and Equity Capitalization

Successful not-for-profit HCOs have accumulated substantial equity. Equity of not-for-profit organizations can increase only from donations and retained earnings. Any HCO must establish a core of equity finance. Equity is also useful in joint ventures, allowing the partners to be rewarded for successful risk taking. For-profit equity investors generally expect returns commensurate with their risk, often several times the return expected by lenders. Tax laws are important in equity finance, from both the point of view of the corporation and that of the investor. They permit not-for-profit organizations to retain tax exemption for their share of the earnings if they hold certain levels of control.

Well-managed not-for-profit HCOs exercise extreme prudence in deploying equity. The bulk of the HCO's investments should be in low-risk debt securities. The HCO can pursue some higher-risk investments limited to amounts that the organization could lose without seriously impairing its mission. The rewards for successful use of equity financing through joint ventures are appealing, and this model will probably grow in popularity.

Borrowing, principally the long-term tax-exempt bonds, will remain an important form of capital finance. The borrowing capacity of an organization depends on the overall level of risk to the lenders. Elements of the business that have tangible independent value, such as real estate and accounts receivable, are attractive to lenders. The typical community hospital holds long-term debt that is about 50 percent of its equity.[19] Well-managed HCOs deliberately manage their debt and investments to attract lenders at advantageous rates.[20] Effective investment of borrowed funds, maintenance of cash reserves, and profitable operations are all important. In the long run, the organization can maintain a favored position only by investing prudently to enhance its own customer base. Unwise borrowing, excess borrowing, or insufficient investment will diminish the chance of success.

Exhibit 13.9 shows a simplified example to clarify the complex financial and operational issues involved in capital funds acquisition. A certain HCO might plan to spend $50 million over the next three years to expand primary care and outpatient services. It anticipates a handsome increase in net income

EXHIBIT 13.9
Implications of Alternative Funding Sources for an Ambulatory Care Project

Scenario ($ in millions)	HCO Equity Investment	Earnings from Project	Bond Interest Paid*	Net HCO Income/ Year**	Return on Equity***
100% from equity	$50	$10	$0	$10	20%
50% bonds, 50% equity	$25	$10	$2	$8	32%
50% bonds, 25% equity, 25% joint venture equity	$12.5	$10	$2	$4	32%

*Bond interest 8%
**(Project earnings – Bond interest) – (HCO equity share)
***Net HCO income as percent of HCO equity

of $10 million per year from the new service, with relatively small risk that the income will fall below that level. It has several sources for the $50 million. It could use cash reserved from prior earnings. It could seek tax-exempt bonds, which are likely to have the lowest cost of capital. It could create a for-profit joint venture with its physicians or with another corporation and raise part of the money from equity investment. Finally, it could combine any or all of these approaches.

The use of debt finance can substantially increase the project attractiveness, and the use of a joint venture partner can reduce the capital requirement. The combination of the two allows the institution to start the project with a minimum investment of its own capital and an appealing return on the capital, if earnings match expectations. If earnings fall short, the bond interest is fixed and the entire drop is borne by the equity investors. Partnership with a physician organization commits the physicians to the project's success and reduces the risk of failure.

The number of questions and assumptions required even in this simple example indicates the complexity and challenge. Obviously, accurate forecasts of volume, costs, revenues, and impact on other services are essential, even though opening is several years away. These matters must be addressed in the proposal for the venture. In addition, assumptions must be made about the following:

- *Price and volume interactions for the new service.* A nuanced understanding of the market tolerance for prices and the risks involved if demand does not meet expectations is essential to evaluate the project and the financing mechanisms.
- *Costs of alternative sources of capital.* Each of the sources has different costs and obligations built into it. The use of retained earnings may impair the organization's ability to meet other needs, such as the replacement of equipment or an increase in market share by the acquisition of competitors. Bonds will have an interest rate dependent on the market at the time of sale, the organization's overall financial position, and federal tax policy. Organizations that have been prudently managed in the past will have advantages for all kinds of capital. They will have more retained earnings, lower bond interest, and more debt capacity and thus will be more attractive to outside investors.
- *Impact of the financing on other strategic goals.* The financing may affect competitors or partners in ways that are advantageous to the organization. A joint venture with primary care physicians may provide an avenue to affiliate them more closely with the organization and may improve the ability to recruit. The result may be higher market share and an increased overall profitability. A joint venture with a potential competitor may reduce risk and expand resources simultaneously.
- *Tax implications.* If ordinary income taxes apply, they will be enough to make substantial differences in the results. (Corporate tax rates were about 35 percent

of earnings in 2009.) A tax adviser may be able to find precedents that establish the tax obligations of the various structures, or it may be necessary to seek a consultation letter from the IRS.

The LRFP financial model will be employed to test outcomes not only for the expected conditions but for a range of possible futures. Each major funding avenue will be explored several times, under varying assumptions. Consultants will advise on approaches, assumptions, and implications. The financial results will be evaluated against the marketing and operational considerations. The final solution can be recommended to the board with widespread support from the participants.

Managing Endowments

Most not-for-profit HCOs have acquired endowments or funds they expect to hold for long periods of time. These funds can be invested for growth or income. The assistance of professional investment managers is advisable. Larger organizations use several different managers. The organization must evaluate its overall investment strategy, weighing its risk against potential earnings. In general, permanently endowed funds return about 5 percent per year, after protecting the corpus against inflation. The return is often dedicated to specific charitable purposes such as research, education, and charity care.

Managing Short-Term Assets and Liabilities

Working capital
The amount of cash required to support operations for the period of delay in collecting revenue.

Any operation requires **working capital**—funds that are used to cover expenditures made in advance of payment for services. The finance system manages these transactions to maximum advantage for the organization. A healthcare system with a nine-week average billing cycle, a biweekly payroll, and a four-week inventory cycle requires about $25 million in working capital for $100 million of annual expenses. The cost of this capital—about $1 million per year in interest paid or forgone from investments—is the equivalent of 10 or 15 full-time employees.

Cash Management

Working capital management deals in terms of days. Income can be obtained by moving assets rapidly. Cash and other liquid assets are placed where they will obtain the highest return consistent with risk and the length of time available. (Large sums of money can be invested for small interest returns on an overnight basis.) Accounts receivable and inventories are minimized because they earn no return. Accounts payable, payroll, and other short-term debts are settled exactly when due (or when discounts can be applied), allowing the organization to use the funds involved as long as possible.

Short-term borrowing is available to HCOs. Bank loans and factoring of receivables are common sources. Short-term borrowing is minimized because it costs money. At the same time, however, costs of borrowing need to be compared to opportunity costs of liquidating assets or failing to meet liabilities in a timely fashion. The objective is to reduce total costs of working capital, rather than to avoid borrowing per se. HCOs can reduce capital needs by leasing equipment, paying extra (in effect an interest rate) for the privilege of deferring payment.

HCOs are paid for their services once they have submitted an invoice—the patient ledger—to the responsible party. Health insurers insist on substantial documentation of the invoice. Most now require a specific diagnosis following the International Classification of Diseases and an attestation by the physician affirming the diagnosis. Because complex diagnoses are more highly paid, entering the correct diagnosis is important to both parties. The HCO should identify all disease but is obviously forbidden to enter nonexistent disease. It is also important to prepare the invoice in a timely fashion. Each day of delay—best practice is to gain payment in less than 50 days—adds to the working capital need. Large HCOs establish a substantial mechanism to prepare invoices promptly, assist the physician to identify all existing diseases, and audit to avoid violating the law.

Revenue Management

Managing Multicorporate Accounting

Many HCOs are now multicorporate structures or healthcare systems. Both for-profit and not-for-profit legal entities are permitted to create or acquire subsidiaries by forming new corporations, purchasing or leasing existing organizations, and investing in other corporations. They can reverse these actions by sale, liquidation, or transfer. The only restrictions on these actions are those established by antitrust laws and regulations that govern tax-exempt status. Investment in a given subsidiary can range from negligible to wholly owned, although to qualify for tax exemption it must be controlled by a not-for-profit board. Any combination of for-profit and not-for-profit entities is possible. The tax obligations of each corporation are considered individually as the structures develop.

Two major types of systems have emerged. First, individual hospitals in the same market have merged, formed joint ventures, or established subsidiaries. These tend to be relatively small—$500 million a year or less. They are essentially the same as individual hospitals. Second, about 100 multimarket systems have become important suppliers of healthcare. Many now exceed $1 billion per year in revenue. Many are religious, and many are for-profit. Kaiser Permanente, by far the largest system, is a nonreligious not-for-profit healthcare system that includes its own insurance operation. These systems have the opportunity to centralize important components and generate returns to scale; finance, for example, can perform many functions in one office and serve dozens of hospitals. The system's member HCOs can also form multicorporate structures.

The major financial benefits of multiple corporate structures are as follows:

- *Capital opportunities.* Subsidiary corporations of either single-market or large systems offer opportunities to dedicate capital and to raise new capital through borrowing, gifts, or equity. Activities attractive to equity capital can be pursued only through a for-profit structure, but a not-for-profit parent corporation can form a for-profit subsidiary. Large systems offer scale and diversification attractive to bond buyers. As a result, they can obtain lower interest rates.
- *Reward.* Separate for-profit corporations allow various groups to invest in activities of interest to them and to receive financial reward for the success of those activities. Joint subsidiaries can reward physicians for loyalty and quality.
- *Risk.* The liabilities and obligations of the owned or subsidiary corporation cannot generally be transferred to the parent. (There are certain exceptions, and the law in this area is changing.) Thus, the parent risks only those assets actually invested in the subsidiary.
- *Taxation.* Not-for-profit corporations can be taxed on certain activities, and for-profit corporations can respond to incentives built into the tax law. Separate corporations can frequently be designed with a view toward minimizing the overall tax obligation.

The finance system has the obligation to identify, evaluate, and recommend these opportunities. They must work within the limits established by accepted accounting practice, Medicare fraud and abuse provisions, and IRS regulations.

A relatively common example is an HCO that is exempt from taxes under Section 501(c)(3) of the Internal Revenue Code forming a for-profit corporation with outside investors and then contracting with that corporation to carry out certain activities. The HCO reduces its capital requirement, retains control of the cost and quality of services, and expects to earn profits from its ownership position. The transactions must be priced at fair market value. Joint ventures and equity arrangements with physicians, like other physician contracts, may not offer financial incentives to refer or admit patients to the parent HCO, except under certain types of managed care insurance. They also may not extend tax exemption to physicians in private practice, and they may not reward physicians for improvement of the profitability of the parent corporation.

Auditing Functions

Any corporate entity is required to maintain control of all its properties for its owners. The governing board and members of management are individually and collectively responsible for the prudent protection of assets. They act as agents for owners and must avoid inurement in not-for-profit organizations. The assets include property, cash, and intangibles such as reputation and established market recognition. In hospital organizations, information is one of the most valuable and at-risk assets. The agency obligation extends through the organization. Asset protection is every associate's responsibility, and specific protection functions are assigned to various units. Assets are further protected by a combination of an internal audit function and a hired external auditor.

Internal Audits

Internal auditing provides an ongoing review of the accuracy of data, the safety of assets, and the systems to protect against misfeasance and malfeasance. The internal auditing function can be outsourced. Many Catholic healthcare systems use the Catholic Healthcare Audit Network, an organization they founded that provides extensive, uniform, and independent auditing.

Information Assets

The organization's data warehouse—the *source of truth*—is protected physically by knowledge management services, which is also responsible for the definition and accurate capture of information. The internal audit function monitors actual compliance to definition—whether the reported measure is calculated and recorded exactly. The split responsibilities are deliberate; division and some duplication of functions is a widely accepted pattern for protection. The accounting information in the warehouse is routinely audited, including cash balances and accounts receivables, supplies, and the accurate posting of payroll and other expenses. Basic statistics, such as discharges by DRG or ambulatory patient group, must be audited to assure third-party payers of the validity of charges. In the process of auditing the medical record information, internal auditing can validate the statistics used in specification and adjustment and in many measures of quality.

Physical Assets

Generally, the protection of the physical assets is considered part of the function of the plant system, assigned to security, maintenance, and materials management. Prudent purchasing practices are included in the responsibilities of materials management. The controller is responsible for the physical protection of cash, securities, and receivables. The risk of misappropriation of assets is probably greater than the risk of theft or destruction by outside sources. Internal audit is responsible for estimating the actual loss of physical property and for reviewing processes that protect against loss. The major risks it guards against are as follows:

- Inurement
- Unjustified free or unbilled service to patients
- Embezzlement of cash in the collections and supply processes
- Bribes and kickbacks in purchasing arrangements
- Diversion or theft of supplies and equipment
- Falsified employment and hours
- Purchase of supplies or equipment without appropriate authorization
- Supervision of financial conflicts of interest among governing board members and officers

All organizations face continuing losses of physical assets, and acceptable performance requires continuing diligence. A sound and well-understood program has been developed for this purpose. It has six parts:

1. Detailed, written procedures govern the handling of the various assets and transactions. These procedures primarily rely on the division of functions between two or more individuals and the routine reporting of checks and balances to protect assets. It is common to assign the responsibility for authorizing the transaction (a payment or charge) to operations managers and the responsibility for collecting or disbursing funds to accounting personnel.
2. Adequate written records and accounting systems document the actual use of assets. The software used in automated systems must conform to FASB accounting rules.
3. Special attention is paid to collections and cashiering. Significant efforts must be made to ensure that third parties and individuals pay promptly and fully. Payment in cash and checks must be protected against embezzlement. Carefully designed systems to ensure prompt collection and protect receivables and cash rely heavily on the principle of division of functions and on calculations designed to verify completion of transactions.
4. Adherence to risk-control procedures and documentation requirements is monitored through internal auditors.
5. The independence of the internal auditor can be ensured by arranging reporting directly to the chair of the board audit committee.
6. Annual outside audits verify adherence to procedure and validity of reported outcome.

Inurement, Fraud, and Abuse

Not-for-profit structure requires that no individual benefit be accrued from service to the corporation beyond any stipulated salary or compensation. *Inurement* is the diversion of funds to persons in governance or management as a result of their position of trust. Under these rules, directors, officers, or trustees are prohibited from engaging in business that allows them to derive financial advantage from their governing board role. The corporation is not enjoined from doing business with a board member if such business and board membership are in the owners' interests. Thus, the key word is *advantage*.

To protect against inurement, the institution must establish, and the internal auditor must enforce, policies that reduce financial conflict of interest. These policies have two parts. First, every governing board member and officer is required to file an annual disclosure statement that identifies all of his or her financial interests and potentially conflicting commitments, including membership on other voluntary boards. Second, members are expected to divorce themselves from any specific decision or action that involves their interests or conflicting affiliations. Well-run organizations achieve this by making the point well in advance of any specific application and by selecting members who understand both the law and the ethics.

The rule applies as well to physicians, but its application is more complex. Physicians cannot gain beyond specified benefits of privilege to avoid inurement and specific prohibitions, called *fraud and abuse*. All physician contracts must be reviewed for compliance (discussed in Chapter 6). Many organizations have an independent compliance officer who is assigned responsibility for the review. The compliance officer should also report independently to the governing board, and his or her activity should be subject to internal audit.

External Audits

Outside auditors certify the financial statements to be correct, usually on a fiscal-year basis. The federal government requires an audit as a condition of participation in Medicare, and many intermediaries have similar requirements. Lenders require annual audits before and during the period of any loan. The external audit is less extensive than the internal, although it now typically includes an assessment of the internal audit. It emphasizes areas of known high risk.

Sampling techniques are commonly used in auditing, with attention focused on proportion to the risk involved. Auditors are expected to maintain a deliberate distance from internal employees being audited, including the internal auditors, and to use objective methods to ascertain the accuracy of reported values for balance sheet items. They are also expected to review accounting processes and to suggest changes that will improve accounting accuracy.

The governing board selects the outside auditors, receives their report and reviews it carefully, and takes action to correct any deficiencies noted. Considerable care in selecting and instructing the auditor is justified.[21] The auditor should be accountable directly to the board's finance committee. The firm should be free of any other financial relationship to the organization. This means that consultants should not be hired from the same firm handling the audit. It is unacceptable to use a firm that is represented on the governing board.

The audit committee of the governing board includes the independent trustees who serve as chair, finance chair, treasurer, or secretary of the board. It may consult with, but should not include, employed associates. The committee formulates instructions to the auditor, revising them annually. The revisions can bring different aspects of the asset-protection system under scrutiny each year. The instructions should be based in part on advice from management but should be confidential between the finance committee and the auditor.

The auditor's report goes directly to the audit committee. Thus, the auditors are free to comment on all levels of management. The auditors' comments on both problems with the accounts and weaknesses identified in the asset-protection policies are included in a document called the management letter, which accompanies the audited financial reports. The audit committee should hear an oral summary and discussion of the management letter. The full board should formally accept both the reports and the letter. The expectation for the management letter is "no deficiencies," and it is usually achieved. Well-run HCOs have little trouble with this system. The success of this system assures all stakeholders of truthfulness and equity, removing those concerns from negotiations.

Continuous Improvement of the Accounting and Finance Functions

In addition to its role managing the financial resources of the HCO, the finance activity is a critical component of evidence-based management, constantly supplying routine and special reports and managing the goal-setting process. It must pursue continuous improvement of all its activities, using its operational performance measures (discussion below) and listening responsively to its many clients.

People

Various professional and skilled personnel work in the finance system of even small HCOs. Many of these people perform tasks that are indistinguishable from those in any other corporation, while others perform tasks that require extensive familiarity with healthcare. On-the-job training is often practical at lower levels, but supervisory people now usually have advanced degrees in accounting or finance.

Professional personnel with healthcare experience are often in short supply. There is a chronic shortage of chief financial officers (CFOs). Recruitment should always be national, health-specific knowledge should be highly prized, and the governing board should be directly involved in the CFO selection. Job specifications for a CFO tend not to depend on the size of the organization. Sustaining qualified, professional financial management in small organizations is a severe problem, one that may underlie more mergers and contract management than is recognized. Contract financial management is available through firms that provide general management.

Chief Financial Officer

The CFO is accountable for the operation of the finance systems, including the financial management functions, and advises the CEO and the governing board on finance issues. The CFO or a deputy also assumes the duties of an employed treasurer in commercial corporations, collections, disbursement, asset control, and management of debt and equity. The HCO's treasurer is frequently a trustee who serves principally as chair of the finance committee.

The CFO of a well-run HCO should have substantial experience that includes exposure to the finance systems of several organizations, familiarity with all functions of the finance system, experience with debt management, and demonstrated ability to assist operating management. Evidence of technical skill is important and can be supported both by specimens of work and by references. Evidence of interpersonal skills—particularly the ability to work with people outside the finance department—is also important and can be supported by references. The credentials for a CFO usually include a master's degree in management or business and may include certification as a public accountant. The larger public accounting firms often assist in finding CFOs and, not surprisingly, are also a major source of supply. The recruitment team should include senior management, senior physician management, and governing board representation.

Other Professional Personnel

The functions of finance and accounting require substantial technical knowledge. The leaders of the activity should have experience in the areas where they are accountable. Specialty certification is available. The Healthcare Financial Management Association provides a professional examination. The Certified Public Accountant examination is required for external auditors, and popular among HCO financial managers;[22] the examination includes mastery of FASB requirements. Certification is also available for managerial accounting.[23] The Institute of Internal Auditors offers training programs.[24]

Organization of the Finance System

Within the Finance Unit

The organization of the finance system is dictated by its functions and has been thoroughly codified, in part because of the use of separation of activities to protect assets. Budgeting, cost accounting, financial management, and auditing require relatively small numbers of people, with the largest numbers of personnel being in various aspects of patient accounting and collections. Exhibit 13.10 shows a typical organization pattern.

EXHIBIT 13.10
Organization
of the Finance
System

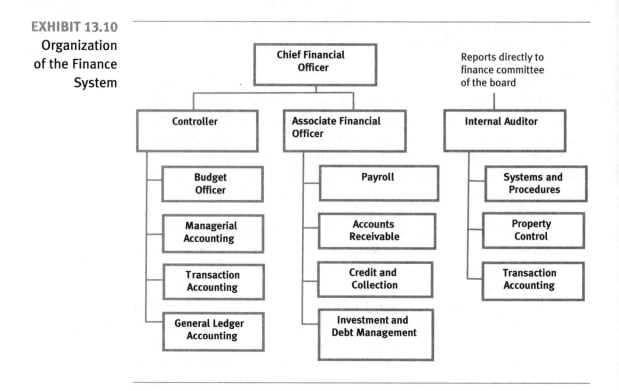

Relation of Finance to Operations

Almost every part of the organization shown in Exhibit 13.10 is in direct daily contact with the rest of the HCO, often over sensitive matters. The key to success is maintaining a professional, productive level of exchange. Clear, convenient systems and forms make routine information gathering as efficient as possible. Orientation and training sessions for finance personnel at all levels help them understand clinical procedures and participate in continuous improvement projects. Well-designed processes and training in consensus building make the interactions effective. It should be universally understood that operations management is responsible for setting, achieving, and departing from expectations. Finance personnel provide data and interpret them; they do not enforce budget discipline.

Relation of Finance to the Governing Board

The finance system relates directly to the governing board through the finance committee, and the CFO often represents the senior management team on the committee. Provision must be made for executive session of the committee, meeting without members employed by the HCO. Reports from the internal and external auditors should first be received in executive session.

In this and preceding chapters, several tasks have been specifically identified for the finance committee of the board:

- Assist in selecting the CFO
- Annually review the LRFP and recommend the final version to the full board

- Recommend the budget guidelines to the full board
- Recommend pricing policies to the full board
- Review the proposed annual budget, and recommend it to the full board
- Set the final priorities, and recommend the capital and new programs budget to the board
- Receive the monthly or quarterly report that compares operations to expectations
- Support the audit committee, supervising both the internal and external audits
- Review major capital expenditure and financing proposals

This list explains why membership on the finance committee is time consuming and intellectually demanding. Members are important at meetings of the full board as well, and overlapping appointments or joint meetings with the planning committee occur. In addition, the finance committee has routine obligations to approve the HCO's banks and financial contracts, real estate transactions, and contracts over predetermined amounts. The list can easily fill 10 or 12 fast-paced meetings each year. Virtually the entire staff work for the finance committee is prepared by finance personnel.

Measures

Quantitative Performance Measures

The finance activity must be measured using appropriate parts of the operational scorecard, with negotiated goals, benchmarks, and continuous improvement. These measures are entirely different from those that measure the organization's financial position. The organization as a whole, not just its finance activity, must be accountable for the financial performance. The finance team is accountable for its operational goals. As for all support activities, the goals must be carefully set, with emphasis on the level of service necessary to support finance's customers. Effectiveness is more important than efficiency. Overemphasizing efficiency presents serious dangers; underperformance in the finance and accounting functions is often difficult to detect and can mount to millions of lost dollars before it is detected.

Costs of accounting and finance, associate satisfaction, and customer satisfaction are measured as in all other activities. The quality of accounting and finance services requires a thorough understanding, but a number of useful measures can be collected and benchmarked. Many of them are derived from financial ratios—relative measures constructed from the financial reports. Measures of demand and output are often problematic. Unlike patient ledger accounting, where the numbers of postings and accounts maintained allow a productivity calculation that can be benchmarked, financial reporting, auditing, and managerial accounting have no readily accessible unit cost. Exhibit 13.11 shows the array of operational measures that can be used to identify OFIs, negotiate goals, and achieve continuous improvement.

EXHIBIT 13.11
Operational Measures of Finance and Accounting

Area and Examples		Goal	Benchmark
Demand Only a few functions—most notably patient ledger accounting—have usable measures of demand		Timely completion of transactions	Rarely available
Cost Number of personnel and labor costs for functions or accountability units		Fully meet customer needs without excess cost	Rarely available
Associate satisfaction Satisfaction, absenteeism, and retention		Retention of all qualified associates	Provided by survey companies
Output and productivity		See *Demand*	Rarely available
Quality Current assets and liabilities	Financial ratios for cash and receivables Earnings from short-term liquid assets Days in receivables Short-term borrowing amounts and cost	Minimize cost of current assets and current liabilities, subject to contractual obligations	Ratios, earnings, days, and short-term debt costs can be benchmarked
Long-term assets and liabilities	Endowment earnings Debt service cost, age of plant, and investments in replacement and new technology	Maintain competitive services for patients and associates	Ratios can be benchmarked
Financial and managerial reports	Internal and external audit reports	Zero defect	Not applicable
Analytic and consultative services	User complaints and corrections Post hoc accuracy of forecasts Service delays Comparison to external consultants	Events must be individually evaluated	Not applicable
Customer satisfaction Surveys of user satisfaction		Develop loyal internal customers	User satisfaction can be benchmarked

Subjective Quality Assessment

As with the governing board, additional insights into OFIs can be gained by systematic collection of opinions. Opinions from associates in the finance committee, internal and external auditors, and customers can be revealing and constructive. Outside consultants can also review performance. The LRFP, other financial analyses, and the budgeting process are particularly likely to benefit from these subjective assessments.

The following are subjectively evaluated criteria met by successful organizations:

- The LRFP, analytic report, or budget package is clear, concise, internally consistent, and consistent with external realities.
- Assumptions and their implications are specified.
- Prudent and reasonable sources have been used to develop external trends, and a variety of opinion has been reviewed whenever possible.
- The plan or report develops contingencies on major, unpredictable future events.
- Unexpected events that require modification are unforeseen by competitors and other external sources.
- The plan or report is well received by knowledgeable board members and outsiders such as consultants, bond rating agencies, and investment bankers.

Similar subjective criteria for all finance and accounting functions are available in textbooks and from consultants.

Managerial Issues

The changes introduced by the movement to population health will create substantial difficulties for some HCO service lines, as they adapt to shifting market pressures. The cost and revenue forecasts supplied by financial management will drive down-sizing, closing, and merging of units, placing stress on the annual goal-setting activities and many PIT agendas. Evidence from the leading HCOs suggests that the approaches outlined in *The Well-Managed Healthcare Organization*—empowerment, continuous improvement, service excellence, and the two planning models, epidemiologic planning and the LRFP—will lead many HCOs to success. Optimizing these tools requires attention to three fundamental issues in financial management: an atmosphere of honesty and transparency; a collegial, blame-free culture; and prompt, careful management of conflict.

Supporting an Atmosphere of Honesty and Transparency

Senior leadership must enforce the discipline to ensure that all the financial functions are fully achieved, creating an atmosphere of honesty and transparency. These functions are unusually susceptible to human failings—denial, avoidance, neglect, deliberate subversion or falsification, and greed. There is a constant risk that the organization will let some matters slide, particularly when addressing them is likely to be unpleasant. The governing board and its audit committee are the first line of defense against this tendency. They must provide full and visible support for the internal and external audit functions, including support for their independence and unique reporting relationship to governance. Senior leadership must accept the challenge as well. The culture must support effective action on identified issues, avoid blame for honest error, and reward individuals who raise hard questions. Any threat to the integrity of the assets or the information must be promptly and forcefully addressed. This level of discipline is essential not simply to ensure integrity but also to reassure all associates and suppliers that their own actions will not be undercut by fraud, distortion, or even carelessness. Contracts will be fulfilled. The data will be reliable. Gaming will not be tolerated.

Maintaining a Collegial, Blame-Free Culture

The functions of finance and accounting are so widespread that interaction between finance and other managers is almost constant. Those interchanges must be perceived by other managers as constructive. Finance personnel must be seen as contributors and colleagues. They have traditionally been viewed too often as adversaries or enforcers. In large part, building constructive relationships is a matter of training and modeling. Finance personnel can be trained to fulfill Sharp HealthCare's 12 behavioral standards and five "Must Haves" (described in Chapter 2) as well as any associate. The CFO and the finance leadership must understand, implement, and model those behaviors.

Managing Conflict Promptly and Professionally

In a disciplined and collegial culture, many of the potential conflicts arise from differences in perspective. Potential conflicts are commonplace from both financial and managerial accounting decisions. They often arise in goal setting. Finance has done its job as it sees it; operations managers either do not understand or see it differently. Prompt resolution is essential. The usual tools—listening, further data gathering and analysis, negotiation, counseling, process revision, and retraining—are appropriate. It is rarely necessary to go beyond them to disciplinary action. Experienced managers become familiar with applying these solutions and can teach them by mentoring and example. What is important is a tradition of prompt but judicious resolution.

Financial Accounting

Revenue accounting is a common source of conflict. Service line managers want the largest possible income from each case, and much income is controlled by the diagnostic codes assigned. Assigning incorrect codes to increase severity, called *upcoding*, is illegal and should be monitored by both internal and external audit. Assigning too few codes or understating the severity of disease is wrong as well, but the fact that the treating physician must attest to the codes under threat of criminal charge causes many physicians to understate severity. The solution is in diagnostic coding assistance, including analysis of diagnostic and treatment orders to ensure capture of all treated diseases. The solution also includes reassurance to the treating physicians. If the audit mechanisms and the criteria for adding diagnoses are understood and reliable and if specific queries are thoroughly discussed and evaluated, physicians will be confident and satisfied. Management's job is to see that both conditions are fully met.

Certain elements of the financial reports—such as allowances for bad debts, reserves for changes in payment from large third parties, reserves for financial restructuring, and reserves for employee pensions—must be estimated. The estimates are subjective and can be deliberately varied within FASB limits to affect net income. In intercorporate accounting, allocations for indirect costs are also subjective. Deliberate distortion beyond FASB limits or for individual gain (such as the distortion of profits to ensure incentive payments to management) is illegal. Well-managed organizations use consistent rules for these transactions. They include these rules in contracts with subsidiaries and audit the contracts to ensure compliance.

Managerial Accounting

The elements of the cost data routinely reported from general ledger transactions, like depreciation costs, charges for central services, and allocated costs, are always a source of contention. Operations managers deserve assurance that the charges are given the same level of scrutiny and rigorous control that their direct costs receive. Senior management should show the following:

1. Costs of generating these services are accurately accounted and benchmarked.
2. Wherever practical, the best possible source of service is selected. This means that outside vendors are used where appropriate.
3. Transfer prices are used whenever feasible. Transfer prices give managers control over quantity and can be compared easily to outside vendors.
4. Allocated costs are used only when necessary and are based on fair, reasonable, and consistent allocations.
5. Specific complaints are addressed promptly and thoroughly, and indicated changes are implemented.

Managerial accounting is also used extensively in performance improvement, to model alternative solutions. These applications are often complex technical exercises. The managerial role is to see that all members of the PIT are comfortable with the assumptions and analyses and understand the implications of the findings. This is usually a matter of clear reporting by the analysts, adequate discussion, and thoughtful response to questions. The operations managers' perspective can lead to important improvements in the modeling. Sensitive response to their questions increases their confidence in the results. (Note that the goal is less ambitious than "understand the analysis." People today comfortably use complex technology that they do not fully understand.)

Goal Setting

Setting the annual goals is never easy. The exercise is designed to force the organization to consider the demands of customer stakeholders, and it is inevitably stressful. Three major activities distinguish excellence:

1. *The budget technology is carefully established.* The packages are fully described and understood by operations managers. Calculations are computerized, allowing managers to focus on the decisions rather than on paperwork. The best organizations train managers in how to use the software to explore the implications of various answers. Hands-on training, support from superiors, and mentoring from experienced peers help first-line managers master their roles.[25]
2. *The board's guidelines are clearly explained.* Each manager understands why the guidelines are important, how they were established, and how they are extrapolated from the organization as a whole to his or her unit. Because all members of the team should understand the guidelines, the manager should be able to explain them to others.
3. *The negotiations to reach the budget should be considerate, fair, and realistic.* This inevitably means that some units that are doing well will be challenged to excel, while others that are struggling are given extra support.

Financial Planning

The assumptions are the critical element of financial planning. Results from the LRFP models are often sensitive to small changes in forecasts for demand and prices of patient services and for costs of purchased items. Because they are forecasts, there is no "right" answer. Management should insist on three specific protections:

1. Forecasts are obtained from respected and unbiased sources if available.
2. An effort is made to obtain alternate forecasts.
3. Sensitivity analysis is used in the model to test the impact of alternative forecasts, and the implications of the results are fully discussed.

The point of these protections is that *ceteris paribus* extrapolations are not enough; critical variables must be thoroughly understood and carefully forecast.

Additional Resources

Cleverley, W. O., P. H. Song, and J. O. Cleverley. *2010. Essentials of Health Care Finance*, 7th ed. Sudbury, MA: Jones & Bartlett Learning.

Finkler, S. A., D. M. Ward, and J. J. Baker. 2007. *Essentials of Cost Accounting for Health Care Organizations*, 3rd ed. Sudbury MA: Jones & Bartlett.

Gapenski, L. C. 2012. *Fundamentals of Healthcare Finance*, 2nd ed. Chicago: Health Administration Press.

Nowicki, M. 2014. *Introduction to the Financial Management of Healthcare Organizations*, 6th ed. Chicago: Health Administration Press.

Young, D. W. 2014. *Management Accounting in Health Care Organizations*, 3rd ed. San Francisco: Jossey-Bass.

Notes

1. Centers for Medicare & Medicaid Services. 2014. "Health Information Privacy." [Online information; retrieved 5/26/14.] www.hhs.gov/ocr/privacy/index.html.

2. U.S. Internal Revenue Service. 2014. "Instructions for Schedule H (Form 990)." [Online information; retrieved 5/26/14.] www.irs.gov/pub/irs-pdf/i990sh.pdf.

3. Prince, T. R. 1992. *Financial Reporting and Cost Control for Health Care Entities*, 289–378. Chicago: Health Administration Press.

4. Cooper, R., and R. S. Kaplan. 1988. "Measure Costs Right: Make the Right Decisions." *Harvard Business Review* 66 (4): 98–106.

5. Player, S. 1998. "Activity-Based Analyses Lead to Better Decision Making." *Healthcare Financial Management* 52 (8): 66–70.

6. Baker, J. J. 1995. "Activity-Based Costing for Integrated Delivery Systems." *Journal of Health Care Finance* 22 (2): 57–61.

7. Finkler, S. A., D. M. Ward, and J. J. Baker. 2007. *Essentials of Cost Accounting for Health Care Organizations*, 3rd ed., 83–97. Sudbury, MA: Jones & Bartlett.

8. Griffith, J. R., and K. R. White. 2003. *Thinking Forward: Six Strategies for Highly Successful Organizations*, 87–117, 153–55. Chicago: Health Administration Press.

9. Voss, G. B., P. G. Limpens, L. J. Brans-Brabant, and A. van Ooij. 1997. "Cost-Variance Analysis by DRGs: A Technique for Clinical Budget Analysis." *Health Policy* 39 (2): 153–66.

10. Berman, H. J., and L. E. Weeks. 1993. *The Financial Management of Hospitals*, 8th ed., 385–585. Chicago: Health Administration Press.

11. Cote, M. J., and S. L. Tucker. 2001. "Four Methodologies to Improve Healthcare Demand Forecasting." *Healthcare Financial Management* 55 (5): 54–58.

12. Abernethy, M. A., and J. U. Stoelwinder. 1991. "Budget Use, Task Uncertainty, System Goal Orientation and Sub-unit Performance: A Test of the 'Fit' Hypothesis in Not-for-Profit Hospitals." *Accounting Organizations and Society* 16 (2): 105–20.

13. Swieringa, R. J., and R. H. Moncur. 1975. *Some Effects of Participative Budgeting on Managerial Behavior*. New York: National Association of Accountants.

14. Clarke, R. L. 2007. "Price Transparency: Building Community Trust." *Frontiers of Health Services Management* 23 (3): 3–12.

15. Lindrooth, R. C. 2008. "Research on the Hospital Market: Recent Advances and Continuing Data Needs." *Inquiry* 45 (1): 19–29.

16. Jencks, S. F., M. V. Williams, and E. A. Coleman. 2009. "Rehospitalizations Among Patients in the Medicare Fee-for-Service Program." *New England Journal of Medicine* 360 (14): 1418–28.

17. Davis, K., and S. Guterman. 2007. "Rewarding Excellence and Efficiency in Medicare Payments." *Milbank Quarterly* 85 (3): 449–68.

18. Cleverley, W. O., and J. O. Cleverley. 2008. "10 Myths of Strategic Pricing." *Healthcare Financial Management* 62 (5): 82–87.

19. Reiter, K. L., J. R. C. Wheeler, and D. G. Smith. 2008. "Liquidity Constraints on Hospital Investment When Credit Markets Are Tight." *Journal of Health Care Finance* 35 (1): 24–33.

20. Wheeler, J. R., D. G. Smith, H. L. Rivenson, and K. L. Reiter. 2000. "Capital Structure Strategy in Health Care Systems." *Journal of Health Care Finance* 26 (4): 42–52.

21. Reinstein, A., and R. W. Luecke. 2001. "AICPA Standard Can Help Improve Audit Committee Performance." *Healthcare Financial Management* 55 (8): 56–60.

22. American Institute of CPAs. 2014. Home page. [Online information; retrieved 5/26/14.] www.cpa-exam.org.

23. Certified Management Accountant Program. 2014. Home page. [Online information; retrieved 5/26/14.] www.imanet.org/cma_certification.aspx.

24. Institute of Internal Auditors. 2014. Home page. [Online information; retrieved 5/26/14.] www.theiia.org.

25. Griffith and White (2003, 164–65).

14 INTERNAL CONSULTING

Critical Issues in Internal Consulting

1. *Maintaining and interpreting factual information that describes the community served:*
   - Identify population, economic, healthcare, and competitor trends.
   - Plan for service and workforce requirements.

2. *Obtaining useful benchmarks and best practices:*
   - Interpret statistical data.
   - Help operators identify improvable variation.
   - Advise on legal and regulatory issues and approve HCO contracts.

3. *Providing performance improvement teams (PITs), planning teams, senior management, and governance with timely and effective knowledge-based support:*
   - Support PIT and other chairs in efficient committee practices.
   - Guide teams in Lean and advanced analysis.
   - Model proposed processes.
   - Conduct tests of proposed processes.

4. *Identifying, evaluating, selecting, and implementing new programs and capital investments that yield returns in improved performance:*
   - Assist individuals in developing feasibility studies and business plans.
   - Assist units in preparing requests for capital.

Questions for Discussion

These questions are about applying the chapter content. It's often helpful to discuss them with classmates or mentors, gaining different perspectives on the issues.

1. Identify a specific community with at least one moderate-sized HCO. Consider the events important to the HCO this year and last year, such as federal or state regulatory changes, changes in health insurance, and shifts in the local economy. What should the governing board have expected about these events in the annual environmental assessment?

2. The operating room supervisor asks internal consulting what to do about demand he is not able to meet. What should internal consulting offer as a plan for developing a solution?

3. If you were planning an initial discussion about goal setting and capital budgeting for newly appointed first-line supervisors, what topics would you include?

4. Review the control chart on cesarian sections (Exhibit 14.6). The obstetrics service notes that it successfully reduced the mean rate 21 months ago and that the remaining variation is well within the usual definition of a controlled process, which is that no report exceeds 3 sigma control limits. Therefore, its staff says, no opportunity for improvement can be found on cesarian sections. The chief medical officer wants to know what further investigation is appropriate before she accepts this as a valid conclusion.

5. An economic recession has increased charity care and bad debts from 4 percent to 6 percent of net revenues. The board asks for "all possible" cost reductions, and one board member notes that the internal consulting activity "consumes more than $1 million a year. Surely we could defer that." What arguments would you assemble to support continuing this activity? What kinds of data should you prepare?

Purpose

The purpose of internal consulting is

to provide information, forecasts, tools, and analyses in support of evidence-based management.

Internal consulting provides support for performance improvement teams (PITs) and planning teams, helping them systematically investigate opportunities, issues, and alternatives. It also supports senior management and the governing board in strategic decisions—fundamental questions about the future of the enterprise. The ideal is to make these operating and strategic decisions in such a way that even with complete hindsight, none would be changed. In reality, organizations fall short, but well-managed organizations come closer than others. They thrive because they collect information exhaustively, forecast carefully, apply tools appropriately, and conduct analyses that allow them to identify the best alternatives. Those are the skills of internal consulting.

Two fundamental concepts underpin internal consulting in high-performing HCOs:

1. Success requires aggressive, far-reaching, unceasing search for improvement. Internal consulting provides the evidence and the analysis for the search, at both the strategic and operational levels.
2. Internal consulting does not make decisions. It supplies facts and analysis to its clients.

Functions

The questions raised by internal consulting clients arise from the dynamic relationship of the HCO to its stakeholders and from specific proposals for the future. The answers can require input from any logistic or strategic support activity and, in many situations, specific medical and nursing knowledge. All answers require forecasting—extrapolation to future environments. Internal consulting must coordinate its own resources, those from other units, and external resources to answer those questions as accurately as possible.

The internal consulting functions shown in Exhibit 14.1 emphasize information assembly, analysis, and integration. They divide the work of internal consulting somewhat arbitrarily into projects for the HCO as a whole, for PITs, and for capital investment proposals. The "any other factual concern" function establishes both the unit's universal breadth and its critical limitation to fact-finding rather than decision making. Internal consulting establishes the facts. Its clients decide the HCO's future.

EXHIBIT 14.1
Functions
of Internal
Consulting

Function	Description	Examples
Supporting the organization as a whole		
Environmental assessment	Annual review of changes and trends that affect future performance	Trends in population size, age, and health insurance coverage
Community-based epidemiologic planning	Forecast of community demographics and disease incidence	Trends in births and high-cost diseases Forecasting physician supply
Benchmarking and identifying best practice	Search for external expertise on clinical or other technical topics	Clinical protocols Collaboratives Environmental control
Statistical analysis	Refinement of data to remove extraneous variation; forecasting; statistical process control	Rates adjusted for patient characteristics Correlation Statistical significance
Legal, regulatory, and ethical review	Compliance with guidelines, regulations, court decisions, and the HCO's own values	Federal and state regulatory requirements Cultural competence
Supporting improvement projects		
Increasing effectiveness of process improvement teams	Training in process analysis Direct consultation Outside consultants	Lean and Six Sigma analyses Assistance in process redesign Assistance in pilot trials
Process modeling	Identifying implications of proposed work processes	Cost–benefit analyses Simulations Staffing models
Evaluating and testing alternative solutions	Design of pilots and sensitivity analyses	Reliability tests Worst-case scenarios
Supporting governance	Identifying and evaluating major new services and forms of organization	Mergers and acquisitions New service lines Revised corporate structures
Supporting the capital investment review		
Assisting operating units to identify and prioritize capital opportunities	Identifying competitive proposals and improvements in operating scorecards	Replacing equipment Expanding clinic locations Adding diagnostic services
Developing formal capital requests	Specifying changes in equipment, facilities, and work processes	Documenting renovation needs Forecasting new cost and quality performance
Implementing and integrating		
Implementing and integrating new programs	Coordinating multi-unit changes in facilities, equipment, or work processes	Monitoring new equipment installation Managing new construction Achieving proposal goals
Responding to any other factual concern relevant to the HCO's continued success		
Improving internal consulting and the continuous improvement process		

As shown in Exhibit 14.2, internal consulting has five major vehicles for helping its clients:

1. *Immediate reply.* Many questions require only a short answer, brief discussion, or short follow-up message.
2. *Just-in-time support.* Internal consulting can arrange training or a specific service, including calling on other logistic and support services. For example, the HCO's electrical power manager can consult on new equipment needs.
3. *Designated team member.* Internal consulting can assign one of its staff members to participate with the PIT, identifying, clarifying, and arranging fulfillment of PIT needs.
4. *Internal consulting project team.* For complex questions, a team of internal experts can be assembled. Members can come from any part of the HCO. The project team for a proposed clinical service line might include expertise in medicine, nursing, epidemiology, accounting, finance, law, and marketing. The team

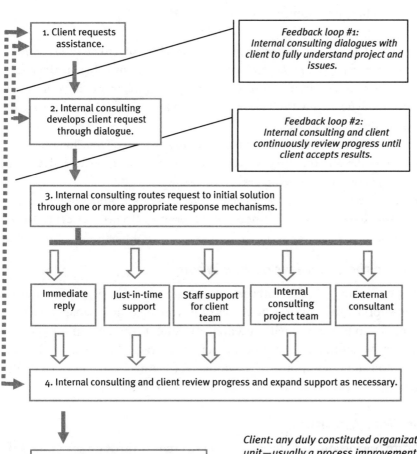

EXHIBIT 14.2
Internal Consulting as a Clearinghouse

differs from the initial PIT in the nature of the charge. It is fact-finding; the PIT is charged with making a recommendation.

5. *External consultants.* Even a large HCO does not have specialists in every field, and small ones can afford only the most limited internal consulting. Internal and external resources can be combined as well. The internal consulting manager can help select, instruct, and coordinate outside consultants.

The approach outlined in Exhibit 14.2 has four important advantages:

1. It provides every client with a point of contact for technical support.
2. It clearly establishes the client's customer position and gives the client final say over the adequacy of the advice and the process.
3. It has two important feedback loops to ensure timely but thorough service.
4. It allows the internal consulting manager to minimize cost and delay by judicious use of the initial conversation, just-in-time opportunities, and coordination of resources.

It also has three important consequences:

1. *Any clinical, logistic, or strategic support activity that can contribute to the client's issue must respond to the internal consulting call.* Knowledge management, human resources, environment services, accounting, and marketing can expect to contribute frequently to PITs. Internal consulting serves to coordinate and integrate these contributions.
2. *Internal consulting controls all outside consulting contracts.* This allows careful selection of the vendor, effective management of the engagement, and full use of less expensive internal resources.
3. *Decision making is assigned to the client.* Internal consulting does not decide. It focuses on the factual foundation needed for others to make evidence-based decisions.

Supporting the Organization as a Whole

In high-performing HCOs, internal consulting provides or coordinates services that support the ongoing activities of governance and management. The major applications are in environmental assessment, the epidemiologic planning model, benchmarking and best practices, statistical analysis, and various legal and ethical reviews, but the commitment to meeting client needs often aggregates these processes and calls on additional sources.

Environmental Assessment

Healthcare organizations reduce risk and uncertainty through scanning activities to forecast expected environmental conditions and design responsive futures.[1] Internal consulting assembles an annual environmental assessment, supporting a detailed quantitative analysis with a written summary high-lighting critical changes and opportunities. In addition to the quantitative analysis—and just as important—is the analysis of qualitative information from boundary-spanning activities. The report is widely circulated among the HCO leadership and provides background information for many PITs and planning activities.

Good environmental assessment takes into account the following:

- *Community demography, epidemiology, and economy.* A thorough quantitative description of the market being served, identification of all major trends in de-mographics and disease incidence, and forecasts of the future are essential to the environmental assessment.

- *Patient and community attitudes.* Trends in total purchases of healthcare, sites of care, sources of payment, satisfaction with care, and market share should be reported with material changes highlighted. Patient surveys, complaints, and household surveys are trended and benchmarked. Many important topics must be reported qualitatively. Results from listening activities, focus groups, direct interviews, and related sources should be summarized in a brief report.

- *Health insurance buyer intentions and health insurance trends.* Trends, prices, and market share of the various insurance products must be examined and fore-cast to develop a complete perspective. The willingness of employers, unions, and governments to pay for care, and the terms they expect to use for payment, generally cannot be quantified, but realistic estimates and a detailed understand-ing of buyer interests are critical. While state and national trends are important, the view of local groups on key matters such as services, debt, price, and ameni-ties is often the final determinant of planning and financial strategy.

- *Trends in clinical practice.* Technology, payment contracts, and the attitudes of practitioners and patients interact to create demands for new services and new modes of delivery. In the 1980s, for example, patients began to prefer outpa-tient over inpatient care. After the passage of the Affordable Care Act, many physicians in independent practice moved to closer affiliation with hospitals. The act's accountable care organization model, backed by changes in the insur-ance payments, opened a new approach to chronic disease management. The implications of many changes like these can be forecast using the epidemiologic planning model. Even describing those that cannot be quantitatively forecast improves decision making.

- *Associate attitudes and capabilities.* Trends in the skills and attitudes of current employees, physicians, and volunteers are important background to planning decisions. Formal surveys are now routinely administered. Compensation levels for major groups should be forecast. Most organizations gain additional insights through focus groups and listening activities.

- *Trends in physician supply and organization.* The number of physicians in prac-tice in the community, by specialty and other characteristics, is a critical indicator of both cost and quality of care. The number and level of affiliation with the HCO determines market share. A database is maintained to support physician–organization planning functions (described in Chapter 6).

- *Trends in other health worker supply.* Well-managed institutions forecast their need for professional associates of all kinds. The lead time allows them to adapt to shortages and surpluses, using advance warning to plan workforce recruitment or reduction.

The planning unit is accountable for a thorough and current database of all of these elements and a written annual review that highlights important trends and developments. It should also be accountable for reporting and, where possible, integrating insights or beliefs regarding future trends offered by members of governance and senior management.

Community-Based Epidemiologic Planning

Internal consulting is the source of truth for demographic, disease incidence, and market demand data. It maintains the databases that support epidemiologic planning (see Chapter 3 and applications in many subsequent chapters). It works with clients to prepare multiyear forecasts of demand for clinical and other services. It produces short- and long-run forecasts for a number of measures derived from clinical demand, such as employment, traffic, and supplies. The forecasts are used in strategic positioning (see Chapter 15), the development of facility and service plans, and expectations for the next budget year.

The reliability of the forecasts and the interpretive advice provided by internal consulting are critical elements in long-term success of the organization. Important forecasts should be offered with **sensitivity analysis**, an exploration of the implications of alternative assumptions about the future. Competent interpretation includes ranges for estimates of incidence rates, advice on specification alternatives, and translation to resource requirements that help operators understand the dynamics of productivity and the uncertainty of forecasts. The epidemiologic planning model is available from national consulting services. The input data requirements are difficult to replicate, even for a large healthcare system. The calculation and presentation software make construction of forecasts, sensitivity analysis, and exploration of alternative scenarios quick and easy. An in-house capability is necessary to retrieve and trend internal data. It also becomes an important resource of expertise on the local situation.

Sensitivity analysis
Analysis of the impact of alternative forecasts, usually developing most favorable, expected, and least favorable scenarios to show the robustness of a proposal and to indicate the degree of risk involved.

Benchmarking and Identifying Best Practice

A large, high-performing HCO needs thousands of benchmarks, and they are not easy to find. Internal consulting provides an expert who knows criteria for evidence and common sources and who can help clients select benchmarks and improve them. Benchmarking requires standard definitions of the measure being benchmarked. Benchmarking should include finding the best practice for a process. The benchmark data identify the best practice; the organization achieving benchmark is often willing to share its procedures and insights in return for reciprocal treatment. Benchmarks are frequently hierarchical—"best in HCO," "best in system," "best in nation," and "world class." Ranking allows celebration of gains as they occur, but the opportunities for improvement (OFIs) are still clear.

Multihospital systems develop benchmarks for their members. The Centers for Medicare & Medicaid Services provides Hospital Compare data, which are useful for benchmarks at the local, regional, and national levels. Commercial companies and consultants offer a variety of cost and quality data sets. National satisfaction surveys include comparative data with their reports. Some comparison sources are voluntary networks that also share best practices. Several successful systems promote direct relationships between associates with similar assignments, forming networks of nurses, purchasing agents, and so forth.[2] Clinical collaboratives, such as those run by the Institute for Healthcare Improvement, offer a way to learn by sharing experiences.[3] Internal consulting assists by collecting the available alternatives and helping the client understand the differences between current and best practice.

Statistical Analysis

Data from the data warehouse and external sources support performance monitoring; the annual environmental assessment; and forecasts that evaluate process improvement proposals, investment opportunities, and make-or-buy decisions. Statistical analysis is essential for all of these applications to identify and deal with sources of variation. A good performance measure removes as much as possible the variation caused by factors outside the associates' control. A good forecast identifies underlying sources of change and incorporates them.

Operating team members and PIT members should be confident of the data in their reports. The question "How do I know these numbers are realistic?" deserves an honest, reassuring, and technically correct answer. The statistical techniques used to get those answers are increasingly sophisticated and should be carried out or reviewed by a professionally trained statistician. The analysis identifies external causes of variation, specifies their impact, adjusts measures to allow for them, and includes them in forecasts.

Identifying External Causes of Variation

Many elements of both clinical and logistic processes are beyond the control of HCOs and their teams. When measures of these processes are used in evidence-based management, the goals should reflect only factors within the team members' control. When measures are forecast, changes in external factors must be included. External causes are identified from the literature or by statistical test and accommodated by specification, adjustment, and carefully designed forecasting models.

The process of *specification* identifies external groups whose performance differs. In marketing, specification is called *segmentation* (see Chapter 15). It examines whether specific groups differ in performance characteristics. Specification usually follows established taxonomies, or ways of subdividing populations. Exhibits 14.3, 14.4, and 14.5 show common taxonomies for specifying patients, payers, and providers, respectively.

The individual forecasts from specification can be aggregated to generate a single *adjusted* forecast by assuming a specific mix of categories. In a simplified example, specific cardiovascular mortality rates for an HCO might be calculated in several different age groups and for men and women. Then, the specific rate for each age and gender group is multiplied by the fraction of the comparison population in that group, and the adjusted rate is the sum of those products. The comparison population is usually the national population or a state population. The adjusted rate holds the population structure constant so that the aggregate performance can be compared over time or across several sites.

Forecasting models identify trends in data and forecast them to future situations. Several different statistical methods are available to prepare forecasts, and many important measures can be forecast subjectively. Forecasts of

EXHIBIT 14.3 Patient-Oriented Specification Taxonomies		
Category	Classifications
Demographic	Age
	Sex
	Race
	Education
Economic	Income
	Employment
	Social class
Geographic	Zip code of residence
	Census tract
	Political subdivision
Healthcare finance	Managed versus traditional insurance
	Private versus government insurance
Diagnosis	Disease classification
	Procedure
	Diagnosis-related group
	Ambulatory patient group
Risk	Health behavior attribute
	Pre-existing condition
	Chronic or high-cost disease

Category	Classifications
Employers	Size
	Geographic location
	Industry
	Ownership
	Income level
	Union organization
	Health insurance benefit
	Health insurance type
Intermediary	Health insurance type
	Ownership or corporate structure
	Size
	Number of health insurance subscribers
	Employer groups covered

EXHIBIT 14.4
Insurance Intermediary and Employer Specification Taxonomies

Category	Classifications
Individual providers	Training, certification, or licensure
	Specialization
	Organizational affiliation
	Location
	Age
Donors	Interest
	Level of contribution
Organized providers	Scope of service
	Geographic location
	Ownership
	Size
	Market share
	Financial strength
	Competitive position

EXHIBIT 14.5
Healthcare Provider Specification Taxonomies

important variables, such as demand for a certain service, are usually composites of several methods. Good forecasts also identify most likely, highest, and lowest values so that the implications of forecast error can be evaluated using sensitivity analysis.

Statistical process control uses the standard deviation of time series data to identify significant variations, that is, not likely to be due to random variation and therefore likely to be correctable. It allows the process manager to identify promising OFIs and avoid futile efforts to correct performance. Any measure reported over time can be graphed as a run chart—a simple line graph of reported values by date. Exhibit 14.6 shows a run chart and the same data in

Statistical Process Control

EXHIBIT 14.6
Run Charts and
Control Charts

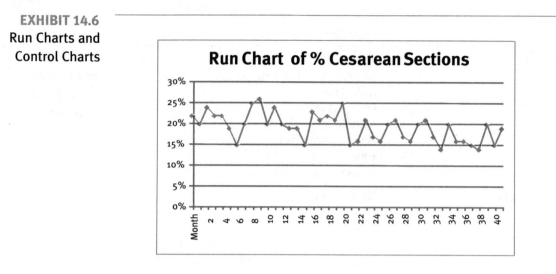

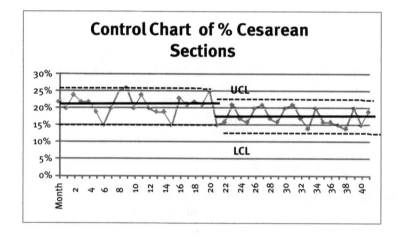

a control chart, with statistical control limits. The control chart shows that there was a statistically significant change in the underlying process at month 21, resulting in both a lower mean and less variation.

Exhibit 14.6 shows that no subsequent month is statistically different from the current mean; the process is "in control." A process in control is not a good OFI unless a benchmark can be found that is significantly better than the current mean. Any measure that is uniformly defined and reported over time can be analyzed with process control, identifying the OFIs most susceptible to study and improvement.

Legal, Regulatory, and Ethical Review

Many performance improvement or planning projects raise complex questions of law and ethics. These questions must be resolved by careful study and authoritative information. Well-managed HCOs organize their response around the input from an ethics committee, a compliance office, and experts in environmental management and human resources management. Many larger HCOs also have an institutional review board (IRB) that addresses questions related to research. Operating teams and individuals are encouraged to use these services as well.

An advisory ethics committee is used in most HCOs to assist caregivers, patients, and families with difficult ethical decisions (described in Chapter 2). The committee's functions should also include "formulating institutional policies to guide the professional staff in making ethical decisions and educating hospital personnel about healthcare ethics in general."[4] Responding to inquiries is a fruitful way to implement all three functions. It improves the consistency and comprehensiveness of protocols and work processes. It catches team members at a teachable moment.

Ethics Committee and IRB

    Similarly, questions important to the rights of patients in research situations are addressed by the IRB, or if necessary by the Office for Human Research Protections (OHRP) of the U.S. Department of Health and Human Services (HHS). IRB approval is mandatory for any research that directly involves human subjects. Concerns sometimes arise regarding whether quality improvement activities are subject to IRB review. OHRP has made clear that

> HHS regulations for the protection of human subjects do not apply to . . . quality improvement activities, and there is no requirement under these regulations for such activities to undergo review by an IRB, or for these activities to be conducted with provider or patient informed consent.

The OHRP definition of quality improvement activities is quite broad:

> [A]ctivities conducted by one or more institutions whose purposes are limited to: (a) implementing a practice to improve the quality of patient care, and (b) collecting patient or provider data regarding the implementation of the practice for clinical, practical, or administrative purposes.[5]

Many proposals for new services or revised processes involve various regulatory and legal constraints. Real estate transactions, construction, compensation agreements, billing practices, and supervision of nonprofessional caregivers are all areas where legal review is advisable. As a result, many PITs and planning committees need advice. Internal consulting coordinates it with other design and fact-finding activities.

Compliance Management and Legal Consultation

    HCOs have created a *compliance officer* position to coordinate and integrate responses on these and other topics that present legal implications. The compliance officer is responsible for issuing guidelines to prevent illegal, improper, or unethical conduct; conducting independent reviews of operations; and responding to all questions of potential or actual violations.[6] In the absence of a designated compliance officer, the questions must be answered by the HCO's general counsel, an attorney appointed to represent the organization on legal matters.

Environmental and Human Resources Management

HCOs must deal with both general environmental management issues and specific ones, such as high-voltage radiation and hazardous waste. They must also comply with laws and regulations governing worker safety, wages and hours, and collective bargaining contracts. Consultation on such questions is arranged through the environmental management and human resources management activities.

Certificate of Need

Many states require a certificate of need (CON) for new services and construction or renovation. CONs are a form of franchise, a government-issued permit to proceed with capital investment. These laws are enforced with varying degrees of rigor, and their importance is diminishing. In states where they remain, CON success depends on timing, well-designed and attractive services, technically well-prepared proposals, and the support of influential persons in the community. Strategies for dealing with CONs vary. The influence of these laws is arguable.[7] The U.S. Department of Justice has opposed the use of CONs.[8] Most well-run organizations have developed strategies and tactics for gaining the approval of all or nearly all their important options and proposals. Obtaining these approvals is usually the responsibility of the compliance officer or the general counsel, but documentation comes from the project itself, prepared by internal consulting.

Supporting Improvement Projects

Internal consulting has several resources to expand the analytic capabilities of PITs and planning teams. These include helping PITs operate more effectively, conducting advanced process analysis, coordinating skills of other logistic services, modeling alternative processes, managing outside consultants, and designing pilots and trials of proposals. In addition, internal consulting often works on strategic initiatives for which its client is the governing board or senior management.

Increasing the Effectiveness of PITs

PITs and planning teams bring specialists together from different areas to focus on a shared OFI. They can easily become ineffective and frustrating for their members. Internal consulting has several devices to help the PITs become more effective, including training for PIT members, direct consultation, and outside consultants.

High-performing HCOs provide basic continuous improvement training to all members of the leadership group. New managers and promotable associates are offered short courses (usually one or two days each) in goal setting, capital budgeting, and process analysis. These courses are generally offered by human resources but are staffed by planning personnel. They supplement programs in supervision and meeting management (discussed in Chapter 11). They emphasize "how to" and actual examples, working simultaneously on analytic skills, interpersonal skills, and self-confidence.

- Goal-setting courses include a full description of the goal-setting process, emphasizing the governing board's role in setting strategic guidelines, the use of benchmarks, the identification of OFIs, the use of PITs to change work processes, and negotiation processes. Hands-on practice with exercises and cases familiarizes people with computerized budgeting tools. Newcomers are often assigned an experienced mentor for their first round.[9]

- Capital budgeting courses describe how expansions and new equipment are planned, explaining the process to prepare a competitive request, the criteria used in judging requests, and the competitive process of capital allocation.

- Basic process analysis courses review the philosophy of continuous improvement and its elementary applications. The advantages of measures and an elementary review of measurement use, reliability, and validity are demonstrated, along with simple concepts of variability. Basic tools for analyzing processes are taught with examples and applications. These include flow process charting; bar, scatter, frequency, and Pareto graphs; fishbone diagrams; and run and control charts.[10] The role and functioning of PITs are described. In *action learning* approaches, teams are formed and address real problems with continuous guidance. The approach develops both analytic and team-building skills.

  The basic course allows analysis of simple issues, but its biggest benefit may be in demonstrating what is meant by evidence-based management. It shows that objective study of work processes leads to new and useful insights; performance really is driven by process.

- Advanced training opportunities in process improvement emphasize process control (Six Sigma),[11] elimination of waste (Lean manufacturing),[12,13] and integration of internal customers (Toyota Production System).[14] The differences between these approaches may be more apparent than real, and no evidence shows that any approach is superior.[15]

This training produces a cadre of managers familiar with the basic approaches of process improvement so that most important PITs have several knowledgeable members.

Advanced Process Analysis

Many key OFIs are too complicated to solve with just the basic tools. Direct consultation can be provided by industrial engineers, accountants, and others with professional training and experience in healthcare applications. Specific needs can be met as they arise by using just-in-time solutions. PITs that address complex problems can have a trained leader assigned to monitor group discussions and coordinate consultation as the issues are raised and understood by the group. The leader can be assisted by a team from internal consulting and other support services. Internal assistance is often preferable to that from outside consultants. Internal consulting brings a comprehensive knowledge of the organization that external consultants lack, and it is more directly invested in the results.

Coordinating Other Logistic Support

Internal consulting becomes a clearinghouse for coordinating improvement efforts, helping the performance improvement council (PIC) to avoid overlapping or missed opportunities among several PITs. It can help other logistic support units codify frequently needed information and establish processes to answer recurring questions. It can design effective contracts and monitor performance of external consultants, improving timeliness, completeness, and cost-effectiveness of service.

Process Modeling

Process modeling allows a much clearer and more detailed picture of proposed improvements. Activity-based cost analysis provides the basis for make-or-buy decisions. Econometric models can indicate price trends. Simulation models allow exploration of hourly operation, testing performance against uncontrollable variation. Markov approaches allow study of complex chains of demand—for example, from the emergency department to the catheterization lab to the operating room. Optimization models allow examination of trade-offs between resources and outputs and help identify critical constraints.

These models expand understanding of the process under study, identify useful solutions, allow sensitivity analysis, and establish realistic performance goals for the ultimate solution. Although they are substantially cheaper than real-world trials, they are costly to develop, often requiring dozens of hours from highly skilled professionals. Even when a basic model has been developed and tested elsewhere, it must be applied using local data. Data needs are usually extensive, requiring either special studies or sophisticated search of patient record and financial accounting information. Internal modeling capability can be supplemented by consortiums or outside consultants.

Outside Consultants

Outside consultants have the advantage of drawing on similar problems elsewhere, and often they have developed specialized tools and solutions that have a demonstrated record of success. They offer the strength of concentrated effort on a single issue. They bring additional resources on a short-term basis. If they are routinely hired through the internal consulting activity, standardized evaluation criteria and contract approaches will increase the value of their services.

Evaluating and Testing Solutions

The improvement cycle calls for a pilot test of any proposed process revision. Simple changes may require only a week or two of experience and a team meeting to review results. Large process redesigns can involve substantial field trials. The trials are usually less rigorous than randomized controlled trials—the gold standard used in clinical processes—but making them as rigorous and objective as possible is important. The planning unit is usually responsible for consulting on the experimental design, measures, and criteria. The unit is often used to analyze the data and make a recommendation because it brings improved objectivity.

Supporting Governance and Senior Management Projects

Important improvement opportunities arise from the governing board and senior management. These often involve relationships with competitors and external stakeholders and have consequences that go beyond the usual PIT. Examples include merger and acquisition opportunities, responses to competitor activity, and corporate restructuring. These opportunities are strategic-level OFIs. They often present special needs for confidentiality and careful development of sensitive information. Although external consultants are usually advisable for such projects, internal consulting can frequently help assemble necessary facts, develop forecasts, and identify implications.

Supporting the Capital Investment Review

Capital investments, such as new programs, facilities, or equipment, represent multiyear commitments to operational processes and programs as well as commitments of limited capital funds. Correct selection of investments is critical to mission achievement.[16] Excellent HCOs have highly developed investment review systems to improve their investment decisions. The review process must promote innovation, making sure that no reasonable opportunity goes unexamined, and wise selection, making sure that the best opportunities are implemented. Reviews must also be efficient to support making the right decisions with little delay and minimal demands on associates' time. Scale and equity are also important. Large HCOs commit tens of millions of dollars annually to capital requests and need a process that is perceived as reliable and equitable.

Checklist for Project Planning

Any investment concept or opportunity needs to be reviewed against several conditions:

1. *The expected contribution to mission achievement.* This is usually measured by changes in operational goals and, for large projects, changes in the strategic scorecard. The contribution to mission need not be in dollars, but it must exceed the investment required.

2. *Physical constraints.* Changes in facilities involve architectural issues like floor loads, radiation safety, and Life Safety Code requirements. Equipment must fit space and utility constraints and must meet safety requirements.

3. *Asset control and cost minimization.* Purchases must be carefully specified and, if possible, competitively bid. The delivered goods must match the specifications.

4. *Implementation.* Even relatively small projects can involve several steps of equipment changes, renovation, process redesign, and retraining. Installation must be scheduled and coordinated with ongoing activities. Large projects require months or years of management.

5. *The actual contribution to mission achievement.* The expected contribution must be built into the appropriate unit's operational goals, and support must be provided to achieve the improved targets.

Using a formal checklist of questions, such as the one in Exhibit 14.7, increases fairness, helps identify impractical projects quickly, and establishes an initial estimate of contribution. Experienced managers soon learn the kinds of projects that gain funding. They drop or modify projects that fall short, reducing the set of proposals to a manageable group. Advice from internal consulting and finance is available to help apply the checklist and identify the contribution.

The issue in applying the checklist is prudent evaluation—that is, diligence in understanding the options and their implications. Well-managed HCOs divide capital investments into strategic and programmatic. *Strategic* opportunities affect several units or service lines. The strategic review process is described in Chapter 15. *Programmatic* proposals focus on a single or small group of accountability units. Both can be reviewed using the checklist in Exhibit 14.7.

Examples of programmatic opportunities are shown in Exhibit 14.8. Well-managed organizations encourage programmatic proposals because they reflect an alert, flexible work attitude and because they provide OFIs. An abundant supply of programmatic proposals minimizes the danger that the best solution will be overlooked. Hundreds of programmatic concepts originate each year in large HCOs. Dozens survive initial review and are formally documented as proposals.

Programmatic Capital Review

The objective of the review process for programmatic capital requests, shown in Exhibit 14.9, is to rank-order the requests into a single list for the HCO. The rank-ordering incorporates multiple competing perspectives. Reaching

EXHIBIT 14.7
Checklist for
Evaluating
Improvement
Proposals

Mission, Vision, and Plan
What is the relationship of this proposal to the mission and vision?
Is this proposal essential to implement a strategic goal in the long-range plan?
If the proposal arises outside the current strategic goals, can it be designed to
    enhance or improve the current plan?

Benefit
In the most specific terms possible, what does this project contribute to health-
    care? If possible, state the nature of the contribution, the probability of
    success, and the associated risk for each individual benefiting and the kinds
    and numbers of persons benefiting.
If the organization were unable to adopt the proposal, what would be the
    implication? Are there alternative sources of care? What costs are associated
    with using these sources?
If the proposal contributes to some additional or secondary objectives, what are
    these contributions, and what is their value?

Market and Demand
What size and segment of the community will this proposal serve? What fraction
    of this group is likely to seek care at this organization?
What is the trend in the size of this group and its tendency to seek care here?
    How will the proposal affect this trend?
To what extent is the demand dependent on insurance or finance incentives?
    What is the likely trend for these provisions?
What are the consequences of this proposal for competing hospitals or
    healthcare organizations?
What impact will the proposal have on the organization's general market share
    or on other specific services?
What implications does the project have for the recruitment of physicians and
    other key healthcare personnel?
What are the promotional requirements of the proposal?

Costs and Resources
What are the marginal operating and capital costs of the proposal, including
    startup costs and possible revenue losses from other services?
Are there cost implications for other services or overhead activities?
Are there special or critical resource requirements?
Are there identifiable opportunity costs associated with the proposal or other
    proposals or opportunities that are facilitated by this proposal?
Are there other intangible elements (positive or negative) associated with this
    proposal?

Finance
What are the capital requirements, project life, and finance costs associated
    with the proposal?
What is the competitive price and anticipated net revenue?
What is the demand elasticity and profit sensitivity?
What are the insurance or finance sources of revenue, and what implications do
    these sources raise?
What is the net cash flow associated with the proposal over its life, and what is
    the discounted value of that flow?

(continued)

EXHIBIT 14.7
Checklist for
Evaluating
Improvement
Proposals
(continued)

Other Factors

What are the opportunities to enhance this proposal or others by combination?

Are there customers or stakeholders with an unusual commitment for or against the proposal?

Are there any specific risks or benefits associated with the proposal not identified elsewhere?

Does the proposal suggest a strategic opportunity, such as a joint venture or the purchase or sale of a major service?

Timing, Implementation, and Evaluation

What are the critical path components of the installation process, and how long will they take?

What are the problems or advantages associated with deferring or speeding up the implementation?

What are the anticipated changes in the operating budget of the units accountable for the proposal? What changes are required in supporting units?

EXHIBIT 14.8
Examples of
Programmatic
Proposals

Proposal	Description	Approximate Cost	Possible Contribution
Renovate ORs	Enlarge operating suite into adjacent inpatient unit, modernize	$10,000,000	Increase attractiveness to ambulatory surgery patients; improve post-op infection rate.
Replace air-conditioning condensers	Replace aging equipment with more reliable and more efficient	$ 500,000	More reliable service; lower unit cost, lower carbon production
Purchase robotic surgery equipment	Machine used for several abdominal surgery procedures	$ 2,000,000	Match competitor's investment; improve patient comfort, speed patient recovery
Replace exercise machines	4 specialized exercise machines to replace worn older models in PT	$ 100,000	Increase patient comfort and reduce chance of service failure

OR: operating room; PT: physical therapy

consensus is rarely easy, but the process is driven by the board's timelines. The final list is presented to the governing board, which identifies how far down the list to fund based on its prior analysis of the long-term financial plan and strategic goals (see Chapter 4). Board review of individual programmatic requests

EXHIBIT 14.9
**Programmatic
Capital Review
Process**

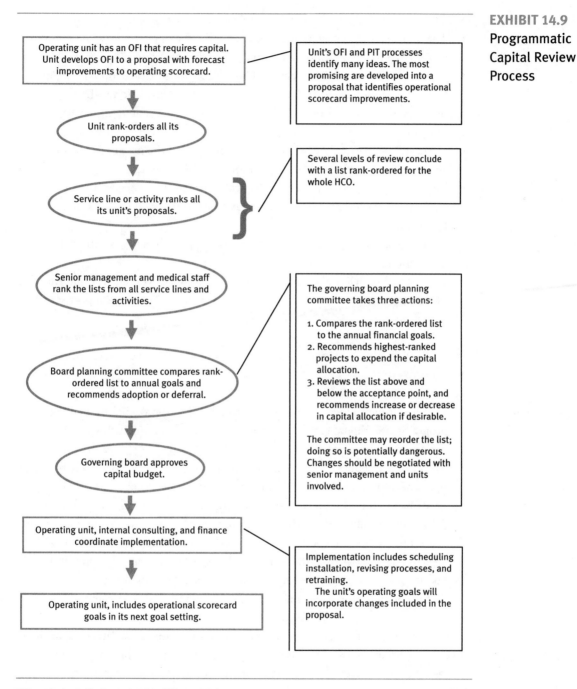

Operating unit has an OFI that requires capital. Unit develops OFI to a proposal with forecast improvements to operating scorecard.

Unit's OFI and PIT processes identify many ideas. The most promising are developed into a proposal that identifies operational scorecard improvements.

Unit rank-orders all its proposals.

Service line or activity ranks all its unit's proposals.

Several levels of review conclude with a list rank-ordered for the whole HCO.

Senior management and medical staff rank the lists from all service lines and activities.

The governing board planning committee takes three actions:

1. Compares the rank-ordered list to the annual financial goals.
2. Recommends highest-ranked projects to expend the capital allocation.
3. Reviews the list above and below the acceptance point, and recommends increase or decrease in capital allocation if desirable.

Board planning committee compares rank-ordered list to annual goals and recommends adoption or deferral.

The committee may reorder the list; doing so is potentially dangerous. Changes should be negotiated with senior management and units involved.

Governing board approves capital budget.

Operating unit, internal consulting, and finance coordinate implementation.

Implementation includes scheduling installation, revising processes, and retraining.
    The unit's operating goals will incorporate changes included in the proposal.

Operating unit, includes operational scorecard goals in its next goal setting.

OFI: opportunity for improvement; PIT: process improvement team

is rare and generally unwise. The board may amend its capital investment guideline, voting either to reduce the investment because the last accepted proposal can safely be deferred until next year or to increase the investment because the benefits of the highest-ranking rejected proposal are compelling.

Well-run organizations emphasize these characteristics:

- The operating unit is clearly responsible for identifying opportunities.
- The unit's senior managers act as advocates for the opportunities and coordinate support from units, including internal consulting and clinical internal customers.
- Internal consulting assistance is readily available to develop proposals. It, in turn, calls on other logistic and strategic support. Information technology, human resources, environmental services, finance, and marketing are routinely involved.
- Costs and benefits are quantitatively documented in the proposal, and the unit agrees to the benefits as future operational scorecard goals.
- The HCO's mission statement and its commitment to evidence-based medicine and evidence-based management are used as the guide to rank new opportunities.
- There is medical and nursing review and ranking of all projects with clinical implications.
- Clinical and nonclinical proposals are judged competitively against one another, in a common review process that includes medical and clinical support service representation.

The result is a process that supports both empowerment and continuous improvement.

- The operating budget is built upon a "same store" approach. Units submitting programmatic capital requests prepare two sets of goals, including and excluding the proposed investment.
- The evidence supporting the claimed contributions is rigorously evaluated. Multiple reviewers comment upon and rank the proposals. Many of the reviewers have proposals of their own and will vigorously criticize competing projects.
- Associates are empowered. The review process not only must identify the best proposals but also must be perceived as predictable and equitable to associates.[17] The approved list is not "what the board said"; it's "what the ranking teams decided."
- Specific goal changes related to accepted capital proposals are implemented. The unit is committed to achieving the goals claimed for the investment.

The role of internal consulting is to encourage a broad search for promising ideas, assist proposal development teams in preparing proposals for competitive review, ensure accuracy in forecasts and claims, and support fair review. The following procedures encourage managers to seek investment opportunities and evaluate them:

- The continuous improvement culture encourages units to seek imaginative ideas. Ideas are respected even when they are unusual.
- Internal consulting team members are readily available to discuss concepts informally, assist with proposals, explain the evaluation process, and identify potential contributions.

- Internal consulting is a source of knowledge about the plans in existence and the discussion that surrounded related proposals. Partnerships with other units often succeed where freestanding proposals fail.

Over time and with internal consulting's help, managers learn to recognize the kinds of proposals that will be successful. Many projects are reshaped, sometimes to entirely new and much more complex ideas. Replacements for physical therapy (PT) exercise equipment look simple, but they should prompt a review of PT's future demand, the clinical outcomes the new machines can achieve, alternative clinical approaches to reach the same outcomes, the desirability of alternative sites for the service, and the possibility of actually expanding PT volume by selling the service to others. The project could move from programmatic to strategic as it raises important issues beyond the original replacement. That will rarely happen, but the possibilities will have been explored. Internal consulting plays an important role in understanding the opportunities and building consensus.

Note that planning staff members never judge the proposals themselves. They provide facts and concepts to managers and let the managers decide. They protect the process of review itself, discouraging attempts to subvert or avoid it and making proposal preparation as efficient and fair as possible.

Implementing and Integrating Recommendations

Once new processes or capital investments are recommended for adoption, two further steps are required:

1. *Implementation.* Many projects require months or years of preparation. Contracts must be let, construction or moving scheduled, installation completed, final reviews passed, and associates trained in new methods before the project is ready for routine use. The benefits of the project are delayed until this work is finished and are impaired if the work is inefficiently managed. Project management is a service in itself. It can substantially reduce both costs and delays. The use of PERT software to coordinate multiple contributions can save millions in large projects.[18]
2. *Integration.* Proposals are accepted because they promise specific performance improvements. Those promises must be built into the operating goals of the units involved. Progress toward them must be monitored, and assistance must be arranged if difficulties are encountered. Internal consulting should continue to monitor progress until the initial goals have been reached or are no longer applicable.

The implementation of projects that require construction or extensive renovation is commonly assigned to environment-of-care management (discussed in Chapter 12). Small projects are often monitored by internal consulting. In any case, internal consulting monitors the goal-setting processes to ensure that the claimed benefits are achieved.

Responding to Any Other Factual Concern

Internal consulting is a knowledge management resource for the HCO. Its purpose requires it to pursue any question or issue where understanding or resolution of the issue will be improved by a stronger grasp of the factual situation. Under the ongoing guidance of internal consulting, the HCO as a whole develops an ability to identify, understand, and react to opportunity that becomes a major competitive advantage. The clearinghouse role of internal consulting is central here. The availability of a consulting resource is a strong bulwark for evidence-based management. Internal consulting's response to inquiries should routinely exceed expectations.

Improving Internal Consulting

As a major supporter of the HCO's continuous improvement effort, internal consulting must itself model the concept. It maintains an operational scorecard (see the Measures section below). It makes a systematic effort to benchmark itself and identify best practices. It identifies, pursues, and implements OFIs within its own operations as it assists others in similar tasks. It sets and achieves improvement goals. In the process, it reviews and improves the role of the PIC and the HCO's overall continuous improvement effort.

People

Team Members

Internal consulting requires trained professionals in several fields, including expertise in statistics, operations analysis, and forecasting plus knowledge management, human resources, environmental services, finance, legal counsel, marketing, and strategic analysis. Clinical knowledge is also important. The most critical role of internal consulting is as a clearinghouse. In a small HCO, a single person might be the internal consulting resource. Her success would depend less on her technical knowledge (she could not conceivably master all the technology required) than on her ingenuity in finding knowledge resources, linking seekers to them, and encouraging exploration. In a large organization, professionals with a foundation in any of the areas or in general management can succeed as much by helping their clients reach a successful conclusion as by having a mastery of their technical field.

Organization

The first three functions of internal consulting—support the HCO, support improvement projects, and support capital investment review—have become so important that it is difficult to imagine an HCO succeeding without solid processes. The effectiveness with which they are done is a major driver of strategic success. Small HCOs—such as clinics, doctors' offices, hospices, and critical access hospitals—have only two choices. One is to affiliate with a larger

HCO, pursuing either vertical or horizontal integration. The other is to purchase service from an external consultant.

Large HCOs must fulfill these functions in a way that makes them a distinctive competency. That requires establishing explicit accountability for each function, with operational measures and goals. One successful structure identifies a senior management team member as the vice president of planning or internal consulting. This individual leads a team responsible for the organization-wide functions and supplies process analysis and statistical capability to improvement and capital investment projects. The team has understood authority to call on all other logistic and strategic support units to assist in its projects or to meet general organizational needs. Another common structure assigns the team to the marketing and strategy vice president. The structure is not as important as the skills of the internal consulting leader and the commitment of senior management to effective processes.

Outside Consultants

Most HCOs use external consultants. Assigning contracting authority to the internal consulting group encourages the appropriate use of existing knowledge and the maximum benefit from the consulting engagement. The keys to successful use of external consultants are as follows:

1. *The assignment should be clearly specified in terms of process, timing, and goal.* The clearer the assignment and the more details of the work specified in advance, the better the chances for success. It is sometimes wise to use consultants for general education and to gain fresh insights into vague, ill-defined problems, but such use should be limited to short-term assignments.
2. *Internal skills and knowledge should be fully used before external consultants are engaged, and internal experts should work directly with external ones.* This minimizes cost and maximizes retention of the external advice.
3. *Consultant firms should be selected on the basis of relevant prior experience.* In the absence of direct experience with a consultant, opinions of other clients should be solicited prior to any major engagement.
4. *Consultant activities should be carefully monitored against the specifications throughout the project.* A timetable and monthly interim achievement checkpoints should be used to monitor progress.
5. *Each consultant must have an explicitly assigned internal supervisor.* Failure to identify a point of contact slows the consultants, adds to their costs, and defeats the possibility of continuous monitoring during the contract period.

Internal Consulting in Multihospital Systems

Healthcare systems that operate in several locations frequently centralize some aspects of internal consulting to improve the technical skills of personnel, provide economies of scale, and ensure transfer of best practices. Much of the functions that support the organization as a whole can be centralized. With Internet connectivity, it does not matter where the calculations are done, and consistent application across a system provides comparative information. Important aspects of the environmental assessment require an established local presence. Small local staffs provide direct support to the line managers, identify important local variations, and rely on the central staff as a consultant resource. On project assistance, the central resource behaves as a favored external consultant.

Measures

The internal consulting activity, as every other part of the well-run organization, has performance measures, short-term goals, and regular reporting of achievement against these. A reasonable set is shown in Exhibit 14.10. These measures follow the usual operations scorecard dimensions. Requests for service are specifically counted. Some, but not all, become *engagements*. The term is used by outside consultants to describe a specific project or contract with a client. It is used here to identify an ongoing commitment to a specific unit or project. Internal consulting staff and other associates can assign their hours to specific engagements, and each engagement can be evaluated for cost, quality, and return on the internal consulting investment.

Internal consulting also may be evaluated on technical proficiency, such as the completeness of data, the availability of analytic software, and the use of correct analytic techniques. Such an evaluation would be arranged by senior management using outside consultants.

Building many of the measures around engagements makes it possible to compare internal consulting performance to alternative sources, such as a retainer arrangement with outside suppliers. The engagement approach supports a service mentality on the part of the team members. They must keep logs of activities, and individual effort must be transfer priced to show costs. Once this is done, the project-specific consulting costs, proposal decisions, projected improvements, realized improvements, and client satisfaction can be tracked. Although some measurements are estimates, even approximations show the unit's success at several different levels:

- Proposal approval rates reflect the ability of the unit to steer clients toward effective projects.
- Cost per project compared to projected contribution shows the effectiveness of specific engagements.
- Cost compared to contribution of implemented projects is an indicator of internal consulting's contribution to mission achievement.
- Total consulting costs compared to the value of all projects implemented also indicates the unit's contribution.

Dimension	Measures	Examples
Demand for services	Counts of user requests Engagements Unfilled or delayed requests	Log of requests and dispositions Engagements and personnel assignments Delays in responding to service requests
Cost	Total direct costs Hours on assigned engagements External consultant costs Data and information acquisition costs	Hours of personnel assigned to engagements External consultant fees Costs of comparative or benchmark information
Human resources	Satisfaction of internal consulting personnel Vacancy rates and turnover	Surveys, personal and group discussions of work environment
Productivity	Total cost as percent of HCO operating cost Cost per support request Cost per project completed Total cost as percent of improvements implemented	"Contribution," actual improvements in operational measures from completed engagements Contribution as a percent of internal consulting direct costs
Outcomes quality	Forecast accuracy: variation from actual Timeliness: projects completed on schedule Improvements achieved	Variation of annual forecasts from actual Accuracy of epidemiologic planning model forecasts Counts of engagements completed on time Counts of engagements achieving expected goals
Client satisfaction	User satisfaction surveys Overall planning service Engagement-specific service Recognition and resolution of problems Supportive attitude	Users' responses to services: "would rehire, would recommend"

EXHIBIT 14.10
Operational
Performance
Measures
for Internal
Consulting

Benchmarking the Exhibit 14.10 data is challenging. Large HCO systems can benchmark performance on engagements against similar units, but "similar units" are elusive. Comparing the internal consulting unit of a high-performing HCO to an HCO with substantial OFIs in its culture or a limited prior effort at process improvement is misleading. The different environment means that the two units are doing different things with clients who have different skill sets. The ultimate judgment that the organization is or is not positioned where it should be in the community is based on the environmental surveillance itself and is inevitably bound up with the judgment of the chief executive officer and the governing board. The decision should focus not on the cost of operation or the cost per engagement, but rather on the value of the contribution.

Managerial Issues

Three managerial issues are known to be troublesome for internal consulting:

1. How can the HCO ensure quality of internal consulting?
2. How much should an HCO spend on internal consulting?
3. How does the HCO protect the empowerment of PITs and operating teams?

Ensuring Quality of Work

Careless or incomplete work by internal consulting can fatally disable an HCO. Successful internal consulting units excel in four areas: (1) They take extra pains to guard against oversights and errors, (2) they use the best comparative data and the most objective forecasts they can obtain, (3) they are rigorous in their evaluation of proposal costs and contribution, and (4) they work consistently to delight their internal customers.

The outcomes quality and customer satisfaction measures on the operational scorecard (Exhibit 14.10) are important indicators of the success; any deterioration is an immediate OFI. Internal reviews, where a work product by one analyst is critiqued by a second, are important and should be routine on all large-scale engagements. An outside review team can be helpful in identifying specific activities that need improvement. Attendance at technical training programs allows analysts to keep and expand their skills. The visible commitment of the senior management leader is important. Individual performance reviews are also useful and can be tied to incentive compensation.

Sizing Internal Consulting

The investment in internal consulting is made to improve mission achievement. The value of the operating improvements from successful proposals must cover the cost of the investment in internal consulting. That value is not simply revenue or profit. It includes contributions to community health. High-performing HCOs achieve value using the service excellence model. The key sizing question is not "How much did internal consulting cost?" but "Did the HCO explore and implement all the OFIs that would substantially improve the balanced scorecard?" If promising projects are being delayed or ignored, internal consulting is too small. If the projects being proposed have only trivial impact on the scorecard, the unit is too big.

The conditions that occur at that optimum are indicated by the operational scorecard (Exhibit 14.10):

1. The client's needs are met without excessive delay.
2. Clients are satisfied with the service received.
3. The value of individual engagements is substantially higher than the engagement cost.
4. Implementation and integration are translated to improved performance on unit scorecards.

And, on the strategic scorecard,

5. The HCO continues to improve and move toward benchmark on all measures.

Failure to meet any of these conditions is an OFI, subject to investigation and improvement by the internal consulting unit, the PIC, and the senior leadership team.

Note that no benchmark exists for the operating cost of internal consulting. As is true of all logistic services, the optimum cost is not what some other HCO pays but the minimum expenditure that yields return on strategic performance.

Protecting Associates' Empowerment

The transformational model explicitly empowers HCO associates to change their work situation to improve mission achievement. Empowerment removes one of the major frustrations of working in a large organization. An empowered worker is entitled to the tools and supplies she needs, knows that she has that entitlement, and uses it effectively to improve her performance. That dynamic is the major component of service excellence. Internal consulting can endanger empowerment through either of two dynamics:

1. *Information asymmetry.* Internal consulting assembles and analyzes a broad range of data that can easily appear arcane and forbidding to clients. With their superior command of the facts, internal consulting associates can easily usurp the operating associates' right and obligation to make the final decision.
2. *Loss of control of the PIT or planning process.* Team review of OFIs can be used as a political device, a graveyard for OFIs that someone in a position of power finds unattractive or inconvenient.

A successful internal consulting operation must take special steps to guard against these risks.

Balancing Information Asymmetry

The key to the information asymmetry problem is careful explanation of the what, why, and how of data and analysis used by internal consulting. Any PIT or operating team member has the right to understand

- what: definition, provenance, and limitations of all the measures that are used in an analysis;
- why: the implications of alternative measures; and
- how: the limitations of the analysis and the implications of alternative analyses.

Making these elements clear to the associates involved in each project is a professional responsibility analogous to the similar obligation of physicians and lawyers. The client is entitled to the fullest possible understanding to support his or her final decision about the course of action. Fulfilling the responsibility is an important assurance of empowerment. The consultant team must be trained to do that. A question on the client survey, "How often did [internal consulting] explain things in a way you could understand?" will monitor performance. (This wording is taken directly from the Hospital Consumer Assessment of Healthcare Providers and Systems patient survey.) Understanding what, why, and how is essential to empowerment and critical in gaining consensus and effective implementation.

Controlling the Planning Process

The processes of programmatic and strategic review are subject to two different risks that require direct management. One is evasion. Some associates may press to evade the review processes, usually under the guise of emergency or inevitability. The other is subversion. The review process is started, but some associates use delays and obstacles to keep the proposal from final review.

Evasion is stopped by effective senior leadership. Rank has no privileges under servant leadership. No capital dollars are spent except through the programmatic or strategic processes. Once it is made clear that special pleading will not work and the review processes are essential to fairly balance the needs of all, the problem is solved. (There may, of course, be true emergencies from unforeseeable events. The governing board and the CEO will need to take special action.)

Subversion is also a deliberate action to defeat the review processes. Opponents of a proposal use the need for more study as a device to prevent action. Like evasion, subversion leads to bad individual decisions, but it also destroys the processes themselves. The PIC and internal consulting can prevent subversion by enforcing three rules. First, the HCO must scrupulously maintain its commitment to the evidence, making sure that all analyses are objective by using the best available data, without concealment or distortion. Second, the PIC must ensure appropriate representation on each PIT or planning committee (no unit with a stake in the outcome can be omitted) and a level playing field among PIT members. Third, the PIC must enforce the timetable so that the PIT proceeds in a timely manner. "Evidence" is always limited and imperfect. The decision about whether it supports a given proposal is always a judgment. Under the programmatic and strategic review processes, the judgment is made and reviewed by a formally designated structure—the PIT, the PIC, the board's planning committee, and the board. While everyone gets a say, no special interest can dominate the decision process.

Additional Resources

Alemi, F., and D. H. Gustafson. 2007. *Decision Analysis for Healthcare Managers*. Chicago: Health Administration Press.

Chalice, R. 2007. *Improving Healthcare Using Toyota Lean Production Methods*. Milwaukee, WI: American Society for Quality.

Harrison, J. P. 2010. *Essentials of Strategic Planning in Healthcare*. Chicago: Health Administration Press.

Iezzoni, L. I. (ed.). 2012. *Risk Adjustment for Measuring Health Care Outcomes*, 4th ed. Chicago: Health Administration Press.

Ozcan, Y. A. 2009. *Quantitative Methods in Health Care Management*, 2nd ed. San Francisco: Jossey-Bass.

Zuckerman, A. M. 2012. *Healthcare Strategic Planning*, 3rd ed. Chicago: Health Administration Press.

Notes

1. Begun, J. W., J. A. Hamilton, and A. A. Kaissi. 2005. "An Exploratory Study of Healthcare Strategic Planning in Two Metropolitan Areas." *Journal of Healthcare Management* 50 (4): 264–75.

2. Griffith, J. R., and K. R. White. 2003. *Thinking Forward: Six Strategies for Highly Successful Organizations*, 241. Chicago: Health Administration Press; Griffith, J. R., and K. R. White. 2005. "The Revolution in Hospital Management." *Journal of Healthcare Management* 50 (3): 170–90.

3. Institute for Healthcare Improvement. 2014. "Collaboratives." [Online information; retrieved 6/18/14.] www.ihi.org/Engage/collaboratives/Pages/default.aspx.

4. Hester, D. M., and T. Schonfeld (eds.). 2012. *Guidance for Healthcare Ethics Committees*. New York: Cambridge University Press.

5. U.S. Department of Health and Human Services, Office of Human Research Protection. 2014. "Frequently Asked Questions About Human Research." [Online information; retrieved 6/16/14.] http://answers.hhs.gov/ohrp/categories/1569.

6. American College of Healthcare Executives. 2014. "Position Description: Chief Compliance Officer." [Online information; retrieved 6/16/14.] www.ache.org/newclub/career/comploff.cfm.

7. U.S. Government Accountability Office (GAO). 1981. "Health Systems Plans: A Poor Framework for Promoting Health Care Improvements." *Report to the Congress by the Controller General of the United States*. Washington, DC: GAO.

8.   Miller, J. M. 2008. "Competition in Healthcare and Certificates of Need." Statement of the Antitrust Division, U.S. Department of Justice. [Online information; retrieved 6/16/14.] www.usdoj.gov/atr/public/comments/233821.htm.

9.   Griffith and White (2003, 174–79).

10. Institute for Healthcare Improvement. "IHI Open School Courses." [Online information; retrieved 6/16/14.] www.ihi.org/education/ihiopenschool/Pages/default.aspx.

11. iSixSigma LLC. 2014. Home page. [Online information; retrieved 6/16/14.] www.isixsigma.com.

12. Lean Enterprise Institute. 2014. Home page. [Online information; retrieved 6/16/14.] www.lean.org.

13. Sproull, R. 2009. *The Ultimate Improvement Cycle: Maximizing Profits Through the Integration of Lean, Six Sigma, and the Theory of Constraints.* New York: Productivity Press.

14. Minoura, T. 2003. "The 'Thinking' Production System: TPS as a Winning Strategy for Developing People in the Global Manufacturing Environment." [Online article; retrieved 10/13/05.] www.toyotageorgetown.com/tpsoverview.asp.

15. Vest, J. R., and L. D. Gamm. 2009. "A Critical Review of the Research Literature on Six Sigma, Lean and Studer Group's Hardwiring Excellence in the United States: The Need to Demonstrate and Communicate the Effectiveness of Transformation Strategies in Healthcare." *Implementation Science* 4 (1): 35.

16. Prince, T. R., and J. A. Sullivan. 2000. "Financial Viability, Medical Technology, and Hospital Closures." *Journal of Health Care Finance* 26 (4): 1–18.

17. Sorensen D., and D. Sullivan. 2005. "Managing Trade-offs Makes Budgeting Processes Pay Off." *Healthcare Financial Management* 59 (11): 54–60.

18. Internet Center for Management and Business Administration. "PERT." [Online information; retrieved 6/18/14.] www.netmba.com/operations/project/pert.

15 MARKETING AND STRATEGY

1. *Marketing is a broad approach to building exchange relationships.*
   - Not limited to patients, it applies to all aspects of the organization's interfaces with the world.
   - The order of the four Ps (product, place, price, promotion) is important.

2. *Markets are segmented.*
   - *Segments* are subgroups with similar needs.
   - Specific segments drive many strategy and marketing decisions.

3. *Listening is fundamental to both marketing and strategy.*
   - The goal is to understand the perspectives of customers, associates, and suppliers.
   - Both qualitative and quantitative approaches are used.

4. *Strategies are framed using the tools of evidence-based management.*
   - Strategies integrate the results of the environmental assessment and include quantitative forecasts.
   - Extensive discussions and listening allow stakeholders to gain understanding and agreement.

5. *Senior management and governance manage strategic discussion and implementation.*
   - Not-for-profit HCOs require a long-term commitment to mission and ongoing use of evidence to achieve excellence.
   - Large healthcare systems can strengthen both the commitment and the evidence-based tools more readily than small organizations can.

Questions for Discussion

These questions are about applying the chapter content. It's often helpful to discuss them with classmates or mentors, gaining different perspectives on the issues.

1. Why are the four Ps ordered as product, place, price, promotion? What sorts of questions would the four Ps prompt for implementing the new Well-Baby Program suggested in Exhibit 15.2? How would you answer those questions in a real HCO?

2. Consider a planning team designing a major renovation or expansion of a patient service. Focus groups and surveys will cost nearly $100,000. How might that expenditure pay off? What is your backup plan if you think that's too much money?

3. How would you justify a hospital's investment in health promotion and palliative care? Successful efforts could mean less income for the hospital and its doctors and even reduced employment. Identify the stakeholder segments that must be sold on the concept, and propose the best arguments for each.

4. The Managerial Issues section in this chapter suggests that the logistic and strategic support functions described in chapters 10 through 15 create a critical competitive advantage for large-scale HCOs. Summarize the arguments you would make to a trustee of a small not-for-profit HCO that an excellent healthcare system could offer substantial advantages to patients, associates, and community over continued freestanding operation. What questions would you expect from the trustee?

5. The second paragraph of the Managerial Issues section is an indictment of U.S. healthcare that concludes, "the typical hospital is not strategically managed; it is simply drifting." Could this be true? Is there a counterargument? If it's true, what should be done about it?

Purpose

The purpose of marketing and strategy is

to identify, evaluate, and respond to changes in stakeholder needs.

In a free-market society, both customer and associate stakeholders "vote with their feet," selecting organizations that meet their needs often without fully expressing what those needs are. An organization thrives because it attracts and retains stakeholders better than competing alternatives. Marketing and strategy are closely linked activities to make the HCO optimally attractive to stakeholders.

Marketing is the deliberate effort to establish fruitful relationships with exchange partners and stakeholders. *Strategy* (see p. 36) is the selection of the profile of stakeholder needs to be met. In successful HCOs, as in other industries, marketing and strategy are intertwined, creating a seamless, continuous activity that monitors the basic direction of the enterprise; modifies the direction as conditions change; and, in some cases, redirects the enterprise through merger, acquisition, or closure.

Marketing
The deliberate effort to establish fruitful relationships with exchange partners and stakeholders.

Success can be more than the sum of its parts; fruitful relationships tend to be mutually reinforcing. Successes produce stronger relationships and support further improvement. Failures weaken the organization and start a cycle that leads to collapse or reorganization. The issues quickly become complex. Success must meet several different and interrelated criteria:

- The services offered attract adequate demand and use processes that are competitive on cost, amenities, and quality.
- The work environment attracts and retains associates who are committed to implementing the strategy.
- The services identify and capitalize on a competitive advantage or "distinctive competency," a reason customers select them over alternatives.
- The constellation of services attracts and builds patient and associate loyalty and fulfills what patients and associates can realistically expect.

Each of these criteria presents a risk of failure. All the criteria require attention to the whole environment. The set of solutions is the organization's strategy—sometimes called the *business model*.

Functions

The functions of marketing and strategy are summarized in Exhibit 15.1.

EXHIBIT 15.1
Functions of
Marketing and
Strategy

Function	Processes	Purpose
Marketing		
Identifying and segmenting customer and associate markets	Surveillance, data analysis, segmentation of market	Understand stakeholder needs and identify participants whose needs are consistent with the HCO mission
Listening to exchange partners' needs	Surveys, focus groups, monitors, personal contact	Gain a clear and complete understanding of what the HCO must do to attract exchange partners in sufficient number
Developing brand and media relations	Communication to establish awareness of HCO and its scope of services	Make the HCO as a whole attractive to the community by emphasizing widely shared goals in a variety of communication methods
Convincing potential customers to select the HCO's services	Communication to patient populations with specific needs	Make potential patients aware of the services and persuade them to select the organization over its competitors
Attracting and motivating capable associates	Communication to target associate populations, advertising, incentives	Ensure a steady stream of qualified applicants, even in areas of personnel shortages
Managing other stakeholder relationships	Surveillance, senior management listening, partnerships to align other stakeholders	Establish constructive relationships with other organizations such as insurance intermediaries, employers, and providers of competing or complementary services
Improving the organization's marketing activity	Marketing plans, goal setting, evaluating marketing effectiveness	Set goals that move toward benchmarks and values for market share
Strategy		
Maintaining the mission, vision, and values	Visioning exercise	Allow multiple stakeholders to consider and comment on mission, vision, and values
Defining the strategic position	Evaluating and selecting alternative approaches to maximizing mission achievement	Position an array of clinical services geographically to achieve a competitive advantage with an identified population
Documenting the strategic position	Maintaining and coordinating strategic plans	Integrate multiple strategic and programmatic responses
Implementing the strategic position	Managing investments and processes that will achieve the strategic goals	Ensure that the HCO responds to opportunities and threats from external events
Improving the strategic process	Establish goals and opportunities for improvement strategy processes	Continuously improve strategy and strategy formulation

Marketing Functions

The term *marketing* has a professional definition that is substantially broader than its common use. Here is one favored by Philip Kotler, a noted professor of marketing:

> the analysis, planning, implementation, and control of carefully formulated programs designed to bring about voluntary exchanges of values with target markets for the purpose of achieving organizational objectives.[1]

Others use a "four Ps" mnemonic to capture the breadth of the concept:

1. *Product*. What exactly is the product or service offered in the exchange? (includes benchmarks and competitive operational standards)
2. *Place*. Where and how does the exchange take place? (includes hours of service, geographic locations, and relations between services)
3. *Price*. What is the total economic value of the exchange? (not only the price paid the vendor but also collateral costs such as transportation and lost income)
4. *Promotion*. What activities are necessary to bring the opportunity to the attention of the stakeholders likely to accept it? (includes publicity, advertising, and incentives)

The order of the four Ps is important. The consequences of bad product design or placement cannot be overcome by low prices or extensive promotion. Marketing applies not just to customers but to all exchanges, including those with competitors, employees, and other community agencies.

Marketing is about relationships. Healthcare marketing must overcome several complexities that affect relationships:

- Intimate, life-shaping services about which people have strong and sometimes irrational feelings
- Delivery mechanisms that have high fixed costs (requires careful adjustment of supply and demand and opens the possibility of differential pricing)
- Providers who are divided into a large number of professions, who often compete between and within their specialties
- Unpredictable customer expenses that fall disproportionately on a few people (must be financed by health insurance, bringing a third party into the transaction; the insurance mechanism raises the need for agreement about what is appropriate)
- Health insurance that is financed largely through taxes and employer contributions, bringing a fourth and a fifth party into the transaction
- Differences of opinion among patients, buyers, providers, and society at large about what is appropriate (even with protocols, optimum treatment is only imprecisely known; evidence-based conclusions may not be satisfactory

to customers; serious disagreements exist about what is necessary or even acceptable).

In such a complex environment, it would be disastrous to think of marketing as a simple or limited activity. Exhibit 15.2 tracks the major functions

EXHIBIT 15.2
Illustration of Marketing Functions

Function	Well-Baby Illustration	HCO Illustration
Identify and segment customer and associate markets	Forecast numbers of babies Identify OFI for mission achievement Segment Well-Baby market	Identify and segment local population Forecast size, age, and disease by segment
Listen to stakeholder needs	Use surveys, focus groups, and other listening activities to identify segment-specific needs	Monitor market share, satisfaction, and qualitative concerns by segment Identify OFIs in market-share growth
Develop brand and media relations	Raise mothers' awareness of Well-Baby services with articles, advertisements, and collaboration with community agencies	Make community aware of HCO's services Maintain relations with community agencies Maintain media relations Manage negative media events
Influence potential customers	Design product, place, price, and promotion to attract and retain mothers in specific market segments	Maintain multiple campaigns for specific HCO services and market segments
Attract and motivate associates	Design product, place, price, and promotion to attract and retain pediatricians, nurses, and other caregivers	Maintain multiple campaigns for specific HCO associate needs
Manage other stakeholder relationships	Identify competitors and collaborators Pursue partnerships to enhance Well-Baby goal	Monitor competitor performance Identify collaboration opportunities Pursue partnerships to enhance mission achievement

OFI: opportunity for improvement

of marketing as they apply to a single project—the Well-Baby Program of care—and to the entire program of a large, established HCO.

Identifying and Segmenting Markets

As Kotler implies, specific targets are the key to marketing. Market **segmentation** differentiates exchange partners into particular subgroups on the basis of groups' exchange need and the message to which they will respond. It is closely analogous to the statistical process of specification (described in Chapter 14) and, in fact, often starts with the same taxonomies. Like listening and branding, it underlies the other marketing functions.

Segmentation
The deliberate effort to separate markets by customer need and the message to which the markets will respond.

Market segmentation makes listening and promotion more efficient. People of different ages and genders have unique healthcare needs and may also carry certain insurance, want certain schedules and amenities, and listen to certain media. To attract a given demographic, the organization should work with that insurance plan, provide those schedules and amenities, and advertise in those media. Efforts that are not targeted are inherently inefficient. Segmentation usually goes well beyond demographics and into economic, cultural, and lifestyle issues as the organization attempts to build demand for specific services.

In the Well-Baby Program example, it is immediately obvious that all mothers are not alike. They and, more important, their approach to child care differ by education, income, culture, employment, and health insurance coverage. The segments have different needs. Several already have their needs met. Others need specific product and placement—locations, hours, and culturally competent caregivers. Several present financial constraints to the HCO, imposed by the Medicaid price. Different segments require different promotions, in their language and through their community networks and preferred radio stations, newspapers, and websites. Similarly, the HCO needs to view its total market by segment. Gains in market share come by identifying segments that have unmet needs and designing responses that meet those needs.

Listening to Stakeholder Needs

Marketing requires listening activities to understand exchange partners' perspectives. Understanding promotes dialogue, identifies and prioritizes needs, suggests paths to improved relationships, and reveals opportunities for improved work processes. Excellent HCOs make listening a major part of their activities. They use formal surveys, electronic health record (EHR)–based measures, focus groups, and a wide variety of personal-contact devices that involve dozens or hundreds of managers. Many of these yield qualitative rather than quantitative information. The marketing unit plays a critical role in assembling and interpreting these data.

The major listening approaches are summarized in Exhibit 15.3.

Formal Surveys

Surveys provide the most reliable quantitative information about relationships and attitudes and are widely used in marketing, journalism, and politics. Sampling techniques allow inference from a relatively small number of contacts, and samples can be stratified to reflect specific population segments. Patients and associates are 100 percent sampled, providing regular reports on both summary attitudes toward the organization and its services and insight into perceptions about specific processes. As discussed in Chapter 5, the Centers for Medicare & Medicaid Services (CMS) mandates and publishes results of Hospital Consumer Assessment of Healthcare Providers and Systems (HCAHPS), a 27-item survey of communication with doctors, communication with nurses, responsiveness, pain control follow-up care, cleanliness, and noise.[2] A similar set—the ambulatory CAHPS—is available from the Agency for Healthcare Research and Quality.[3] Household surveys are also commonly used; they provide data on community attitudes and conditions as opposed to populations of people affiliated with the organization.

Surveys have become highly sophisticated instruments. The questions, timing, method of contact, response rate, and specification of the population can all affect the results so that professional design and analysis are almost always necessary. Surveys for patients and associates are now provided by commercial companies, which handle these statistical issues and also provide trend, comparative, and benchmarking data.

EHR-Based Measures

Statistical monitors can be constructed around standardized events like CMS's quality measures, reported on the web at Hospital Compare[4] and Why NotTheBest.org.[5] They are derived from the diagnostic codes mandated on Medicare hospitalization insurance claims and are required by most insurers. They cover a limited set of events, but one that is relatively free of reporting bias and can be benchmarked and trended. Their most important use is to validate the subjective reporting processes.

Qualitative Reports

HCOs use a variety of reports generated by the associates, patients, and family to identify situations where results fall short of expectations or exceed expectations. Leading HCOs now use "unexpected event" reports and service recovery generated by associates, various complaint vehicles, and cards to recognize exceptional effort by associates. The trigger in each of these is the subjective sense that a reportable event has occurred. Underreporting is a serious issue. Associates are trained to report service-recovery situations

EXHIBIT 15.3
Major Listening
Activities

Activity	Description	Application
Formal Surveys		
Patient satisfaction	Telephone, web, or mail survey	Assesses patient satisfaction with both amenities and perceived quality of care; usually provided by a national survey firm using CAHPS (Chapter 5) questions and others and rigorously sampling various patient categories. Forms the basis for the loyal patient estimates.
Associate satisfaction	Telephone, web, or mail survey	Offered to various categories of associates; usually provided by a national survey firm, which supplies comparative data and evaluates reliability; forms the basis for the loyal associate estimates.
Community	Telephone or mail survey	Estimates market share, prevalence of insurance, travel patterns, and other characteristics not in the decennial census; can be used to update census data; can be focused on specific population segments.
Monitors		
Incident (unexpected event) reports	Associate-generated written reports	Associates are encouraged to report any event that represents a serious failure, such as a fall, a clinical error, or an unacceptable delay.
Service recovery	Written reports of actions to correct failures	Associates are authorized to offer gifts or benefits in cases where processes have egregiously failed; the incident and the recovery must be reported in writing.
Complaints	Written, oral, or electronic reports from patients or associates	Patients are offered "bounce-back" cards, and both patients and associates are encouraged to communicate directly with organizational authorities.
"Caught in the act"	Written reports of exceptional behavior by associates	Cards for catching someone in the act of doing good are publicly available; the events reported are judged by a panel, and prizes are awarded.
Statistical process control	Counts of untoward events documented in the patient record	The electronic record can be surveyed for evidence such as diagnoses, specific drug orders, progress notes, or treatments reflecting adverse events such as infections, falls, treatment errors, and complications. These can be tracked and monitored either as sentinel events—all cases investigated—or using statistical process control (Chapter 14).

(continued)

EXHIBIT 15.3
Major Listening
Activities
(continued)

Personal Contact

Focus groups	Small groups of current or potential customers meeting face-to-face	Focus groups are encouraged to speak candidly about existing services and explore what is important about proposed services; they provide insight to specific process opportunities that do not arise in surveys.
"On-call" managers	24/7 designated contact official	A senior manager is always accessible to patients or associates for prompt attention to complaints or difficulties arising; allows direct intervention and service recovery in complex situations.
Walking rounds	Regularly scheduled senior management visits	Front-office managers maintain personal contact through visits to actual work sites, which encourage questions, explain positions, reward efforts, validate public pronouncements, and humanize.
Shadowing and walk-throughs	Observation of a single patient through a complex process	Shadowing allows associates to understand both the process and its impact on patients; walk-throughs actually duplicate patient activity.
Mystery shopping	Observation of a competitor's process	Mystery shoppers were initially used to discover competitors' prices. In healthcare, they reveal competitors' processes and competitive advantages.

CAHPS: Consumer Assessment of Healthcare Providers and Systems

and clinical errors whenever they occur. Follow-up rewards reporting, avoids blame, and focuses on prevention. The events can be coded by type, location, and severity to indicate trends and processes or units that need attention.

Personal Contact

Leading HCOs supplement survey, EHR, and event data with deliberate personal contact. They encourage senior leadership to be highly visible in the organization by rounds and on-call responses. They encourage process improvement teams to observe and walk through the processes they are studying. They sometimes hire agents to observe and report on competitors' processes. They assemble focus groups—small groups of actual or potential customers who are encouraged to discuss factors in product, placement, and price that are important to them. These personal-contact activities yield only qualitative and highly subjective information, but they accomplish three important goals:

1. They show leadership's commitment to continuous improvement and put a human face on policies and work requirements.

2. They improve leaders' empathy with team members in their work environment.

3. They provide detailed information that is often valuable in resolving specific situations.

Personal-contact programs have some important limitations. Managers must be trained to avoid blame in their responses and to stress process analysis and improvement. Personal contact works best when the organization has developed sound work processes and uses the contact to supplement measurement, process analysis, and goal setting. It cannot be effective in situations where the basic work processes are inadequate. Too many requests to solve specific problems is evidence that issues must be addressed systematically rather than episodically.

Developing Brand and Media Relations

Marketing deliberately works to improve the HCO's image, people's impression of it, by branding activities and media relations.

Branding

The **branding** function maintains the overall reputation or image of the organization so that it remains attractive to most members of the community at large. Branding usually begins as a community-wide communications effort to convey the mission and

Branding
A community-wide communication effort to convey the mission and the competitive advantage of the organization.

the competitive advantages of the organization. Branding activities include public and community relations, image advertising and promotion, maintenance of an attractive website, and media relations. A deliberate program includes descriptive information for various media, relationships with other influential community agencies such as schools and the faith community, and sponsorship of community events such as health fairs and athletic teams. It also includes personal appearances by management and caregivers, deliberate contacts with influentials and opinion leaders, and damage control for negative media events.

Obviously, success begins with having a good story to tell. An increasing number of HCOs release specific information about finances, service, and quality to the public. Image promotion is far from a panacea. It takes a large number of exposures to increase name recognition, and changing the HCO's attractiveness is hard, although increases in quality may be linked to improved branding.[6] Community surveys allow the organization to monitor two dimensions of branding. Familiarity is measured by consumers' ability to recall the name without prompting or to recognize it in a list. Attractiveness uses survey questions to assess how the HCO compares to competitors and which attributes are most attractive. The implication is that an established reputation—being among the first two or three names people independently recall for healthcare—is a valuable asset, hard to replace, and well worth protecting.

Media Relations

Most organizations are acutely aware of what is said about them in the media, but the evidence suggests that the public at large is quite resistant to media statements. Nonetheless, the media can portray the organization favorably or unfavorably, and the result often depends on the quality of information supplied by the organization. Media communication is either HCO or media initiated. HCO-initiated communication is the planned release of information as part of branding. Attractive and thorough press releases, strong visual elements (e.g., photos, videos), knowledgeable and articulate spokespersons, and newsworthy information all assist in improving the coverage. A deliberate program of regular information releases and efforts to draw media attention to favorable events promote a positive image. The more information released, the more likely the community's familiarity with and attraction to the HCO will increase.

Media-initiated communication is often related to major news events, such as healthcare to prominent individuals or a healthcare crisis. A crisis is anything that suddenly or unexpectedly has adverse effects on an HCO or its patients, associates, or community. In the worst case, media-initiated communication arises from unfavorable events, such as lowered bond ratings, civil lawsuits, or criminal behavior by associates. Investigative journalism is an aggressive effort to dig out all the public might want to know, with emphasis on what the HCO might want to hide. Effective handling of media initiatives begins with preventing events that will draw investigation. It is supported by a strong branding program that releases positive, newsworthy information about the HCO. When unfortunate issues arise, the HCO should anticipate reporters' questions and prepare detailed, candid responses. Spokespersons should be identified and equipped with thorough, convincing replies to questions. The organization should have a plan in place for communicating when a media crisis occurs.[7]

Convincing Potential Customers

HCOs are a respected source of information on health matters, and they communicate often with patients and others in their community. Leading organizations work hard to retain respect, tying their branding activities to specific communications about three principal goals:

1. Convince patients to select this provider and services.
2. Encourage wellness and disease prevention.
3. Adjust patient expectations about care.

Reaching the public effectively is challenging. Healthcare messages are often on topics people would rather avoid. Commercial retailers spend far larger sums than not-for-profit organizations are comfortable with. "Clutter"—the sheer volume of consumer messages—makes registering the HCO on the customers' minds difficult. Despite this, communications programs can reinforce branding and build demand for effective healthcare.

Influence Patient Selection of Providers and Services

The key to attracting and retaining patients is service, more than promotion. Loyal or delighted patients—those who will return when necessary and refer others—are obtained by maintaining service and quality. The most effective way to manage patient satisfaction is to identify service weaknesses and meet them through continuous improvement. Service recovery can supplement but not replace continuous improvement. Beyond performance and recovery, explicit promotion activities play a small role. An HCO may explicitly promote a new or expanded service or a service where a portion of the market could realistically be shifted to or from a competitor. Such a campaign would include website postings, press releases, advertising, and incentives such as giveaways and performance events. Customer reactions would be carefully monitored.

Influence Healthy Behavior

HCOs with a community health mission join in the wellness promotion movement to encourage healthy lifestyles and cost-effective prevention behaviors. General promotional campaigns to the well members of the population are an important branding opportunity. They use all media, including print and video material in schools and work sites. More important, the healthcare experience often becomes a *teachable moment*—a window of increased receptivity when messages from healthcare professionals are well received. Messages must overcome complex motivations to pursue the unhealthy behavior. Campaigns repeat the message over and over and use a variety of vehicles to convey and reinforce it. Wellness promotion becomes an ongoing activity that consumes a specific budget and is constantly studied for opportunities to improve cost-effectiveness.

Manage Patient Expectations

One aspect of patient satisfaction relates to initial expectations about care. These can be unrealistic. Media reports frequently emphasize dramatic, curative medical intervention and may overstate the power and value of high-tech care. Drug companies overtly hype branded prescriptions of dubious worth.[8] Countering these and restoring realistic expectations are important. In reality, self-treatment and family care are effective in many conditions. In the case of self-limiting disease and terminal disease, there is often nothing healthcare professionals can add.

Similarly, the appropriate use of substitute professionals, such as nurse practitioners in place of physicians or primary physicians in place of specialists, offers advantages in quality, cost, and effectiveness. The marketing approach begins with the attractive provision of the lower-cost service. Promotion helps build awareness of alternatives and provides reassurance to make people comfortable with them, such as reassurance about the availability of technologically advanced care when needed. HCOs promote the use of less skilled professionals; the use of walk-in clinics in place of emergency departments (EDs), ambulatory instead of inpatient care, generic instead of brand name drugs, and equally effective substitutes for high-cost intervention; and improved management at the end of life. All of these can reduce the cost of care while sustaining or improving the quality.

Sophisticated targeting can focus directly on specific patient expectations. For example, advance description of elective surgical procedures can identify many common complications or variations in the recovery pattern and provide instructions or reassurance about them. It can prepare the patient to accept the usual outcomes and, in some cases, convince patients that the rewards of the procedure are not worth the pain, risks, and cost. The HCO may deliberately emphasize activities that are designed to provide symptomatic relief, such as the deliberate use of chiropractic services in place of back surgery in certain cases of low-back pain.[9] Many elements of healthcare—prostatectomies, breast cancer examinations, and high-cost drugs are notorious examples—have been oversold. HCOs with a community health mission have an obligation to counter with sound explanations of the effectiveness of less costly care.

Improve Patient Communication

Successful patient communication is a sophisticated combination of advertising, persuasion, and education. Three approaches improve its effectiveness:

1. *Messages should be carefully targeted to specific population segments where change is desired.* The logic used in prevention and diagnostic testing applies to promotion as well—funds spent communicating to populations who are not involved or are nonresponsive are wasted. While branding usually aims to reach a broad spectrum of the community, promotion should almost always be targeted to specific groups.

2. *Advance plans for promotional campaigns should specify* **reach** *(the focal audience for the campaign),* **frequency** *(how often individuals in the focal audience are contacted), media, cost, and measures of expected outcome.* Quantifying the campaign in advance establishes explicit goals and encourages careful review of alternatives.

Reach
In advertising, an estimate of the number of people who will see or hear a specific advertisement.

Frequency
In advertising, the average number of times each person is reached by a specific advertisement.

3. *Campaigns should explicitly involve community partnerships and coalitions.* Building networks to improve health and healthcare offers several advantages. The costs can be shared. Collaboration also builds on the respect these organizations have, bringing familiar faces to the target audiences. The use of sites and agencies other than healthcare allows more complete and candid discussion of the complex issues. For example, on issues of prevention and end-of-life care, churches, congregate-living centers, and senior recreational facilities can hold educational discussions. On other issues, schools and employers can strengthen communication. The collaboration has listening aspects as well. Specific needs can be identified and addressed. The HCO's own associates can participate as partners. Promotion that reaches both patients and staff will improve staff understanding and acceptance as well.

Attracting and Motivating Associates

Although much of the communication to associates is managed by the accountability structure and human resources, many promotional activities also reach the associates. Websites and signage are seen more by associates than customers. Publicity and advertising attract associate attention. The service excellence program (discussed in Chapter 2) can be described as collaboration with associates to realize the mission and vision of the HCO.

Most large HCOs promote themselves directly to clinical professionals in short supply.[10] Programs to attract physicians who seek locations to practice primary care medicine are commonplace; considerable care and expense is justified in light of the importance of the decision on both sides.[11] Many organizations advertise routinely in nursing, physical therapy, and pharmacy journals to attract new professionals.

Strategic affiliations to recruit personnel are also common.[12] Affiliation with teaching programs enhances recruitment and retention of graduating students. Programs to assist students with summer and part-time work affect not only the students directly involved but also their classmates, who learn by word of mouth. Some institutions reach several years below graduation. Working with inner-city high schools to encourage young people to enter healing professions is popular. Like many promotional activities, it reaches two audiences—the students and the community at large. North Mississippi Medical Center operates a program beginning with "Let's Pretend Hospital, a tool to educate first graders in health care careers."[13] Current nonprofessional associates are also an important source for more skilled opportunities. Scholarships and scheduling assistance to permit further education are common.

Managing Other Stakeholder Relationships

Seek Collaborative Opportunities

One aspect of marketing is the deliberate management of relationships with other organizations. To understand the issues, it is useful to consider healthcare as a large set of component functions and services. These include inpatient and outpatient service lines, primary care sites, and long-term care facilities. They also include support activities, such as pharmacies and meals-on-wheels, and preventive activities, such as exercise programs, health education, immunization, and screening. A cottage model of healthcare has all of these activities operating as independent units that deal directly with the patient and relate to each other as competitors or independents, with occasional brief contracts. Several vendors compete in each function. The growth of healthcare systems is moving healthcare away from the cottage model toward comprehensive care. All services can be provided under a single corporate umbrella. Some large healthcare systems, such as Kaiser Permanente, Intermountain Healthcare, Catholic Health Initiatives, and the New York City Health and Hospitals Corporation, have incorporated large parts of the array.

An HCO must consider both horizontal (integrating competing or similar services) and vertical integration (integrating complementary services). With which services does it collaborate, with which does it compete, and on what terms? The optimum arrangement provides the community with safe, efficient, patient-centered, timely, efficient, and equitable care, but finding that arrangement can be a substantial challenge.

Many contract suppliers, such as emergency physicians, information services, and housekeeping companies, are effective horizontal collaboration examples. The hospital system movement through 2012 was largely horizontal. Many of the smaller systems are formerly competing acute hospitals. Significant and largely untapped opportunities also lie in vertical integration. Most primary and acute physician care is delivered by small group practices that are independent private corporations, although a growing trend is for physicians to be employed by health systems. Although many systems include long-term care facilities, hospices, and home care, most long-term care is delivered by horizontally integrated or independent organizations.

Manage Collaborative Opportunities

Exhibit 15.4 shows some important healthcare components. It suggests that the question about each is "Would this service be improved if it were

1. moved to a tighter ownership/management relationship? or
2. moved to a more independent relationship in direct exposure to market forces?"

The improvement must lie in mission achievement. Closer affiliations may offer an opportunity. The HCO's logistic and strategic support services, its culture as "the best place to give care," and its ability to coordinate care across a spectrum of patient need are valuable resources that can be efficiently shared. But **transaction costs**—loss

Transaction costs
The costs of maintaining a relationship, including the costs of communication, negotiation, and loss of flexibility.

EXHIBIT 15.4
Examples of
Alternative
Collaborative
Structures for
HCO Services

Service or Function	Common Current Arrangement	Possible Alternative Structure
Primary care	Independent physician groups	Joint venture with physician owners Acquire and own practices
Ambulatory services (e.g., oncology, specialty surgery, urgent care)	Independent or horizontally integrated provider	Own or joint venture with physicians Joint venture with competing provider Contract or strategic partnership with horizontally integrated provider
Integrated service line	Owned	Joint venture
Logistic/strategic support (e.g., finance, human resources, knowledge management)	Owned	Contract with strategic partners Centralize in multihospital healthcare organization
Clinical support services	Owned	Strategic partnership with horizontally integrated provider
Health promotion and preventive activity	Independent or not offered	Strategic partnership with community agencies
Long-term services (e.g., home, hospice, nursing home care)	Independent or horizontally integrated providers	Own Joint venture with competing acute care provider Strategic partnership with specialty provider
Low-volume specialty care (e.g., mental, long-term acute care)	Independent or horizontally integrated providers	Joint venture with competing acute care provider Contract or joint venture with current provider

of flexibility, reduced incentives, and conflicting values among participants—differ with each structure and must be carefully evaluated as well.

Large organizations succeed because they invent collaborative mechanisms that are more effective than market forces.[14] The goal-setting and performance terms, agreements for sharing information, sharing of capital investment, and market exclusivity define the collaboration. One implication of the pair of questions is that any component of the existing organization can be sold to or merged with another organization or replaced by a contract relationship. Conceptually, an HCO could be a governing board that manages a large set of relationships with independent companies just as easily as it could be a corporation that owns the full array of services. When the benefits of collaboration exceed the transaction costs, closer affiliation is in order, and vice versa.

Most modern HCOs now collaborate on several major services, of which physician organizations may be the most important. The networks they have created require constant relationship management. Exhibit 15.5 suggests the range of levels of collaborative activity:

- *Agreements and contracts include patient referrals, purchases, temporary worker contracts, or consulting engagements.* These are simple and short-term. Performance standards are set by the market and are often implicit rather than explicit.
- *Strategic partnerships include health insurance participation agreements, physician–hospital privileging, supplier contracts, or outsourcing contracts.*[15] The contract attempts to specify performance characteristics, including continuous improvement and incentives, and is written for a year or more. The standards are negotiated regularly, as with owned units. The intent is to keep the partnership in place. The arrangement can be abrogated, however, if desired by either partner.
- *Joint ventures involve capital investment by both partners, such as ambulatory treatment centers or shared high-cost, low-volume equipment.* Joint ventures usually have joint governance or management teams. The capital investment makes them more difficult to terminate, and they are usually expected to be permanent.
- *Mergers replace the capital, governance, and management of prior corporate entities with a new combined entity.* Mergers are generally irreversible.

EXHIBIT 15.5
Spectrum of
Potential
Relationships
with
Organizations

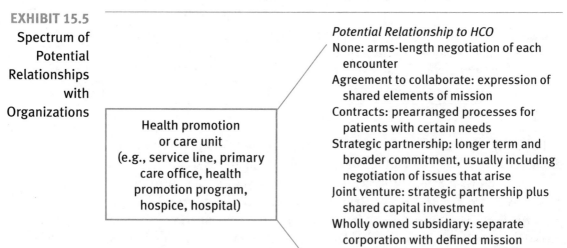

Potential Relationship to HCO
None: arms-length negotiation of each
    encounter
Agreement to collaborate: expression of
    shared elements of mission
Contracts: prearranged processes for
    patients with certain needs
Strategic partnership: longer term and
    broader commitment, usually including
    negotiation of issues that arise
Joint venture: strategic partnership plus
    shared capital investment
Wholly owned subsidiary: separate
    corporation with defined mission
Unit of parent corporation: participates in
    annual goal setting and all appropriate
    programs

Health promotion
or care unit
(e.g., service line, primary
care office, health
promotion program,
hospice, hospital)

- *Acquisitions are where one existing entity totally acquires another.* The acquiring company owns the capital and continues governance and management. Acquisitions are generally irreversible.

Improving the Marketing Activity

Marketing functions are difficult to evaluate, but annual review, identification of opportunities for improvement (OFIs), and deliberate improvement plans are still critical. Specific promotional campaigns for branding, influencing patient behavior, or specific communication to associates can be quantitatively assessed (see the Measures section below). More general activities, such as external relations and ongoing associate relations, must be measured by the strategic scorecard. Market share and satisfaction data measure performance. The epidemiologic planning model is useful to compare an HCO's market share with competitor HCOs to analyze the effectiveness of the marketing strategy and to revise the strategy, as needed. Qualitative indicators from listening are important.

Strategic Functions

Strategy—the placement of the organization in its environment—can be said to pick up where marketing leaves off, but more accurately, the two are seamlessly connected. If marketing is about relationships, strategy is the selection and prioritization of relationships. The organization identifies its strategy through its governance processes (discussed in Chapter 4) and implements it through its operations. The strategic functions (Exhibit 15.1) are the specific activities that help the organization maintain an effective strategy in a dynamic environment.

Maintaining the Mission, Vision, and Values

The mission, vision, and values represent the most central desires of the owners and stakeholders and, as such, become the cornerstone for all subsequent planning decisions. To fulfill that function, they should be as permanent as possible, but even the most carefully set mission may lose its relevance in a dynamic environment. Even though major change is infrequent in the mission and even rarer in the vision, well-run organizations review the need for change annually. Periodically, the organization should undertake a broad-scale review—sometimes called *visioning*. Actual revisions are developed by extensive listening and discussion among large numbers of stakeholders. Several task forces (often involving hundreds of people) are established to attract representation from most of the organization's stakeholders in the debate about possible revisions. The review process not only develops consensus positions but also increases stakeholder understanding of others' viewpoints and the reasons for specific wording. Marketing must manage the task forces, keep track of proposed changes, and arrange for the resolution of serious disagreements. The final changes require formal governing board adoption.

Defining the Strategic Position

As discussed in Chapter 1, the mission, vision, ownership, scope of services, location, and partners of the organization define its *strategic position*. Strategic positioning establishes broad understanding—what service lines our HCO is operating, where, and on what affiliation terms—so that the leadership team can implement effectively and respond to external challenges and opportunities. Successful strategic positions are constructed by identifying alternatives (what-ifs), testing the alternatives extensively with simulations and pilots, and evaluating the tests in task forces or committees of the most knowledgeable stakeholders.

Identify Strategic Opportunities

Strategic alternatives are identified through an ongoing review directed by the senior management team and presented to the governing board for discussion, amendment, and approval. The governing board reviews strategy whenever necessary, but always at the time of the annual environmental review. The fact-finding and analysis are done by marketing, internal consulting, and finance associates, often with assistance from other units.

The review begins by assessing performance on each of the major dimensions of the strategic balanced scorecard—financial, operational, customer, and learning (Exhibit 3.4).[16] Achievements are compared to the prior year's expectations, benchmarks, competitor achievements, and best practices from the literature or other communities. Changes in external conditions are noted in the environmental assessment and often flagged as "threats" or "opportunities." Specific areas of each dimension are often categorized as strengths or OFIs, creating a profile that tests both the organization's goals and its performance. The resulting display (called a SWOT [strength, weakness, opportunity, threat] analysis) is checked against the mission and vision and used to identify what the organization could be.

A key part of the review is the study of overall patterns and identification of the interrelationship between the performance dimensions. Study of high-performing organizations is helpful. Innovative thinking that transcends traditional boundaries helps identify truly creative opportunities.[17] Porter's framework for evaluating strategy is useful, both to improve the balanced scorecard measures and to identify important questions. The framework goes beyond SWOT, raising questions from "five forces" or external domains:[18]

1. *Buyers and customers.* What are buyers', patients', and the community's needs? Are there opportunities for improvement revealed by the profile of quality, cost,

access, and satisfaction performance? Are there unique or emerging economic or epidemiologic characteristics that suggest specific strategic responses?

2. *New technology and substitutes.* What are the implications of new diagnostic and treatment technology? What are other leading HCOs doing? What opportunities exist to reduce the cost of technology, such as by substituting less expensive protocols or changing processes to use less skilled personnel? What opportunities for improvement are presented by new operational technology, such as the EHR?

3. *Resource availability.* What funds are available for investment in expansion or renovation? How will market and regulatory forces change expected revenues? What human resources are required, and how will they be acquired? What opportunities exist to improve retention and service excellence? What land is required? What additional knowledge management?

4. *Competitor activity.* What actions are competitors taking, and what are the implications of those actions for our strategy? What opportunities exist to advance stakeholder goals by collaborating with competitors?

5. *Potential competitors and regulatory impact.* What new models of healthcare delivery are being developed elsewhere? Which stakeholder groups might start competing organizations, and why? What changes are likely in regulatory protections and constraints? What incentives are offered to encourage innovation? What actions might the organization take to forestall competition?

The strategic review is not secret; all of the leadership team is expected to participate. It helps them understand the organization's profile of needs and achievements and the possible improvements. The result is that the strategic position is not secret. In the words of Intermountain Healthcare planner Greg Poulsen, "It's in our competitors' portfolio tomorrow morning."[19] The Intermountain approach is to win not on secrecy but on sound selection and effective implementation. Timeliness and thoroughness are both important.

Evaluate Strategic Opportunities

The opportunities determined by the review are identified and roughly prioritized. Various ways to improve the institution's position—usually called *scenarios*—are proposed and evaluated against the agenda of opportunities. Some die quickly, as major flaws appear. Others receive detailed and quantitative review, and models of their implications are constructed. Models—also called *business plans*—consist of a narrative that describes the alternative as clearly as possible and identifies how it differs from current practice; they also include a quantitative simulation that forecasts the changes in key strategic scorecard measures. The models and their results are evaluated by teams of associates and stakeholders to test the proposal for contribution to mission, synergy with existing programs, risk of failure, fit with the environment, and fit with accessible resources.

Various devices can be used to stimulate discussion and understanding of alternatives. A matrix that allows two dimensions of desirability to be considered is sometimes useful. There are several alternatives for defining the axes. The versions by the Boston Consulting Group[20] and by General Electric[21] are popular. Both lead to a display such as that illustrated in Exhibit 15.6, where the axes are market attractiveness (opportunities for growth or profit) and organizational advantage (internal resources, sometimes called *competencies*). Expanding an existing competency is generally easier than developing new competencies, but ignoring the market is perilous. The display is useful to focus attention on these trade-offs. For example, expanded ambulatory services like accountable care organizations are very "attractive" as a result of changes in Medicare and private insurance. An HCO might find itself with strong resources in primary care delivery, a solid joint venture with most of its primary care practitioners (Situation A in Exhibit 15.6). Expanding its primary care activities would be a strong strategic priority, because expansion is both attractive and resource supported. Another HCO, in Situation B, would work to strengthen its ambulatory care resources but would inevitably be a step behind. A high-tech service, only infrequently needed and requiring

EXHIBIT 15.6
Matrix of Market Attractiveness and Advantage

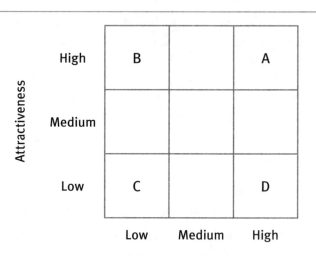

Situation A, where the market is attractive and the hospital has a strong advantage, is one that would be selected for further investment.

Situation B, where the market is attractive, but the hospital faces a large or difficult investment, would be judged on its importance to overall market share.

Situation C, where both market and advantage are low, would be phased out or avoided.

Situation D, where the attractiveness is low, but the hospital has an advantage, would be supported but expanded only to the extent market support could be foreseen.

specialists who are difficult to recruit (Situation C), would be avoided. A service operating near benchmark across its scorecard but with potentially falling demand, such as a well-managed ED (Situation D), would not be expanded but might provide the organizational foundation for developing urgent care centers.

Strategic Theories

Theories for corporate strategy are common, but they do not transfer easily to the complexities of healthcare. Eastaugh[22] has modified four corporate archetypes designed by Miles and Snow[23]—prospector, analyzer, reactor, and defender—to fit hospitals. The differences between the archetypes are two dimensional, as shown in Exhibit 15.7. One dimension—willingness to seek innovation outside the traditional parameters—is external and tends to higher risk. The other dimension—concentration on meeting quality and cost standards in the core business—is internal, analytic, and risk averse. The evidence suggests that prospectors and defenders do badly; too much risk and too little action are both dangerous. Analyzers do better than defenders; carefully selected innovation is better than sticking too closely to established models. Reactors do worst.

Other strategic philosophies have been built around the concept of distinctive competencies—market success depends on excelling in some characteristic that is attractive to customers.[24] They reflect various approaches to defining the competency. Porter's "cost leadership versus [quality] differentiation"[25] is blunted in healthcare by the insurance mechanism, which protects both patients and physicians from cost differences, but quality and service

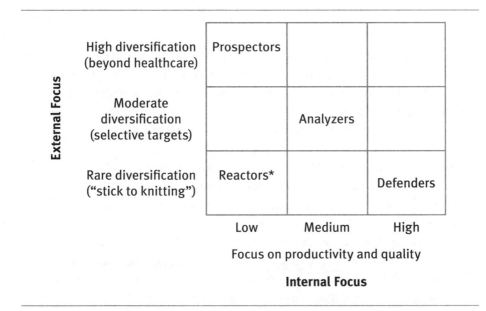

EXHIBIT 15.7
Miles and Snow Typology of Strategic Types

*Reactors do not have a strong strategy in either direction. They respond passively to competitors.

are important differentiators. Not surprisingly, Baldrige-recipient HCOs are significantly superior to average HCOs on HCAHPS scores—at 4 standard deviations.[26] Miller and Friesen's "adaptive, dominant, giant, conglomerate, and niche innovator" philosophy describes different approaches to strategic opportunities as well as different corporate cultures.[27] Niche strategies deliberately seek highly specialized services that include factors that are difficult for competitors to copy. Specialty hospitals that serve children, the mentally ill, cancer patients, and the like are following niche strategies. Small, rural HCOs that offer primary care and limited hospitalization are also niche strategists, and so are independent home care and hospice organizations.

The specialty hospital movement—independent, usually for-profit doctor-owned facilities that provide a single service line—is a niche strategy.[28,29] CMS has procedures in place for enrolling specialty hospitals with an emphasis on the provision of emergency care, transparency in hospital investment, and an enforcement of Stark and anti-kickback rules regarding improper investment (physician self-referral).[30]

The high-performing HCOs used as models by *The Well-Managed Healthcare Organization* have pursued comprehensive rather than niche strategies. They have used transformational management, evidence-based management, and the service excellence model to build community-wide customer and provider brand loyalty. They have countered niche competition with service lines and joint ventures that offer niche services in integrated settings. Those with community health missions explicitly pursue a "conglomerate" strategy; they seek comprehensive coverage of market needs and are willing to explore multiple corporate and collaborative structures. They have been growing rapidly, often by acquisition of smaller surrounding HCOs.[31]

Document the Strategy

Many strategy elements take several years to implement. Implementation processes and new strategies must be coordinated with those in preparation as well as those in place. The decisions that result from the strategic analysis process are incorporated in a set of documents sometimes called the *long-range* or *strategic plans*. The documentation includes the following parts:

- *Environmental forecasts.* These are derived from the environmental assessment, cover about five years, and identify potential directions of change for a second five years. They are updated annually but serve as a central resource and database for the planning activities of all units.
- *Services plan.* This specifies the clinical services and other major activities in which the institution will engage, with annual forecasts of the expected volume and achievement of goals for cost, quality, worker satisfaction, and customer satisfaction.
- *Long-range financial plan.* This summarizes the expected financial impact on income statements, cash flow, long-term debt, and balance sheets (Chapter 13).

- *Information services plan.* This describes the future capability and hardware array of information service, including plans for collection, standardization, communication, and archiving of data (Chapter 10).
- *Human resources plan.* This shows the expected personnel needs, terminations, and recruitment requirements and succession plans (Chapter 11).
- *Medical staff plan.* This is a part of the human resources plan that focuses on physician and related caregiver replacement and recruitment (Chapter 6).
- *Facilities master plan.* This details the construction and renovation activities (Chapter 12).

Although the plans may be separate documents, the processes that generate the decisions must be integrated. In general, mission and vision drive services and finances, and these, in turn, drive facilities, human resources, and information needs. Thus, the plans have a hierarchical relationship. Internal consulting is responsible for coordinating the strategic plans. The other technical and logistic support services are responsible for their components.

Implementing the Strategic Position

The consensus that emerges from the review of scenarios and the governing board's actions is a set of approved projects to be implemented, with timetables and specific strategic scorecard goals for the next several years. Implementation involves many activities that must be coordinated. The changing environment may open important opportunities or threats. Thus, a critical part of implementation is rechecking the basic strategy against the environment and making adjustments. Implementation is managed by senior management, internal consulting, and the operating teams involved. Most projects have management teams that meet regularly to monitor progress and adapt to occurring changes. Major projects have direct senior management participation, and progress is reported to the board.

People

Associates

Marketing processes are increasingly sophisticated. A master's degree in business or health administration is a useful beginning, but neither degree emphasizes the details of advertising or public relations. Experience with a commercial agency or a successful healthcare marketing team is highly desirable for the senior marketing team.

Consultants are available for most marketing functions. Advertising is purchased from agencies with experience in design, campaign development, and media contracts. Market studies and customer surveys are often contracted to consultants. The consultant should be able to achieve better results and lower costs than if the HCO did the surveys itself. The database that results from continuing study of a market is a valuable proprietary resource. Even if much of the data collection is delegated to consultants, the organization should make an effort to retain the data in their entirety. Consultants can assist in strategic marketing by providing data collection and by undertaking sensitive inquiries. Senior staff, consultants, and trustees can be as effective as negotiators, intermediaries, or mediators in sensitive negotiations. Final approval can be reserved to the CEO or governing board.

Strategy is learned by practice. A business or health master's degree is a sound beginning. Experience in marketing, finance, or internal consulting is helpful to improve judgment. Several years' participation with an excellent team is important.

Organization

Large HCOs and healthcare systems have a formal hierarchy for marketing activities with employees or contracts for each function, as shown in Exhibit 15.8. Linking marketing, strategy, and internal consulting is common. In Exhibit 15.8, internal consulting is organized by the functions described in Chapter 14. The dividing lines between marketing, planning, and internal

EXHIBIT 15.8 Formal Hierarchy for a Large Marketing and Internal Consulting Operation

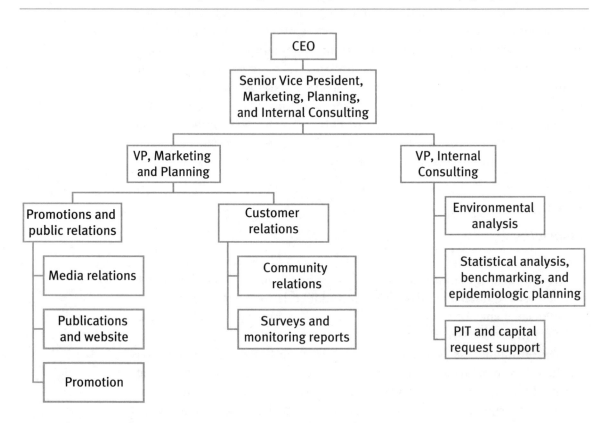

PIT: process improvement team

consulting are flexible; the activities can be combined in various ways, including a single unit. Many real projects call for teams from several of the marketing, planning, and consulting areas. In multihospital systems, a central unit can offer an in-house consultant service, another potential advantage to large-scale HCOs. In smaller organizations, most of the specific accountability centers disappear and consultants are used extensively. The cost per project is higher, and problems of coordination increase.

Strategic support is an activity of the entire senior leadership team. Planning, marketing, and internal consulting units generally provide technical assistance, and outside consultants are frequently used. A voice in senior management is essential. In Exhibit 15.8, it is provided by the senior vice president. The role includes monitoring progress on the various marketing and strategic planning activities and keeping the strategic opportunities before the team.

Measures

Measurement of marketing and strategy is challenging but useful. Strategic strength itself can be assessed inferentially from the strategic scorecard. Operational goals can be established for marketing teams and strategic teams. Specific promotions can be measured and compared to goals. Audits by outsiders can often identify specific OFIs. Operational success does not guarantee strategic success, although it certainly contributes to it.

Assessing Strategic Activity

Strategic success is measured by the strategic scorecard (exhibits 1.10 and 4.3). Repeated failure to meet scorecard goals is a serious danger signal. These key indicators from the scorecard apply to the HCO as a whole and to individual service lines:

- *Quality of care.* Any HCO consistently and substantially below benchmark on outcomes quality measures should be merged or closed.
- *Market share.* Market share should be stable or growing. Although growth is desirable in many situations, it should not be a universal goal. When stable, high-performing HCOs compete, individual growth cannot reasonably improve community-wide performance. Declining market share is a critical signal; if it is not reversed, it suggests that the HCO should be closed, merged, or substantially restructured.
- *Financing.* Most HCOs should operate profitably most of the time. The business cycle or other unusual situation may temporarily impair profits. Safety-net HCOs and others that operate in impaired economies may have chronic difficulty. The long-term expectation must be for sufficient cash flow (profits plus depreciation) to manage debt and meet replacement needs. An HCO that cannot meet that expectation requires substantial restructuring.

- *Investment in human capital and associate satisfaction.* The service excellence model depends on associate satisfaction—"a good place to give care." Failure to provide adequate staffing levels and attract and retain qualified associates is a signal that requires prompt correction. Chronic failure should lead to closure.
- *Overall HCO goal achievement.* A medium-sized HCO sets several thousand specific goals each year. Its service lines have several hundred each. The expectation is that all the goals will be achieved. A failure rate of more than 5 percent is an important signal, and one that is more than 10 percent threatens survival. If failure persists, the HCO should be closed or merged with an effectively managed one.
- *Surprises.* One purpose of strategy is to protect the organization by foreseeing external change in time to adapt to it. Thus, a goal of the strategic activity should be "no surprises"—no unforeseen foreseeable events. Certainly, each major surprise is a sentinel event that is worthy of critical review to understand if it could have been prevented and how.

While interpreting these measures is not as straightforward as many other performance evaluations, the senior management team is accountable. The member of senior management charged with marketing and strategic services is obligated to monitor performance and report routinely, keeping the strategic scorecard prominent in all discussions.

Operational Measures

The units shown in Exhibit 15.8 should have operational scorecards. Total expenditures, although difficult to benchmark, are certainly a focus for goal setting. Client satisfaction, error rates, unfinished assignments, and service delays are useful measures.

Promotional campaigns for branding or for specific services should have built-in pre- and postcampaign evaluations. Campaigns identify specific goals, such as market share or behavior change in population segments. Their costs can be estimated, expectations established about outcomes, and actual results compared to expectations. Expectations can be set about exposures (reach times frequency), response rates (demand), costs, costs per exposure and per response, process quality, timeliness, and changes in customer satisfaction and target market share.

Surveys and statistical analysis of behaviors can evaluate the impact of the promotion. For example, an organization might identify several strategies to expand market share using several service lines, centers of excellence in certain referral specialties, and an expanded availability of primary care physicians. Each of these has specific measures that can be evaluated by surveying the community to gauge recognition of the promotional material and responses and by analyzing trends in new registrants for the various services. Expectations for improvement in these measures can be established and performance evaluated, as shown in Exhibit 15.9. Campaigns may take several years, but interim progress can be evaluated annually.

Establishing Strategic, Marketing, and Internal Consulting Expenditures

Senior management must recommend expenditure goals for strategic, marketing, and consulting activities, and defend them to the board and to questioning associates. The judgment of what's "enough" investment in strategy and marketing is challenging. Benchmarking of strategic expenditures is not appropriate; each HCO's needs are different and expenditures are not

EXHIBIT 15.9
Measures for Specific Campaigns

Campaign	Actions	Measures
Centers of excellence in orthopedics, cardiology	Preparation of data on cost per case and quality of results Publication of original research in peer-reviewed journals, distribution of reprints Direct sales to managers of local HMOs, PPOs Competitive bid for Medicare, Medicaid contracts Presentations to primary care physicians Feature stories in local media Media promotion	Increase in listings or contracts with intermediaries Change in total demand, market share Change in cost per case Change in profit per case Cost of campaign per new case Number of public relations appearances, audience size Number of exposures, exposures/target audience member, cost/exposure by medium Survey of awareness and attractiveness Number of subscribers, percent of total market, cost per subscriber Surveys of patient satisfaction
Increased primary care access	Direct mailing to physicians in primary care fellowships Coordination with presently affiliated physicians Meetings with local physicians affiliated with competitors Program of practice acquisition, expansion Introduction of nurse practitioners Media advertising and public relations Program of office support	Number of new responses Number of new physicians recruited Number of nurse practitioners placed, demand for nurse practitioner services Patient visits/physician Delay for emergency, routine, and preventive office visits Patient satisfaction Program cost per new physician, per new visit

HMO: health maintenance organization; PPO: preferred provider organization comparable. Senior management and governance should be convinced that an adequate environmental assessment is being performed and that progress on major strategic agendas is appropriate to long-term market needs. The test is "How would additional expenditure (or a reduction) affect our strategic scorecard over the next several years?" Answering it is not easy, and the stakes are high. The operational measures for consulting, marketing, and strategy are often helpful in revealing OFIs, where added investment will pay off. The evidence from Baldrige recipients suggests that they do not stint. Their core strategy always optimizes associate satisfaction and associate performance. When opportunities arise, funds and human resources are available to meet them.

Audits

Auditing—systematic review by an outside observer team—can supplement these measures, both with increased understanding of accountabilities and evaluation of more subjective marketing activities. An audit performed by an outside consultant might review quantitative results, pointing out comparable values from other organizations. (True benchmarking is unlikely because other communities are not strictly comparable.) A consultant can conduct or validate surveys or analyses that show results. A consultant can review practices, goals, and organization structures and can suggest OFIs. Even without a consultant, an internal 360-review process can accomplish many of the same objectives by systematically surveying associates in the unit and users of the service. Periodic supplementation by an independent outsider improves the reliability of internal review.

Managerial Issues

Success in strategy is an ability to identify and implement the right changes, at the right time. It requires technical and cultural skills and effective senior leadership. Success feeds on itself. Because it meets needs, it attracts support, and the support provides resources for further expansion.[32] On the other hand, studies of the failures of HCOs usually reveal that strategic errors were made several years before the ultimate crisis, often repeatedly.[33] Unfortunately, excellence is extremely rare.[34]

Hospitals and their associated physicians fall alarmingly short on safety,[35] quality,[36] effectiveness,[37,38] patient satisfaction,[39] and cost.[40,41] Studies of trends in available national measures of performance suggest that the typical hospital is not strategically managed; it is simply drifting.[42,43,44]

Skills for Successful Strategy

Successful strategic positioning depends on two factors: (1) the ability to identify promising strategies quickly and accurately from a broad range of alternatives and (2) the ability to implement the selected strategies effectively. Hamel and Prahalad point out that corporations that thrive in competitive markets have greater ambition and follow a rigorous program of focused, complementary innovation.[45] In healthcare, provider logic, rather than customer logic, has traditionally driven innovation—that is, new products and services are often driven from the perspective of a technological challenge rather than the perspective of what the customer might want given a full understanding of the options. (Cesarean sections, circumcisions, prostatectomies, and executive physicals are among the more glaring examples.) Missing, so far, are creativity, role-playing, and breakthrough innovation oriented around customer realities. There are methods and styles of delivering healthcare we have not yet dreamed of.

The hospitals that are now well managed speak of "a journey."[46] They have made a series of changes that, over a period of a few years, has moved them from drift to excellence. Governance and senior management commitment are essential to start the journey and to sustain it. Excellence requires breaking old habits, learning new skills, and building a new culture. Strategic issues require weighing core values. The rewards and penalties of strategic issues are often deferred, while the immediate decisions are difficult and sometimes painful. Denial is always tempting, particularly when things are going at least tolerably well. Governance and senior management must support, encourage, teach, and reassure for the change to succeed. The journey is completed by building a strong technical foundation. What begins as commitment is translated to a way of life by tools that make addressing the issues easy and denying them hard.

Strategic Leadership Requirements

In the future, excellent senior leaders will spend most of their time negotiating relationships. The commitment to mission and the evidence-based approach will provide the foundation for dialogue; the leadership role will be building consensus around the meaning of the evidence. A sound tradition of transformational leadership will make the negotiations fruitful. The governing board will establish and control the general direction of the organization through its function of selecting the executive, the mission, the strategic position, and the annual goals. Its role in negotiations will emphasize agenda setting.

Evidence of Commitment to Community Needs

Evidence that the HCO contributes to the whole community is a powerful negotiating tool. Individuals seek their personal betterment, but evidence that the organization meets broader needs suggests both fairness and long-term stability, strengthening the case for a constructive relationship. It is not an accident that associates want to work at excellent organizations or that success feeds on itself. Excellent HCOs are rewards based rather than adversarial.

The foundation of their posture toward associates, competitors, and the community at large is collaboration to achieve mutual goals. Potential associates and partners can approach the negotiations recognizing that the organization fulfills healthcare, employment, and financial goals well and that strengthening the organization benefits the community and its citizens.

A Consensus-Building Process

A strong consensus-building process must underpin the negotiations. The evidence from the leading organizations suggests that consensus building has three parts: (1) acceptance of the mission and the evidence-based approach, (2) careful and sensitive listening, and (3) due process. The first preselects, so those who do not accept the validity of the mission and the evidence-based approach need not open discussions. The second provides flexibility and room for innovation. It promotes dialogue to identify innovations and prevents disputes by promptly addressing potentially threatening issues. The third protects the rights of the parties and shows respect. Appeal processes, rules to balance power asymmetries, and mediation and techniques for conflict resolution are available, although experience suggests they will not often be needed.

Trustee Education and Continuous Improvement of Governance

In high-performing HCOs, the trustees are focused on the core strategic decisions that determine the organization's future. The board's governance processes make evading their responsibility difficult. The strategic scorecard and benchmarks help them understand objectively the needs of the organization and the community. Calendars, careful preparation of alternatives, prior work by task forces and committees, and consent agendas structure the decision processes. Guidance from more experienced colleagues helps new members learn responsibilities. The evidence-based approach helps them understand the choices they must make. Strict adherence to conflict-of-interest rules helps them make decisions in the owners' best interest. The best boards now use both individual self-assessment and annual review of the board's decisions and processes to improve their performance.

Multihospital System Contribution

The technical and leadership requirements for strategic excellence suggest a powerful advantage for large, multisite healthcare systems. Catholic Health Initiatives,[47] SSM Health Care,[48] Intermountain Healthcare,[49] and North Mississippi Health Services[50] have exploited this possibility and can document their superiority on the strategic scorecard. Effective healthcare systems can develop expertise in the tools and, in fact, promote learning across their member organizations.

The successful large healthcare system provides four critical contributions:

1. *Shaping the mission, vision, and values to a comprehensive stakeholder perspective and emphasizing those commitments in day-to-day decisions.*[51] The discipline to recognize that long-run success must be mutual success should be the first commitment of the central organization. Catholic Health Initiatives and SSM Health Care show clearly that the discipline can be effectively and productively enforced.

2. *Insisting that the performance of centralized processes be benchmarked.* Moving from purely local healthcare to centralized models is progress only if the measured performance improves. Decisions to centralize are a variant of the make-or-buy decision; they should be made on objective criteria, and implementation should achieve the initial goals. The healthcare system can ensure that this happens.

3. *Maintaining a listening and collaborative environment.* Authoritarian behavior on the part of central managers is profoundly destructive. Sensitive listening, using all the marketing tools to identify both patient and associate needs at the local sites, and responding to those needs make centralization viable. Central leaders must also support a culture of empowerment and transformational management in the local sites.

4. *Maintaining an evidence-based learning environment.* Systems can and should focus on evidence-based, ongoing education for HCO leaders and trustees. They can reduce the cost of training with centralized learning tools. They can implement succession planning and management development, based on competency assessment tools and plans for addressing deficiencies. They can and do promote mentoring and peer learning across their organization, based on what high-performing HCOs have proven to be successful.

The models for the twenty-first century are with us today. They are too little recognized, too seldom copied, and too often ignored in favor of short-term, single-stakeholder advantage.

Additional Resources

Fortenberry, Jr., J. L. 2010. *Health Care Marketing: Tools and Techniques*, 3rd ed. Boston: Jones & Bartlett Learning.

Ginter, P. M. 2013. *The Strategic Management of Health Care Organizations*, 7th ed. San Francisco: Jossey-Bass.

Hillestad, S. G., and E. N. Berkowitz. 2012. *Health Care Market Strategy: From Planning to Action*, 4th ed. Boston: Jones & Bartlett Learning.

Kotler, P., and G. Armstrong. 2013. *Principles of Marketing*, 15th ed. Englewood Cliffs, NJ: Prentice-Hall.

Kotler, P., J. Shalowitz, and R. J. Stevens. 2008. *Strategic Marketing for Health Care Organizations: Building a Customer-Driven Health System*. San Francisco: Jossey-Bass.

Thomas, R. K. 2015. *Marketing Health Services*, 3rd ed. Chicago: Health Administration Press.

Notes

1. Kotler, P., and R. N. Clarke. 1987. *Marketing for Health Care Organizations*, 5. Englewood Cliffs, NJ: Prentice-Hall.

2. Centers for Medicare & Medicaid Services. 2014. "HCAHPS." [Online information; retrieved 6/18/14.] www.hcahpsonline.org/home.aspx.

3. Agency for Healthcare Research and Quality. 2014. "CAHPS." [Online information; retrieved 6/18/14.] https://cahps.ahrq.gov/.

4. Centers for Medicare & Medicaid Services. 2014. "Find a Hospital." [Online information; retrieved 6/18/14.] www.medicare.gov/hospitalcompare/search.html.

5. WhyNotTheBest.org. 2014. Home page. [Online information; retrieved 6/18/14.] www.whynotthebest.org.

6. Snihurowych, R. R., F. Cornelius, and V. E. Amelung. 2009. "Can Branding by Health Care Provider Organizations Drive the Delivery of Higher Technical and Service Quality?" *Quality Management in Health Care* 18 (2): 126–34.

7. Society for Healthcare Strategy and Market Development (SHSMD). 2002. *Crisis Communications in Healthcare: Managing Difficult Times Effectively*, 7. Chicago: SHSMD.

8. Conrad, P., and V. Leiter. 2004. "Medicalization, Markets and Consumers." *Journal of Health and Social Behavior* 45 (Suppl.): 158–76.

9. Curtis, P., and G. Bove. 1992. "Family Physicians, Chiropractors, and Back Pain." *Journal of Family Practice* 35 (5): 551–55.

10. Buerhaus, P. I., K. Donelan, L. Norman, and R. Dittus. 2005. "Nursing Students' Perceptions of a Career in Nursing and Impact of a National Campaign Designed to Attract People into the Nursing Profession." *Journal of Professional Nursing* 21 (2): 75–83.

11. Pathman, D. E., D. H. Taylor Jr., T. R. Konrad, T. S. King, T. Harris, T. M. Henderson, J. D. Bernstein, T. Tucker, K. D. Crook, C. Spaulding, and G. C. Koch. 2000. "State Scholarship, Loan Forgiveness, and Related Programs: The Unheralded Safety Net." *Journal of the American Medical Association* 284 (16): 2084–92.

12. Cleary, B., R. Rice, M. L. Brunell, G. Dickson, E. Gloor, D. Jones, and W. Jones. 2005. "Strategic State-Level Nursing Workforce Initiatives: Taking the Long View." *Nursing Administration Quarterly* 29 (2): 162–70.

13. North Mississippi Medical Center. 2006. Malcolm Baldrige National Quality Award Application. [Online information; retrieved 6/18/14.] www.baldrige.nist.gov/Contacts_Profiles.htm.

14. Chandler, A. D. 1977. *The Visible Hand: The Managerial Revolution in American Business*. Cambridge, MA: Belknap Press.

15. Roberts, V. 2001. "Managing Strategic Outsourcing in the Healthcare Industry." *Journal of Healthcare Management* 46 (4): 239–49.

16. Kaplan, R. S., and D. P. Norton. 2000. "Having Trouble with Your Strategy? Then Map It." *Harvard Business Review* 78 (5): 167–76, 202.

17. Stacey, R. D. 1992. *Managing the Unknowable: Strategic Boundaries Between Order and Chaos in Organizations*, 80–100. San Francisco: Jossey-Bass.

18. Porter, M. E. 1980. *Competitive Strategy: Techniques for Analyzing Industries and Competitors*, 4. New York: Free Press.

19. Griffith, J. R., V. Sahney, and R. Mohr. 1995. *Reengineering Healthcare*, chap. 4. Chicago: Health Administration Press.

20. Abell, D. F., and J. S. Hammond. 1979. *Strategic Market Planning: Problems and Analytic Approaches*. Englewood Cliffs, NJ: Prentice-Hall.

21. Thomas, H., and D. Gardner. 1985. *Strategic Marketing and Management*. New York: Wiley.

22. Eastaugh, S. R. 1992. "Hospital Strategy and Financial Performance." *Health Care Management Review* 17 (3): 19–31.

23. Miles, R. E., and C. C. Snow. 1978. *Organizational Strategy, Structure and Process*. New York: McGraw-Hill.

24. Mintzberg, H., and J. B. Quinn. 1995. *The Strategy Process: Concepts, Contexts, and Cases*, 3rd ed. Paramus, NJ: Prentice-Hall.

25. Porter, M. E. 1980. *Competitive Strategy: Techniques for Analyzing Industries and Competitors*. New York: Free Press.

26. Griffith, J. R. 2015. "Understanding High Reliability Organizations: Are Baldrige Recipients Models?" *Journal of Healthcare Management* 60 (1): 44–61.

27. Miller, D., and P. H. Friesen. 1984. *Organizations: A Quantum View*. Englewood Cliffs, NJ: Prentice-Hall.

28. Herzlinger, R. 2004. *Consumer-Driven Health Care: Implications for Providers, Payers, and Policy-Makers*. San Francisco: Jossey-Bass.

29. Porter, M. E., and E. O. Teisburg. 2004. "Redefining Competition in Health Care." *Harvard Business Review* 82 (6): 64–76, 136.

30. Centers for Medicare & Medicaid Services. 2014. "Specialty Hospital Issues." [Online information; retrieved 6/18/14.] www.cms.gov/Medicare/Fraud-and-Abuse/PhysicianSelfReferral/specialty_hospital_issues.html.

31. North Mississippi Health Services. 2012. Malcolm Baldrige National Quality Award Application, p. i. [Online information; retrieved 7/15/14.] http://petapsco.nist.gov/Award_Recipients/PDF_Files/2012_North_MS_Application_Summary.pdf.

32. Griffith, J. R., and K. R. White. 2005. "The Revolution in Hospital Management." *Journal of Healthcare Management* 50 (3): 170.

33. See, for example, Burns, L. R., J. Cacciamani, J. Clement, and W. Aquino. 2000. "The Fall of the House of AHERF." *Health Affairs* 19 (1): 7–41; Walshe, K., and S. M. Shortell. 2004. "When Things Go Wrong: How Health Care Organizations Deal with Major Failures." *Health Affairs* 23 (3): 101–11; Weber, T., C. Ornstein, M. Landsberg, and S. Hymon. 2004. "The Troubles at King/Drew—5-Part Series." *Los Angeles Times*. [Online information; retrieved 10/21/05.] www.latimes.com/news/local/la-kingdrew-gallery,1,6594064.storygallery.

34. Griffith, J. R., and J. A. Alexander. 2002. "Measuring Comparative Hospital Performance." *Journal of Healthcare Management* 47 (1): 41–57.

35. Leape, L. L., and D. M. Berwick. 2005. "Five Years After 'To Err Is Human': What Have We Learned?" *Journal of the American Medical Association* 293 (19): 2384.

36. Jha, A. K., Z. Li, E. J. Orav, and A. M. Epstein. 2005. "Care in U.S. Hospitals—the Hospital Quality Alliance Program." *New England Journal of Medicine* 353: 265–74.

37. Casalino, L., R. R. Gillies, S. M. Shortell, J. A. Schmittdiel, T. Bodenheimer, J. C. Robinson, T. Rundall, N. Oswald, H. Schauffler, and M. C. Wang. 2003. "External Incentives, Information Technology, and Organized Processes to Improve Health Care Quality for Patients with Chronic Diseases." *Journal of the American Medical Association* 289 (4): 434–41.

38. McGlynn, E. A., S. M. Asch, J. Adams, J. Keesey, J. Hicks, A. DeCristofaro, and E. A. Kerr. 2003. "The Quality of Health Care Delivered to Adults in the United States." *New England Journal of Medicine* 348 (26): 2635–45.

39. Sofaer, S., and K. Firminger. 2005. "Patient Perceptions of the Quality of Health Services." *Annual Review of Public Health* 26: 513–59.

40. Reid, P. P., W. D. Compton, J. H. Grossman, and G. Fanjiang (eds.). 2005. *Building a Better Delivery System: A New Engineering/Health Care Partnership.* Washington, DC: National Academies Press.

41. Jha, A. K., E. J. Orav, A. Dobson, R. A. Book, and A. M. Epstein. 2009. "Measuring Efficiency: The Association of Hospital Costs and Quality of Care." *Health Affairs* 28 (3): 897–906.

42. Griffith, J. R., J. A. Alexander, and D. A. Foster. 2006. "Is Anybody Managing the Store? National Trends in Hospital Performance." *Journal of Healthcare Management* 51 (6): 392–406.

43. Ryan, A. M., B. K. Nallamothu, and J. B. Dimick. 2012. "Medicare's Public Reporting Initiative on Hospital Quality Had Modest or No Impact on Mortality from Three Key Conditions." *Health Affairs* 31 (3): 585–92.

44. Fung, C. H., Y.-W. Lim, S. Mattke, C. Damberg, and P. G. Shekelle. 2008. "Systematic Review: The Evidence That Publishing Patient Care Performance Data Improves Quality of Care." *Annals of Internal Medicine* 148 (2): 111–23.

45. Hamel, G., and C. K. Prahalad. 1993. "Strategy as Stretch and Leverage." *Harvard Business Review* 71 (2): 75–84.

46. Ryan, M. J. 2004. "Achieving and Sustaining Quality in Healthcare." *Frontiers of Health Services Management* 20 (3): 3–11.

47. Griffith, J. R., and K. R. White. 2003. *Thinking Forward: Six Strategies for Highly Successful Organizations.* Chicago: Health Administration Press.

48. Griffith and White (2005); Ryan, Sr., M. J. 2004. "Achieving and Sustaining Quality in Healthcare." *Frontiers of Health Services Management* 20 (3): 3–11; SSM Health Care. 2005. Home page. [Online information; retrieved 2005.] www.ssmhc.com/internet/home/ssmcorp.nsf.

49. Bohmer, R., A. C. Edmondson, and L. R. Feldman. 2002. *Intermountain Health Care,* Case 9-603-066. Boston: Harvard Business Publishing; Intermountain Health Care. 2005. *Intermountain Health Care Annual Report.* Salt Lake City, UT: Intermountain Health Care.

50. Anonymous. 2013. "Together, Joint Commission Hospital Requirements and Baldrige Performance Excellence Criteria Support Quality and Safety Improvement Efforts." *Joint Commission Perspectives* 33 (7): 17–18.

51. Young, D. W., D. Barrett, J. W. Kenagy, D. C. Pinakiewicz, and S. M. McCarthy. 2001. "Value-Based Partnering in Healthcare: A Framework for Analysis." *Journal of Healthcare Management* 46 (2): 112–32.

GLOSSARY

360-degree or multi-rater review. Formal evaluation of performance by subordinates, superiors, and peers of the individual or unit.

ACA. See *Patient Protection and Affordable Care Act*

Accountable care organization (ACO). A set of healthcare providers—including primary care physicians, specialists, and hospitals—that work together collaboratively and accept collective accountability for the cost and quality of care delivered to a population of patients. The patient-centered medical home is an accepted model for achieving the ACO goals.

Accountability. See *Agency*

Accountability center. The supervisor of an accountability center. Also called a primary monitor or first-line supervisor.

Accountability hierarchy. A reporting and communication system that links each operating unit to the governing board, usually by grouping similar centers together under middle management.

ACO. See *Accountable care organization*

Ad hoc committee. A committee formed to address a specific purpose for a specified time period.

Adjustment. A statistical technique to aggregate values from specified population subsets, allowing comparison of samples from populations with differences in the relative size of subset populations. See also *specification*.

Affordable Care Act. See *Patient Protection and Affordable Care Act*

Agency or accountability. The notion that the organization can rely on an individual or a team to fulfill a specific, prearranged expectation.

Associates. People (employees, trustees and other volunteers, and medical staff members) who give their time and energy to the HCO and its activities.

Bad debt. Cost for patients who were expected to pay for care but did not.

Benchmark. The best known value for a specific measure, from any source.

Big data. Large and complex data sets that may be analyzed for patterns.

Branding. A community-wide communication effort to convey the mission and the competitive advantage of the organization.

Business plan. A model of a specific strategy or function that guides design, operations, and goal setting.

Case manager. A health professional who advocates for the patient to receive the most appropriate treatment with acceptable quality in the most effective manner and appropriate setting at the best price.

CEO. See *Chief executive officer*

Certificate of need. Certificate or approval for new services and construction or renovation of hospitals or related facilities; issued in many states.

Chief executive officer (CEO). The agent of the governing board who holds formal accountability for the entire organization.

Clinical staff bylaws. A formal document of the governance procedures for physicians and licensed independent practitioners in the organization; approved by the governing body; sometimes called *medical staff bylaws.*

Clinical staff organization. The organization of an HCO's clinical staff members that provides a structure to carry out policies, expectations for quality of clinical care, and communication from physicians to the governing body.

Community benefit. Current law requires hospitals to satisfy the community benefit standard in order to qualify as tax-exempt charities under section 501(c)(3) of the Internal Revenue Code. The standard addresses charitable care, educational services, and other benefits HCOs provide to their communities.

Community needs assessment. A process for identifying and quantifying opportunities for improvement in a community.

Competency. Having requisite or adequate ability or quality that results in effective action and/or superior performance in a job.

Compliance programs. Programs designed to meet statutory and regulatory requirements; may be based on legislation or voluntary efforts such as accreditation.

Consent agenda. A group of agenda items passed without discussion unless a member requests a review; used to focus attention on priority matters.

Credentialing. The process of validating a professional's eligibility for medical staff membership and/or privileges to be granted on the basis of academic preparation, licensing, training, certifications, and performance.

Critical access hospitals. Rural community hospitals that receive cost-based reimbursement.

Cultural competence. A set of complementary behaviors, practices, and policies that enables a system, an agency, or individuals to work and effectively serve pluralistic, multiethnic, and linguistically diverse communities.

Database management system. A system for aggregating and disaggregating electronic data designed to facilitate the recovery and use of data.

Data warehouse. Web-accessible library of work processes, protocols, and performance measures available to all associates.

Emergency Medical Treatment and Active Labor Act (EMTALA). The act requires all HCOs providing emergency care to accept all patients, regardless of ability to pay, until they are stabilized and can be safely moved.

Empowerment. The ability of an associate to control his or her work situation in ways consistent with the organization's mission.

EMTALA. See *Emergency Medical Treatment and Active Labor Act.*

Epidemiologic planning model. A statistical analysis and forecast of the health needs of the community served.

Ethics committee. A standing multidisciplinary committee that is concerned with biomedical ethical issues and decision-making processes, formulation of policies, and review and consultation of medical ethical issues.

Evidence-based management. Relies heavily on performance measurement, identification of best practices, and formal process specification.

Exchange. A mutual or reciprocal transfer that occurs when both parties believe themselves to benefit from it. It results in a relationship between an organization and its environment, such as employment, sales, donations, purchases, etc.

External auditor. A certified public accounting firm that attests that the accounting practices followed by the organization are sound and that the financial reports fairly represent the state of the business.

Facilities master plan. A document that begins with an estimate of the space needs of each service or activity proposed in the services plan.

Federally qualified health center. Services for underserved areas or populations that offer a sliding fee scale, provide comprehensive services, have an ongoing quality program, and seat a board of directors; funded with grants under section 330 of the Public Health Service Act.

Fellows. Residents who pursue advanced study, usually in a subspecialty.

Financial budget. Expectation of future financial performance; composed of income and expense budget, budgeted financial statements, cash flow budget, and capital and new programs budget.

Fiscal intermediary. An outside contractor that processes claims for U.S. government programs such as Medicare and Medicaid.

Frequency. In advertising, the average number of times each person is reached by a specific advertisement.

Functional protocols. Formally established, scientifically based expectations that specify how and by whom specific care activities are carried out.

General ledger. Technically, the record of all the firm's transactions; the term often refers to the fixed and collective assets, such as depreciation, that must be allocated to operational units.

Governance bylaws. A corporate document that specifies quorum rules of order, duties of standing committees and officers, and other procedures for the conduct of business.

Gross revenue. An entry to the patient ledger of the charge for a specific healthcare service; no longer a meaningful measure. See also *Net revenue.*

Group purchasing. Alliances that use the collective buying power of several organizations to leverage prices downward.

Healthcare system. A corporate or governmental structure including one or more hospitals and often other HCO services.

Health systems. Healthcare organizations that operate multiple service units under a single ownership.

Homeostasis. A state of equilibrium with one's environment.

Horizontal integration. Integration of organizations that provide the same kind of service, such as two hospitals or two clinics.

Hospitalists. Physicians who manage broad categories of hospitalized patients.

Interdisciplinary plan of care (IPOC). A documented process that includes the patient, the family, and all clinical disciplines involved in planning and providing care to patients, from system point of entry, throughout the entire acute care episode, and to the next level of care.

Internal customers. Associates and teams who rely on other associates and teams within the HCO.

IPOC. See *Interdisciplinary plan of care*

Joint Commission, The. A voluntary consortium of professional provider organizations that evaluates and accredits a wide range of different HCOs.

Joint venture. A corporation jointly owned by two or more independent corporations. Joint ventures always have capital investment by both partners, and usually have joint governance and management teams.

Leadership succession plan. A written plan for replacing people who depart from management positions.

Legacy system. Outdated computer software that lacks the features found in more current versions.

Licensed independent practitioners (LIPs). Caregivers granted legal status to provide specific kinds of healthcare.

Long-range financial plan (LRFP). An ongoing projection of financial position showing earnings, debt, and capitalization for at least the next seven years.

Management letter. Comments of external auditors to the governing board that accompany their audited financial report.

Managerial accounting. A process of restructuring transaction data to support monitoring, planning, setting expectations, and improving performance of accountability centers.

Marketing. The deliberate effort to establish fruitful relationships with exchange partners and stakeholders.

Meaningful use. Measurement thresholds that range from recording patient information as structured data in the EHR to integrating the information across care providers and demonstrating value in exchange for incentive payments from CMS.

Mission. A statement of purpose—the good or benefit the HCO intends to contribute—couched in terms of an identified community, a set of services, and a specific level of cost or finance. Missions were frequently vague, such as "Excellence in care." Now many leading HCOs are moving to population health missions, explicitly accepting responsibility for the broader goal.

Multi-rater review. See *360-degree or multi-rater review*

Net revenue. Income actually received, as opposed to that initially posted; equal to gross revenue minus adjustments for bad debts, charity, and discounts to third parties.

Nonoperating revenue. Income generated from non-patient-care activities, including investments in securities and earnings from unrelated businesses.

Nurse anesthetist. A registered nurse who has advanced education and certification to administer anesthesia without direct physician supervision.

Nurse midwife. A registered nurse who has advanced education and certification to practice uncomplicated obstetrical care, including normal spontaneous vaginal delivery, without direct physician supervision.

Nurse practitioner (NP). A registered nurse who has advanced education and certification to carry out expanded healthcare evaluation and decision making regarding patient care; boundaries of independent practice are set by state laws; nurse practitioners are certified in primary care or acute and specialty care.

Nursing diagnosis. A standardized statement about the health of a client for the purpose of providing nursing care; identified from a master list of nursing diagnosis terminology.

Nursing process. A system of assessing patients, diagnosing individual nursing care needs, planning care, implementing plans, and evaluating care.

Operational scorecard. Performance report for a single work unit or an aggregate of several related units, reporting three dimensions of inputs or resources—demand for service; physical resources or costs; and status of resources, such as the satisfaction and commitment of the unit's associates—and three dimensions of results—output and productivity (ratio of resource to output), quality of service or product, and customer satisfaction. The actual measures can differ by unit, but enough common measures must be used to allow similar units to be aggregated into service lines.

Operating budget. The aggregate of accountability-center expenditure budgets and the corporate revenue budget.

Opportunities for improvement (OFIs). Result of comparing actual outcome against goal and goal against benchmark; also arise from qualitative assessments, including listening.

Patient care guidelines. Formally established, scientifically based expectations that specify what must be done, by whom, how, and when, subject to the caregiver's judgment regarding the individual patient.

Patient care protocols. Guidelines that have been tested and accepted for use by a specific HCO.

Patient-centered care. Care that is respectful of and responsive to individual patient preferences, needs, and values.

Patient-centered medical home. A mechanism for organizing primary care to provide high-quality care across the full range of individuals' healthcare needs.

Patient ledger. Account of the charges rendered to an individual patient.

Patient management protocols. Formally established expectations that define the normal steps or processes in the care of a clinically related group of patients at a specific institution.

Patient Protection and Affordable Care Act (ACA). A federal law (P.L. 111-148) providing for a fundamental reform of the U.S. healthcare and health insurance system, signed by President Barack Obama in 2010.

Peer review. Review of professional performance by professionals with similar training and experience.

Performance improvement council (PIC). A formal coordinating structure composed of representatives from all major activities or activity groups; the PIC's first job is to prioritize the OFIs.

PIT. See *Process improvement team*

Population health. The health outcomes of a defined group of individuals.

Position control. A system of payroll control that identifies specific positions created and filled.

Prevention. A direct intervention to avoid or reduce disease or disability.

Preventive maintenance. The care and servicing by personnel for the purpose of maintaining equipment and facilities in satisfactory operating condition by providing for systematic inspection, detection, and correction of incipient failures either before they occur or before they develop into major defects.

Primary care practitioners. Initial contact providers, including physicians, nurse practitioners, midwives in family medicine, general internal medicine, pediatrics, obstetrics, and psychiatry; often a longitudinal relationship.

Primary prevention. Activities that take place before the disease occurs to eliminate or reduce its occurrence.

Pro forma. A forecast of financial statements establishing the future financial position of the organization for a given set of operating conditions or decisions.

Procedures or processes. Actions or steps that transform inputs to outputs.

Process improvement team (PIT). A group that analyzes processes and translates OFIs to actual performance improvement.

Programmatic proposals. Proposals for new or replacement capital equipment or major revisions of service.

Protocols. Agreed-on procedures for each task in the care process.

Providers. Institutional and personal caregivers, such as doctors, hospitals, nurses, etc.

Rapid response team. Care providers with advanced training in critical care management and emergency treatment protocols; deployed when a patient's condition suddenly worsens.

Reach. In advertising, an estimate of the number of people who will see or hear a specific advertisement.

Reserved powers. Decisions permanently vested in the central corporation of a multicorporate system.

Residents. Licensed physicians who pursue postgraduate education in a medical specialty.

Root causes. The underlying factors that must be changed to yield consistently better outcomes.

Rounding. A planned and thoughtful practice where managers are visible on patient care units and HCO work areas to visit with associates and patients about positive experiences as well as concerns that can be addressed in real time.

Scenarios. Alternative approaches to improving the profile of opportunities reflected in the environmental assessment.

Secondary prevention. Activities that reduce the consequences of existing disease, often by early detection and treatment.

Segmentation. The deliberate effort to separate markets by customer need and the message to which the markets will respond.

Sensitivity analysis. Analysis of the impact of alternative forecasts, usually developing most favorable, expected, and least favorable scenarios to show the robustness of a proposal and to indicate the degree of risk involved.

Servant leadership. The leader's obligation to be sensitive and responsive to associate needs.

Service excellence. Concept whereby associates anticipate and meet or exceed customer needs and expectations on the basis of the mission and values.

Service lines. Patient care teams organized and coordinated around a set of similar diseases or patient needs.

Shared governance. A nursing model in which staff nurses share the authority and accountability for practice decisions and other activities that influence their work environment.

Specialist practitioners. Licensed independent practitioners who care for patients referred by primary care practitioners on a limited or transient basis; likely to manage episodes of inpatient care.

Specification. A statistical analysis that identifies values for a measure by defined subsets of a population, to allow accurate comparisons for each specified group.

Stakeholders. Individuals or groups who have a direct interest in the organization's success.

Standing committee. A permanent committee established in the bylaws of the corporation or similar basic documents.

Statistical process control. A method of identifying significant changes in measures subject to random variation.

Strategic opportunities. Opportunities that, when narrowed for use in business plans, involve quantum shifts in service capabilities or market share, usually by interaction with competitors, large-scale capital investments, and revisions to several line activities.

Strategic positioning. The set of decisions about mission, ownership, scope of activity, location, and partners that defines the organization and relates it to stakeholder needs.

Strategic protection. Activities to safeguard the assets of the organization.

Strategic scorecard. Measures of overall enterprise performance grouped in major dimensions—customers, associates and suppliers, operations (quality and cost), and finance. The strategic scorecard is reported to the governing board and is appropriate for service lines, the HCO as a whole, or its major components.

Strategy. A systematic response to a specific stakeholder need.

Succession plan. See *Leadership succession plan*

Sustainability. The quality of not being harmful to the environment or depleting natural resources, thereby supporting long-term ecological balance.

Telemedicine. The use of medical information exchanged from one site to another via electronic communications to improve a patient's clinical health status.

Tertiary prevention. Activities that reduce or avoid complications or sequellae in existing disease or disability.

Transaction costs. The costs of maintaining a relationship, including the costs of communication, negotiation, and loss of flexibility.

Transfer price. Imputed price for an item of goods or service transferred between two units of the same organization, such as housekeeping services provided to nursing units. The transfer price is based on cost of individual units.

Triage. A method of sorting patients according to the urgency of their need for care.

Trustees. Members of the governing board of not-for-profit HCOs who volunteer their time to the organization; their only compensation is the satisfaction they achieve from their work. The title reflects their acceptance of the assets in trust for the community; also may be called *directors*.

Value-based purchasing. Linking financial incentives to the quality of care provided.

Values. An expansion of the mission that expresses basic rules of acceptable conduct, such as respect for human dignity or acceptance of equality.

Vertical integration. The affiliation of organizations that provide different kinds of service, such as hospital care, ambulatory care, long-term care, and social services.

Vision. An expansion of the mission that expresses intentions, philosophy, and organizational self-image.

Working capital. The amount of cash required to support operations for the period of delay in collecting revenue.

INDEX

ABOUT THE AUTHORS

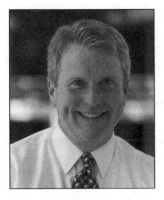

Kenneth R. White, PhD, APRN-BC, FACHE, FAAN, holds the University of Virginia Medical Center Endowed Professorship in Nursing and is the associate dean for Strategic Partnerships and Innovation at the University of Virginia School of Nursing. He also holds appointments in the University of Virginia McIntire School of Commerce and the Darden School of Business.

From 1994 to 2013, Dr. White served on the faculty of Virginia Commonwealth University (VCU) and in leadership positions in the graduate programs in health administration and also as the inaugural Charles P. Cardwell, Jr., Professor and the Sentara Healthcare Professor of health administration. Dr. White is also visiting professor at the Luiss Guido Carli University in Rome, Italy.

Dr. White received a PhD in health services organization and research from VCU, an MPH in health administration from the University of Oklahoma, and an MS in nursing from VCU and a post-master's acute care nurse practitioner certificate from the University of Virginia. He has more than 40 years of experience in healthcare organizations in clinical, administrative, governance, academic, and consulting capacities. Dr. White is a registered nurse, an adult-gerontology acute care nurse practitioner, and a Fellow and former member of the Board of Governors of the American College of Healthcare Executives and a Fellow of the American Academy of Nursing.

He is coauthor (with John R. Griffith, LFACHE) of this and several prior editions of *The Well-Managed Healthcare Organization*, *Thinking Forward: Six Strategies for Highly Successful Organizations*, and *Reaching Excellence in Healthcare Management*; coauthor (with J. Stephen Lindsey) of *Take Charge of Your Healthcare Management Career: 50 Lessons That Drive Success*; and a contributing author to the books *Human Resources in Healthcare: Managing for Success*, *Managerial Ethics in Healthcare: A New Perspective*, and *Evidence-Based Management in Healthcare* (all published by Health Administration Press). Dr. White is also a contributing author to the books *Advances in Health Care Organization Theory* (Jossey-Bass), *Peri-Anesthesia Nursing:*

A Critical Care Approach (Saunders), *On the Edge: Nursing in the Age of Complexity* (Plexus), and *Introduction to Health Services* (Delmar).

Dr. White has received ACHE's James A. Hamilton Award (2012), Exemplary Service Award (2011), Distinguished Service Award (2009), Edgar C. Hayhow Award (2006), and two Regent's Awards (1999 and 2010). He has also received the Virginia Nurses Association award for Virginia's Outstanding Nurse (1999), the VCU President's Award for Multicultural Enrichment, and numerous teaching awards.

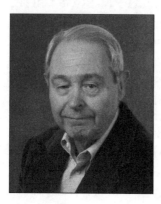

John R. Griffith, MBA, LFACHE, is professor emeritus in the Department of Health Management and Policy at the School of Public Health, the University of Michigan, Ann Arbor. A graduate of the Johns Hopkins University and the University of Chicago, he was director of the Program and Bureau of Hospital Administration at the University of Michigan from 1970 to 1982 and was the chair of his department from 1987 to 1991.

He has served as chair of the Association of University Programs in Health Administration (AUPHA), as a commissioner for the Accrediting Commission on Education in Health Services Administration, and as senior adviser to the board of the National Center for Healthcare Leadership.

Professor Griffith received the Gold Medal Award from the American College of Healthcare Executives (ACHE) in 1992. He has also been recognized with the John Mannix Award of the Cleveland Hospital Council, ACHE's Edgar C. Hayhow Award (in 1989, 2003, and 2006) and Dean Conley Award, the Filerman Award for Educational Excellence from AUPHA, and citations from the Michigan Hospital Association and the Governor of Michigan. He received the Excellence in Teaching Award from the University of Michigan School of Public Health in 2009. He was an examiner for the Baldrige Performance Excellence Program from 1997 to 1998.

In 2014, Professor Griffith was inducted into *Modern Healthcare*'s Health Care Hall of Fame.